PSYCHOPHARMACOLOGY OF CLONIDINE

PROGRESS IN CLINICAL AND BIOLOGICAL RESEARCH

RECENT TITLES

See pages 321–322 for previous titles in this series.

PSYCHOPHARMACOLOGY OF CLONIDINE

Editors

HARBANS LAL
Department of Pharmacology
Texas College of Osteopathic Medicine
Fort Worth, Texas

and

STUART FIELDING
Department of Biological Sciences
Hoechst-Roussel Pharmaceuticals, Inc.
Somerville, New Jersey

ALAN R. LISS, INC. • NEW YORK

Address all Inquiries to the Publisher
Alan R. Liss, Inc., 150 Fifth Avenue, New York, NY 10011
Copyright © 1981 Alan R. Liss, Inc.
Printed in the United States of America.

Library of Congress Cataloging in Publication Data
Main entry under title:
Psychopharmacology of clonidine.

   (Progress in clinical and biological research;
v. 71)
   Includes bibliographies and index.
   1. Clonidine — Congresses. 2. Psychopharmacology
— Congresses. I. Harbans Lal. II. Fielding,
Stuart. III. Symposium on Psychopharmacology of
Clonidine (1980 : Anaheim, Calif.) IV. Series.
[DNLM: 1. Clonidine — Psychodynamics — Congresses.
W1 PR668E v. 71 / QU 65 S989p 1980]
RM666.C56P78   615′.7822   81-14275
ISBN 0-8451-0071-8   AACR2

Contents

Contributors

Mario D. Aceto, PhD [243]
Department of Pharmacology, Medical College of Virginia, Virginia
Commonwealth University, Richmond, VA 23298

Regina C. Casper, MD [197]
Research Department, Illinois State Psychiatric Institute, Chicago,
IL 60612

G. Clincke, MS [177]
Department of Pharmacology, Janssen Pharmaceutica, B-2340
Beerse/Belgium

John M. Davis, MD [197]
Research Department, Illinois State Psychiatric Institute, Chicago,
IL 60612

Janice K. Elder, BS [197]
Research Department, Illinois State Psychiatric Institute, Chicago,
IL 60612

Irl L. Extein, MD [285]
Department of Research, Fair Oaks Hospital, Summit, NJ 07901

Stuart Fielding, PhD [xi, 1, 225]
Department of Biological Sciences, Hoechst-Roussel Pharmaceuticals,
Inc., Somerville, NJ 08876

J. Fransen, BS [177]
Department of Pharmacology, Janssen Pharmaceutica, B-2340
Beerse/Belgium

Mark S. Gold, MD [285, 299]
Department of Research, Fair Oaks Hospital, Summit, NJ 07901

Steven J. Grant, PhD [5]
Department of Psychiatry, Yale University School of Medicine,
New Haven, CT 06510

Louis S. Harris, PhD [243]
Department of Pharmacology, Medical College of Virginia, Virginia
Commonwealth University, Richmond, VA 23298

The bold face number in brackets following each contributor's name indicates the
opening page number of that author's paper.

W. Hoefke, MD [75]
C.H. Boehringer Sohn, D-6507 Ingelheim/Rhein, West Germany

Martin Hynes, PhD [259]
Lilly Research Laboratories, A Division of Eli Lilly and Company,
Indianapolis, IN 46285

Lawrence Isaac, PhD [29]
Department of Medical Pharmacology, University of Illinois College of
Medicine, Chicago, IL 60612

H.M. Jennewein, MD [75]
C.H. Boehringer Sohn, D-6507 Ingelheim/Rhein, West Germany

Herbert D. Kleber, MD [285, 299]
Department of Psychiatry, Yale University School of Medicine,
New Haven, CT 06510

Michael J. Kuhar, PhD [41]
Department of Neuroscience, Johns Hopkins School of Medicine, Baltimore,
MD 21205

Harbans Lal, PhD [xi, 1, 99, 225, 259]
Department of Pharmacology, Texas College of Osteopathic Medicine, Camp
Bowie at Montgomery, Fort Worth, TX 76107

Philip J. Langlais, MA [211]
Brain Tissue Resource Center, McLean Hospital, Belmont, MA 02179

Robert G. Mair, PhD [211]
Neurology Service, Veterans Administration Medical Center, Providence,
RI 02908

Jeffrey B. Malick, PhD [165]
Biomedical Research Department, ICI Americas Inc., Wilmington,
DE 19897

William J. McEntee, MD [211]
Neurology Service, Veterans Administration Medical Center, Providence,
RI 02908

A. Carter Pottash, MD [285]
Department of Research, Fair Oaks Hospital, Summit, NJ 07901

D. Eugene Redmond, Jr., MD [5,147]
Department of Psychiatry, Yale University School of Medicine,
New Haven, CT 06510

Richard B. Resnick, MD [277]
Department of Psychiatry, New York Medical College, New York,
NY 10029

R. Francis Schlemmer, Jr., PhD [197]
Research Department, Illinois State Psychiatric Institute, Chicago,
IL 60612

Gary T. Shearman, PhD [99, 259]
Department of Pharmacology, Texas College of Osteopathic Medicine, Camp
Bowie at Montgomery, Fort Worth, TX 76107

Theodore C. Spaulding, PhD [225]
Department of Pharmacology, Hoechst-Roussel Pharmaceuticals, Inc.,
Somerville, NJ 08876

David C. U'Prichard, PhD [53]
Department of Pharmacology, Northwestern University School of Medicine,
Chicago IL 60611

Arnold M. Washton, PhD [277]
Division of Drug Abuse Research and Treatment, Department of Psychiatry,
New York Medical College, New York, NY 10029

A. Wauquier, PhD [177]
Department of Pharmacology, Janssen Pharmaceutica, B-2340
Beerse/Belgium

W. Scott Young III, MD [41]
Department of Neurology, University of Virginia, Charlottesville, VA 22908

Preface

This monograph is based on a special symposium held in April 1980 at the Federation of American Societies for Experimental Biology meeting in Anaheim, CA, and includes generous contributions from some researcher-authors who could not participate at the symposium. Clonidine was chosen as the subject of this book because of its broad, multifaceted pharmacological effects in both animals and man. In addition to the presentation of experimental data, contributors were invited to speculate on the future, to point out the most promising areas of research, and to focus on those fields of psychopharmacology to which new theraputic benefits may come through the development of specific analogs of this particular drug, leading the way to new therapeutic applications.

Clonidine came to prominence for its potent antihypertensive activity on account of its interaction with α-adrenergic receptors. Clonidine's use in biochemical research led to the recognition of a new type of α-adrenergic receptor, now known to be the α_2-receptor. In recent years, central α_2-adrenergic receptors have been implicated in a number of physiological functions which become deranged in several disease states. Depression, schizophrenia, dementia, heroin and alcohol dependence, and anxiety are some examples. Because of clonidine's specificity and potency in stimulating α_2-receptors in the brain, numerous possibilities exist for continued use of this drug as a tool to help ascertain the pathogenesis of many psychiatric illnesses as well as to investigate avenues for development of new psychotropic drugs.

One particular area of investigation currently being pursued is the physiology of the locus coeruleus. This brain site has been shown to contain high concentrations of endorphin and α-adrenergic receptors besides being a junction for many other neurotransmitter inputs. Clonidine's effects on the locus coeruleus and limbic areas may be related to its anti-anxiety effects as well as its ability to block opiate withdrawal. Other areas of current research involving clonidine include hunger regulation, drug addiction, anxiety-related behaviors, dementia, schizophrenia, and analgesia.

The availability of radioisotopically labeled clonidine has permitted anatomical mapping of clonidine binding sites and alpha-2 binding sites. Brain areas which display a high density of clonidine binding are the nucleus tractus solitaris of the hypothalamus, substantia gelatinosa in the spinal cord, raphe nucleus, periventricular nucleus of the thalamus, and the arcuate nucleus of the median eminence. These anatomical areas have been associated with various pharmacological actions associated with clonidine, eg, antihypertensive, antinociceptive, and endocrine effects.

We were privileged to be the recipients of the thoughts of the scientists, each an authority in his/her field, who accepted our invitation to state the major issues, and their hypotheses and findings. This book will be a valuable reference source for physiologists, pharmacologists, psychologists, as well as clinicians and other health professionals interested in new developments in psychotropic functions. We will be amply rewarded if the material is instrumental in stimulating new research and assists in clarifying many issues that are still foggy.

We gratefully acknowledge the American Society of Pharmacology and Experimental Therapeutics for sponsoring the symposium, and Boehringer Ingelheim for an educational grant which assisted in its organization. Wendy Parker, Marylene Lewis, Latrese Killpack, and Judy Ford provided secretarial and other services. Drs. Debra Bennett, Senka Yaden and Gary Shearman were of immense assistance in many areas. The Texas College of Osteopathic Medicine, the University of Rhode Island, and Hoechst-Roussel Pharmaceuticals, Inc., provided office and other facilities for most of the organizational as well as editorial work. Alan R. Liss and his staff through their hard work made the publication of this monograph possible. We are deeply indebted to all of those individuals and institutions.

Harbans Lal
Stuart Fielding
October 1, 1981

Psychopharmacology of Clonidine, pages 1-3
© **1981 Alan R. Liss, Inc., 150 Fifth Avenue, New York, NY 10011**

Psychopharmacology of Clonidine: An Introduction

Harbans Lal and Stuart Fielding

Clonidine is the dichlorophenyl derivative of an imidozaline compound. Its structural formula is shown in Figure 1.

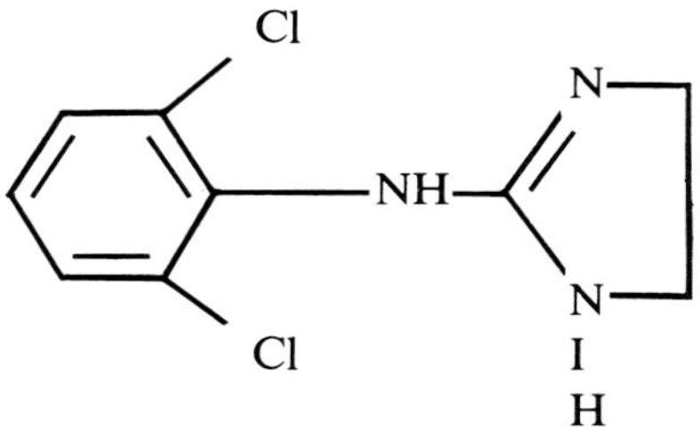

Fig. 1.   2-[(2,6-dichlorophenyl)amino]-2-imidazoline

While imidazoline derivatives generally are known for the wide variety of their pharmacological actions, clonidine came to prominence because of its potent antihypertensive activity related to interaction with α-adrenergic receptors. It was the use of clonidine in biomedical research that led to the present recognition of a new type of α-adrenergic receptors, now known as α_2 receptors. These receptors are pharmacologically similar to the classical α-receptors except that they are visualized in presynaptic locations (autoreceptors) and are therefore considered primarily responsible for the modulation of norepinephrine (NE) release. Recent research has shown that α_2-receptors are also located postsynaptically, where they are inversely coupled to adenylate cyclase since the pharmacological effects on body functions they mediate appear to be opposed to those mediated by α_1 receptors. Besides their presence in the brain, α_2 receptors have been identified in many peripheral tissues including blood platelets, so that stimulation or inhibition of their activity can be expected to produce effects in various organ systems.

Clonidine has been shown to bind to NE sites in a saturable fashion, displaying single-site binding characteristics. Alpha agonists are competitive inhibitors of clonidine binding, yielding linear, rapid-dissociation curves. Yohimbine and piperoxan, two α_2 antagonists, are much more potent than prazosin (α_1 antagonist) in inhibiting clonidine binding, which suggests that clonidine acts preferentially on α_2 receptors rather than on α_1 receptors. Apart from receptor interaction data, a significant drug-potency correlation has been established between clonidine and α_2 receptor-mediated effects on neurotransmitter release in the rabbit duodenum and on cat cardioaccelerator nerves and brain slices, and these findings, too, suggest that the pharmacological effects of clonidine are due to modulation of α_2 receptors.

It is now widely accepted that most of the known pharmacology of clonidine revolves around various manifestations of its interaction with α_2-adrenergic receptors in the brain and in peripheral tissue. The drug acts primarily as an agonist, although some antagonist actions can be demonstrated. Its derivative p-aminoclonidine is a more potent and selective agonist for α_2 receptors. However, the usefulness of this latter drug in psychopharmacology is limited by its very restricted ability to penetrate into the central nervous system.

Clonidine has been extensively studied with respect to its centrally mediated antihypertensive actions. In the brain, clonidine stimulates the anterior portion of the hypothalamus. Activation of this site results in inhibition of excitatory cardiovascular neurons. The rate of neuronal firing in the nucleus tractis solitarii, which inhibits sympathetic outflow from the vasomotor center, is thus effectively increased. In the posterior hypothalamus, clonidine decreases excitation of excitatory input to the sympathetic nervous system, and thereby appears to enhance the excitatory vagal cardiac reflex and the inhibitory baroreceptor reflex. All of these actions result in a diminished sympathetic outflow from the CNS, which translates clinically into decreased arterial blood pressure. Action of these sites ensures the absence of orthostatic hypotension in contrast to the action of classical α-adrenergic blocking agents, which can produce this side effect. Higher doses of clonidine produce a) an increased vagal response to carotid sinus stimulation with a resultant decrement in heart rate; b) inhibition of renin release; c) stimulation of growth hormone release; d) induction of prostaglandin E synthesis, resulting in antagonism of antidiuretic hormone; and e) stimulation of platelet aggregation.

More recently, clinical applications of the effects of clonidine on gastrointestinal physiology have been suggested. Clonidine is a potent antidiarrheal and inhibits gastric acid secretion.

Because of the central role of α_2-adrenergic receptors in modulating brain neurofunctions, a drug such as clonidine may find many uses in CNS dysfunctions. Effects of clonidine that may be of interest in psychiatry, neurology, and behavioral pharmacology have not as yet been investigated. It may be noted that the sedative effect of clonidine was first recorded in the same volunteer whose response brought to light the antihypertensive properties of this drug. Since then, central α_2 receptors have been found to play a role in various brain functions and disease processes. Depression, schizophrenia, dementia, heroin and alcohol withdrawal symptoms, and anxiety are examples.

The specificity and potency of clonidine in stimulating α_2 receptors in the brain thus enables it to be used as a tool for exploring the pathogenesis of many psychiatric illnesses as well as for investigating approaches to the development of new psychotropic drugs. It is this aspect of clonidine that prompted us to compile the present monograph. The sole purpose of this undertaking has been to review critically the most recent research on clonidine and to disseminate its results as an aid in the formulation of future research strategies. If the information here presented proves useful in this respect, we will feel amply rewarded.

The editors wish to thank the American Society for Pharmacology and Experimental Therapeutics for financial support. The monograph represents for the most part papers presented at symposia of the Federation of American Societies for Experimental Biology, sponsored and programmed by the American Society for Pharmacology and Experimental Therapeutics, on April 17 and 18, 1980, in Anaheim, California.

Psychopharmacology of Clonidine, pages 5–27
© 1981 Alan R. Liss, Inc., 150 Fifth Avenue, New York, NY 10011

The Neuroanatomy and Pharmacology of the Nucleus Locus Coeruleus

Steven J. Grant and D. Eugene Redmond, Jr.

I. INTRODUCTION TO THE LOCUS COERULEUS

A chapter on a tiny blue (coerulear) streak in the dorsolateral tegmentum of the pons [Reil, 1809] may seem a strange beginning for a volume on the psychopharmacology of a drug having effects throughout the central nervous system. Surprisingly, many of these effects may be mediated by this tiny but influential streak of cells, now known as the nucleus locus coeruleus (LC). Early workers considered the cells of the LC to be a part of the reticular formation, central gray, or mesencephalic tract of the trigeminal nerve. Russell [1955] was the first to conclude that the neurons of the LC comprised a distinct nucleus with a similar shape and position in a number of species. Its important catecholaminergic specialization remained unknown until the advent of the Falck-Hillarp histofluorescent technique for the visualization of catecholamine neurons and their fiber systems. In a series of studies, the LC was found to be the largest and most compact of a number of norepinephrine (NE)-containing cell groups scattered throughout the pons [Anden et al, 1966; Fuxe et al, 1970; Olsen and Fuxe, 1971; Ungerstedt, 1971]. This discovery of specialized catecholamine-containing cells in the brain has led to the generation of an enormous body of literature that has been thoroughly reviewed [Moore and Bloom, 1979; Fuxe et al, 1978; Amaral and Sinnamon, 1977; Bloom, 1975; Szabadi, 1979; Redmond, 1979] and is beyond the scope of this chapter. The present review will try to interpret the interaction of clonidine with noradrenergic nuclei such as the LC in relation to the drug's psychopharmacological properties.

A. Descriptive Anatomy

The LC contains more than 40% of all NE neurons in the brain of the rat [Swanson and Hartman, 1975] and 70% of those in the monkey [Graver and Sladek, 1975]. The remaining NE neurons are distributed among several smaller groups, collectively referred to as the lateral tegmental (LT) group [Moore and Bloom, 1979]. The LC is remarkably similar in appearance and composition across a wide range of mammalian species. In most species it consists of a small, compact group of cells located bilaterally in the central gray of the isthmus on the floor of the fourth ventricle, medial to the mesencephalic tract of the trigeminal nerve (see Fig. 1). The LC ranges in size from 1.0 mm in the rostral-caudal dimension, 0.25 mm in width, and 0.5 mm in the dorsal-ventral direction in the rat [Swanson and Hartman, 1975; Grzanna and Mollevier, 1980] to 3.0 mm $\times$ 0.5 mm $\times$ 1.0 mm in primates [Hubbard and DiCarlo, 1973; Battista et al, 1972; German and Bowden, 1975; Garver and Sladek, 1975; Demjirian et al, 1976]. LC neurons are more widely distributed in the cat than in other species, and do not form such a compact cell group [Chu and Bloom, 1974; Jones and Moore, 1974]. Each LC contains approximately 1,500 neurons in the rat [Swanson, 1976] and 19,000 in stump-tailed macaques [Garver and Sladek, 1976]. In most species it is composed entirely of NE-containing neurons [Swanson and Hartman, 1975; Grzanna and Mollevier, 1980; Hubbard and DiCarlo, 1973; German and Bowden, 1975]. However, a few serotonin-containing neurons in the LC of neonatal rhesus monkeys have been detected [Sladek and Walker, 1977]. In Nissl and silver-stained preparations, LC neurons appear as medium-sized cells, 20–40μ in diameter. A prominent feature of these cells is their extensive dendritic arborization and axon collateralization [Swanson, 1976; German and Bowden, 1975]. A more diffuse group of slightly larger NE-containing cells is continuous with the ventral border of the compact portion of the LC (see Fig. 1). However, because of their morphology and projec-

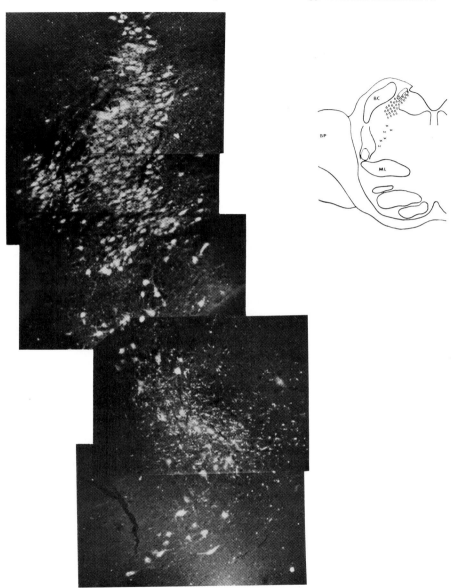

Fig. 1. Histochemical fluorescent staining identifies catecholamine (norepinephrine)-containing cells of the locus coeruleus and subcoeruleus area in the pontine tegmentum of the primate brain (Macaca arctoides). Inset illustrates location of the locus coeruleus neurons (6) and subcoeruleus neurons (SC) in relation to surrounding brainstem structures. BC = brachium conjunctivum, BP = brachium pontis, ML = medial lemniscus. Photograph courtesy of Dr. John Sladek.

tions, the question has been raised whether these subcoeruleus neurons should be considered part of the LC system [cf Moore and Bloom, 1979].

B. General

The neurophysiological and neuropharmacological characteristics of LC neurons have been most extensively studied in the rat. Only a few studies have been performed in the cat [Chu and Bloom, 1973; Hobson et al, 1975] and the monkey [German and Fetz, 1976; Huang et al, 1975; Foote et al, 1978]. The following discussion is therefore based largely on studies in the rat. Extracellular recordings of LC neurons appear as long-duration (1–2 msec), biphasic (positive-negative) action potentials [Nakamura, 1977; Faiers and Mogenson, 1976]. The conduction velocities of LC axons are relatively slow, in the range of 0.3–1.4 m/sec. A step or notch is often seen midway on the ascending limb of the action potential, suggesting somatic and axonal components. In anesthetized rats most LC neurons fire spontaneously at a slow but regular rate of 0.5–4.0 spikes/sec [Nakamura, 1977; Graham and Aghajanian, 1971; Svensson et al, 1975; Cedarbaum and Aghajanian, 1977; Segal, 1979]. Cells that fire with a rhythmic pattern, at relatively fast rates, or in synchrony with respiration have also been reported [Cedarbaum and Aghajanian, 1976], primarily in the caudal pole of the LC. In awake, paralyzed preparations LC neurons fire at a faster rate (5–30 spikes/sec) and often exhibit bursting patterns of firing [Svensson et al, 1975; Pohorecky and Brick, 1977]. Rates of 5–15 spikes/sec have also been reported in awake, unrestrained rats [Foote et al, 1980], cats [Chu and Bloom, 1973], squirrel monkeys [Foote et al, 1980], and rhesus monkeys [German and Fetz, 1976].

C. Neuropharmacology

In the past decade, considerable advances have been made in understanding the pharmacology of NE neurons, largely owing to the use of iontophoretic techniques, which allow substances to be applied directly in the vicinity of LC neurons. Although such studies have to date been conducted exclusively on LC neurons, norepinephrine- and epinephrine(E)-containing neurons in other parts of the brain would presumably also be affected by systemically administered agents acting upon the LC.

In the peripheral nervous system, NE has been found to regulate its own release via α-2 adrenergic receptors located on the presynaptic terminals [Stjarne, 1975]. Alpha receptors also regulate NE release in projection areas such as the cerebral cortex [DeLangen et al, 1979; Wemer et al, 1979; Bauman and Koella, 1980]. Since the application of NE, E, or adrenergic agonists leads to inhibition of the firing of LC neurons [Svensson et al, 1975; Cedarbaum and Aghajanian, 1976, 1977], it appears that a similar negative feedback mechanism modulates the neuronal firing rate under normal conditions. Clonidine is the most potent of these agonists, completely inhibiting LC neurons at extremely low systemic doses (6–10 g/kg IV) [Svensson et al, 1975] (Fig. 2). The relative potency of the agonists in the LC (clonidine > > α-methylnorepinephrine > = epinephrine = norepinephrine > > phenylephrine) is similar to that found for the peripheral α-2 type of adrenergic receptor [Cedarbaum and Aghajanian, 1976, 1977]. This inhibition can be blocked by the α antagonists piperoxane and yohimbine, but not by the β antagonist sotalol. In addition, administration of α antagonists alone greatly increases the firing rate of LC neurons, which therefore appear to be under tonic feedback inhibition by "autoreceptors" in the vicinity of the neurons. It should be mentioned that the selectivity of clonidine for these α-2 receptors is dose-dependent; if more than 100 μg/kg is administered intravenously, clonidine also acts at α-1 receptors [Bolme et al, 1972; Anden et al, 1970; Anden and Strombom, 1976; Rogawski and Aghajanian, 1980a]. Biochemical studies showing that clonidine decreases and piperoxane increases the outflow of 3-methoxy-4-hydroxy-phenethylene glycol (MHPG), the principal metabolite of brain NE, provide further evidence that α-2 receptors regulate LC impulse flow and NE release [Maas et al, 1977]. There is also histological evidence of the existence of NE autoreceptors on LC neurons. Electron micrographs of areas in the vicinity of the soma of LC neurons show synaptic terminals filled with vesicles of the type thought to contain catecholamines [Hokfelt, 1967], which concentrate exogenous H3-NE

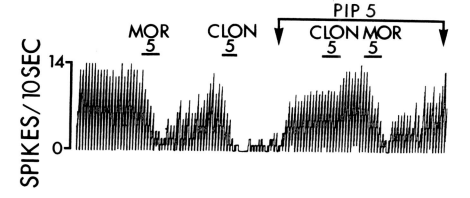

Fig. 2. Effects of microiontophoretically applied clonidine and morphine on the firing of LC neurons. Piperoxane (PIP) selectively blocked the inhibition produced by clonidine, whereas the response to morphine after piperoxane was virtually identical to the original response. The records represent average rate histograms generated by the analog output of an electronic counter (10 sec reset time). Periods of microiontophoretic ejection are indicated by bars above the rate records; the numbers above bars give ejection currents in nAmp. Courtesy of G.K. Aghajanian [1978].

[Descarries and Droz, 1970]. Recently, autoradiographic labeling with tritiated clonidine permitted visualization of α-2 receptor sites in the LC [Young and Kuhar, 1979]. However, in addition to an autoreceptor function, these α-2 receptors in the LC may be activated by input from E-containing neurons [Bolme et al, 1972; Hokfelt et al, 1974].

Alpha-2 receptor mechanisms appear to underlie the characteristic response of LC neurons to sensory stimulation as well as to stimulation of a number of central and peripheral afferents to the LC. As discussed below, LC neurons respond to sensory or afferent stimulation with a short burst of activity followed by a longer quiescent period before normal spontaneous activity is resumed. Prolonged stimulation causes an initial increase in activity which quickly falls off to a lower level [Cedarbaum and Aghajanian, 1977; Segal, 1979]. A similar transient response follows antidromic activation of the LC by stimulation of the cingulum or the main rostral efferent pathway of the LC, the dorsal bundle [Nakamura, 1977; Watabe and Satoh, 1979; Aghajanian et al, 1977]. The post-stimulus inhibition is blocked by the α antagonist piperoxane, but not by the β antagonist sotalol [Aghajanian et al, 1977; Cedarbaum and Aghajanian, 1978]. In addition, destruction of the axons of LC neurons, following injection of the catecholamine neurotoxin 6-hydroxydopamine (6-OHDA) into the dorsal bundle, abolishes both the antidromic activation and the poststimulus inhibition of these neurons [Aghajanian et al , 1977]. By contrast, administration of the serotonergic neurotoxin 5,7-dihydroxytryptamine does not disrupt the response to dorsal bundle stimulation. Finally, poststimulus inhibition can occur at current intensities too low to initiate antidromic spikes. These findings strongly suggest that the suppression of LC firing following afferent stimulation is mediated by inhibitory NE autoreceptors activated by recurrent axon collaterals within the LC.

A number of pharmacological agents are thought to interact with α-2 receptors in the LC. For example, amphetamine slows the firing of LC neurons, presumably through its ability to release catecholamine [Graham and Aghajanian, 1971; Engberg and Svensson, 1979]. On the other hand, tricyclic antidepressants and amfonelic acid (a non-amphetamine stimulant) slow LC neurons by blocking the reuptake of NE, thus increasing its availability at autoreceptor sites [German et al, 1979; Nyback et al, 1975]. In contrast, chlorpromazine accelerates the firing of LC neurons, presumably through α-1 receptor blockade [Graham and Aghanjanian, 1971; Peroutka et al, 1977] and a decrease in the tonic inhibition at the autoreceptors.

LC neurons are also sensitive to transmitters other than E and NE. Only a few agents excite LC neurons, notably glutamate, substance P, and acetylcholine [Guyenet and Aghajanian, 1977, 1979]. Substance P-containing nerve terminals of unknown origin have been observed near catecholamine-containing dendrites in the LC [Pickel et al, 1979]. However, many agents including both dopamine [Cedarbaum and Aghajanian, 1977] and serotonin [Segal, 1979] suppress LC firing. Fibers that stain positively for tryptophan hydroxylase, the enzyme for the synthesis of serotonin, have been seen in close proximity to NE neurons in the LC [Pickel et al, 1977]. However, these processes, which are probably axons originating in the raphe nucleus [Pasquier et al, 1977], rarely form classical synaptic contacts. The inhibitory amino acids glycine and γ-aminobutyric acid (GABA) also attenuate LC firing [Cedarbaum and Aghajanian, 1977, 1978; Guyenet and Aghajanian, 1979]. Nearly half of the terminals in the LC are capable of taking up exogenous GABA [Iversen and Schon, 1973]. In addition, a substantial number of these terminals stain positively for glutamic acid decarboxylase (GAD), the enzyme involved in the synthesis of GABA [Fuxe et al, 1978]. The source of this GABA input is unknown. The GABA-ergic input to the LC may underlie the depression of LC firing following systemic administration of benzodiazepines [Grant et al, 1980]. Recent evidence has indicated that benzodiazepines facilitate the action of GABA at several sites in the nervous system [Tallman et al, 1980; Costa and Guidotti, 1979]. These findings have important implications for an NE hypothesis of alarm or anxiety [Redmond, 1979, 1981; Redmond and Huang, 1979].

The LC has one of the densest concentrations of opiate receptors in the brain, as visualized by autoradiography [Pert et al, 1975]. In addition, enkephalin-containing terminals have been observed in the LC in close apposition to NE-containing dendrites [Pickel et al, 1979]. These studies have revealed an anatomical basis for the powerful inhibition of LC neurons by morphine, met-enkephalin, and the opiate agonist levophranol [Korf et al, 1974; Guyenet and Aghajanian, 1979; Bird and Kuhar, 1977]. This inhibition is due to specific opiate receptors in the LC since it can be blocked by naloxone, but not by the inactive stereoisomer of levophranol, dextrophan. A recently described β-endorphin pathway originates in the vicinity of the arcuate nucleus of the hypothalamus and projects through the central gray [Bloom et al, 1978]. Stimulation of the arcuate nucleus in the cat causes inhibition of LC firing, which is enhanced by systemic administration of morphine, but not dextrophan, and is blocked by naloxone [Strahlendorf et al, 1980]. These interactions between endorphinergic systems and the LC — believed to be a component of the opiate withdrawal syndrome on the basis of LC stimulation in the monkey [Redmond et al, 1976, 1978; Redmond, 1977] — may explain some of the antiwithdrawal effects of clonidine administration in humans [Gold et al, 1978; Redmond, 1981]. A neurophysiological correlate of this treatment was subsequently demonstrated in rats [Aghajanian, 1978]. Chronic administration of morphine resulted in tolerance to the effects of iontophoretically applied morphine in the LC and an increase in firing when withdrawal was precipitated by naloxone. This increase was reversed by clonidine via an α-2 rather than an opiate receptor mechanism.

II. AFFERENTS TO THE LOCUS COERULEUS

A. Anatomy

Early studies of afferents to the LC by retrograde degeneration methods suggested that the LC receives projections from the principal sensory and mesencephalic nucleus of the trigeminal nerve, of which it was considered to be a part [Russell, 1955]. In addition, inputs from the underlying reticular formation, adjacent central gray, the dorsal longitudinal fasciculus of Schutz, and the commissure of the lateral lemniscus were described. Recent studies using modern histochemical methods have demonstrated afferents to the LC from the reticular formation [Shimizu and Imamoto, 1970], the fastigial nucleus [Snider, 1975], serotonergic neurons of the raphe nuclei [Conrad et al, 1974; Pasquier et al, 1977], and some forebrain and hypothalamic areas [Conrad and Pfaff, 1976a, b; Saper et al, 1976; Swanson, 1976]. Functional connections from the LT group [Levitt and Moore, 1979] and E neurons [Hokfelt et al, 1974] have also been demonstrated. A study with localized injection of HRP (horseradish peroxidase) into the LC of rats has disclosed afferent projections to the LC from all levels of the central nervous system [Cedarbaum and Aghajanian, 1978b]. Projections from the forebrain include the insular cortex, the bed nucleus of the stria terminalis, magnocellular and lateral preoptic areas, the medial preoptic area, and the central nucleus of the amygdala, which also receives dense NE innervation from the LC [Pickel et al, 1974]. Hypothalamic nuclei also contribute afferents from the paraventricular nucleus, the dorsomedial nucleus, and the ventromedial nucleus. Midbrain neurons that project to the LC are located in the central gray substance, especially in and around the dorsal raphe nucleus, two areas in the solitary tract nucleus, the vestibular nucleus, the fastigial complex, reticular formation, and the lateral reticular nucleus. Afferents from the spinal cord arise from neurons in the marginal zone of the dorsal horn. A study in the cat using HRP suggested the existence of a number of additional afferent projections [Sakai et al, 1977], but the diffuseness of the LC in the cat [Jones and Moore, 1974] and the resultant inclusion of non-NE neurons in the uptake of HRP make precise identification of afferents to the LC difficult in this species.

Since the LC is one of the most highly vascularized areas in the brain [Finely and Cobb, 1940; Shimizu and Imamoto, 1970], it can also receive afferent stimulation through nonneural pathways. In the LC (and other monoamine-rich nuclei), capillaries abut directly on the soma and denrites of the neurons without the perivascular glial sleeve normally found in the brain [Felten and Crutcher, 1979]. Thus the access of blood-borne substances to the LC such as hormones or systemically administered compounds would be accentuated, and they may have effects in these areas without otherwise crossing the blood brain barrier [Medina et al, 1969]. The close proximity of the LC to the fourth ventricle provides a second route by which substances circulating in the CSF may influence the activity of NE neurons.

B. Neurophysiology

Functional afferent projections to the LC also arise from a wide variety of sensory pathways. The response of LC neurons to sensory stimulation is similar to their response to antidromic stimulation, viz, a short burst of activity followed by a prolonged quiescent period. This contrasts with the inhibition of spontaneous activity that dopamine and serotonin neurons undergo following such stimuli [Hommer and Bunney, personal communication; Segal, 1979]. In anesthetized animals, LC neurons respond only to relatively deep pressure or noxious stimuli, such as a foot or tail pinch and electrical stimulation of peripheral nerves [Korf et al, 1974; Segal, 1979; Igarashi et al, 1979; Takigawa and Mogenson, 1977; Aghajanian and Cedarbaum, 1978a; Huang et al, 1975]. In general, contralateral stimulation produces larger responses than ipsilateral stimuli. The parameters of the response of LC neurons to stimulation of the sciatic nerve have been investigated by Cedarbaum and Aghajanian [1978a]. After a single shock of the sciatic nerve, there is a moderate-latency (mean = 28 msec) initial burst followed by a period of reduced activity (mean = 50 msec), which culminates in a prolonged period (500 msec) during which the neuron is completely quiescent. The response to subsequent shocks is markedly attenuated during this period. However, no decrement in response to repetitive stimulation is observed if low frequencies of stimulation (< 0.5 stimuli/sec) are used. If higher frequencies of stimulation (20 Hz) are maintained over prolonged periods (30 sec), the response quickly drops off from an initial peak to a lower level, which eventually returns to the baseline rate of firing. The rate of decay of the response can be decreased by the α antagonist piperoxane, which blocks autoreceptor inhibition. Piperoxane also decreases the duration of the inhibitory period following single shocks. These results indicate that the transient response of LC neurons to afferent stimulation is largely shaped within the LC by the autoreceptor system, as discussed above.

In awake animals the pattern of response is identical, but the range of stimuli evoking responses is much more diverse. In unanesthetized, paralyzed animals, LC neurons respond to innocuous stimuli such as light, touch, and sound [Korf et al, 1974]. In awake, unrestrained animals, almost all sensory modalities evoke responses in the LC [Foote et al, 1980]. As in the anesthetized preparations, sensory stimulation causes a transient activation of moderate latency (20–60 msec) followed by a longer quiescent period. However, the responses habituate when the stimuli are presented at regular intervals (10–15 sec). Unfortunately, the responses of LC neurons to aversive stimuli, which might be expected to cause more persistent effects, have not yet been evaluated.

LC neurons are also influenced by the circadian rhythm of the sleep–wake cycle. In awake, unrestrained rats [Foote et al, 1980] and cats [Chu and Bloom, 1973, 1974; Hobson et al, 1975], neurons in the LC were found to fire faster during periods of waking than during slow-wave sleep. During rapid eye movement (REM) sleep, most LC neurons in the rat and some neurons in the cat ceased firing, only to resume at a very high rate just before the end of the REM phase. Other neurons in the cat fired at a high rate throughout the entire REM period. These results have been interpreted to mean that decreases in LC activity may trigger REM episodes by the disinhibition of REM generator neurons [Hobson et al, 1975], but the diffuse nature of the LC in the cat makes it likely that some of the neurons that were studied may not have been of the NE-containing kind.

Circadian variations in NE receptors have also been reported in the rat [Kafka et al, 1981]. Interestingly, α-receptor binding was highest in the afternoon, which is the beginning of a rat's period of greatest activation and the time of increasing activity in the LC. However β-receptor binding was highest in the morning, which is the end of a rat's nocturnal activation period and the time of decreasing activity in the LC. These observations suggest that the time of drug administration may be a more important parameter than previously thought in studies involving pharmacological manipulation of brain NE systems.

III. EFFERENTS FROM THE LOCUS COERULEUS

A. Anatomy

Efferents from the LC form one of the most diffuse projection systems in the brain (Fig. 3) [for more details, see Moore and Bloom, 1979; Fuxe et al, 1978; Amaral and Sinnamon, 1977]. Axons of LC neurons have a characteristic morphology: thin (0.5–1.5μ), unmyelinated, and with weakly fluorescing varicosities [Lindvall and Bjorklund, 1974; Levitt and Moore, 1979]. Upon reaching their terminal fields, LC axons collateralize to form a diffuse plexus of fine fibers regularly interspersed with intensely fluorescing varicosities. As in the peripheral nervous system, LC terminals contain numerous dense core vesicles [Descarries and Lapierre, 1973; Lapierre et al, 1973; Descarries et al, 1977]. Surprisingly, only 5% of the NE-containing terminals in the cerebral cortex [Descarries et al, 1977] and fewer than 20%

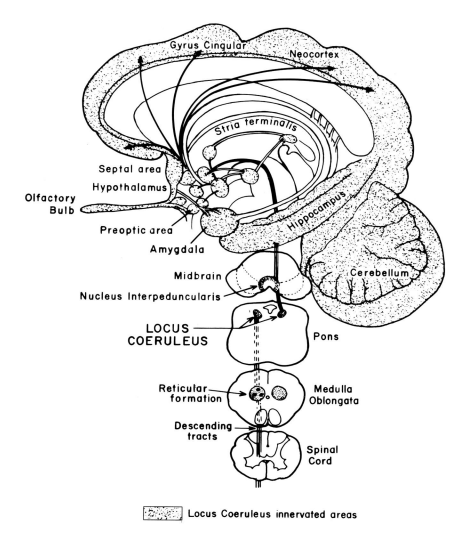

Fig. 3. Areas that receive complete or partial norepinephrine innervation from the locus coeruleus are schematically illustrated in primate brain. Afferent projections to the locus coeruleus (not shown) come from many of these same areas, as well as from most sensory nuclei and the spinal cord.

of the NE terminals in the hippocampus make synaptic contact with post-synaptic elements [Koda and Bloom, 1977]. This may indicate that NE release is not restricted to synaptic contacts, but is diffusely distributed within the terminal field. This explanation is supported by a recent study that demonstrated that β-receptor binding, unlike α-receptor binding, does not correlate with NE distribution in the rat hippocampus [Crutcher and Davis, 1980]. The authors suggested that many hippocampal β receptors may not be apposed to NE terminals. An alternative but not exclusive possibility is that NE terminals are in a constant state of flux, continually breaking and reforming synaptic contacts [Descarries et al, 1977; Moore et al, 1971]. This suggestion is consistent with the remarkable ability of LC neurons to sprout new axons and reinnervate terminal areas after the induction of chemical lesions in both adult and neonatal animals [Levitt and Moore, 1980; Bjorklund and Lindvall, 1979] or after transplantation of LC neurons to other brain areas [Bjorklund et al, 1979].

Both descending and ascending pathways arise from the LC. Although catecholamine fibers were observed at all levels of the spinal cord in the initial fluorescent studies [Dahlström and Fuxe, 1964], a specific projection from the LC to the spinal cord has been demonstrated only recently [Kuypers and Maisky, 1975; Nygren and Olsen, 1977]. Fibers from the LC descend in the central tegmental bundle through the brainstem to the ventral portion of the lateral column of the spinal cord. After damage to the LC, catecholamine fluorescence declines in the ventral column, the intermediate gray, and the ventral half of the spinal cord. LC neurons projecting to the spinal cord are mainly clustered in the caudal pole of the LC [Satoh et al, 1977; Guyenet, 1980]. A recent HRP study in the monkey suggests that the LC primarily innervates parasympathetic nuclei of the spinal cord, whereas the LT group projects to sympathetic nuclei and somatic motor areas [Westlund and Coulter, 1980].

Nuclei of the brainstem receive considerable NE innervation; however, the terminal fields of the LC are distinct from the terminal field of the LT group [Levitt and Moore, 1979]. The LC projects primarily to sensory and associational nuclei in the brainstem. Heavy LC projections have been found in the superior and inferior colliculi, the interpeduncular nucleus, pontine nuclei, sensory nuclei of the trigeminal nerve, and the cochlear nucleus. The LC also sends a massive projection to the cerebellum, which terminates in the molecular layer in close proximity to Purkinje cell dendrites [Olson and Fuxe, 1971; Bloom and Battenberg, 1976]. By contrast, the LT group primarily innervates motor and visceral nuclei, including the nucleus tractus solitarius and the dorsal nucleus of the vagus as well as other monoamine cell groups such as the raphe nucleus [Levitt and Moore, 1979].

The primary route of the rostral ascending fibers leaving the LC is the dorsal bundle, which begins as a compact group of fibers in the central gray, joins the medial forebrain bundle at the caudal hypothalamus, and eventually splits into several pathways in the forebrain to innervate telencephalic terminal fields [Fuxe et al, 1970; Olsen and Fuxe, 1972; Ungerstedt, 1971]. Although the dorsal bundle is the largest and most compact of the NE fiber tracts, other NE tracts have been described. A ventral bundle, composed of fibers from the LT group, travels in the mesencephalic tegmentum to the medial forebrain bundle on its way to terminal fields in the basal forebrain. More controversial is a third fiber system, intermediate in position between the two larger tracts, which may be composed of fibers from the subcoeruleus.

Axons of the LC ascend through the dorsal bundle to innervate widespread areas of the forebrain [Dahlström and Fuxe, 1964; Kobayashi et al, 1975; Segal et al, 1973: Freedman et al, 1975; Ungerstedt, 1971; Fuxe et al, 1970; Lindvall and Bjorklund, 1974; Pickel et al, 1974; Levitt and Moore, 1979; Fallon et al, 1978; Fallon and Moore, 1978; Olsen and Fuxe, 1972; Loisou, 1969; Swanson et al, 1977; Shimizu et al, 1974]. Terminal fields of the LC include portions of the hypothalamus, thalamus (including the geniculate bodies and dorsal nuclei), olfactory bulb, anterior olfactory nucleus and pyriform cortex, septal nuclei, and amygdala. Some of these areas, including the amygdala, septal nuclei, and hypothalamus, also receive substantial input from the LT group [Moore and Bloom, 1979]. The LC provides exclusive NE input to the ipsilateral cerebral cortex [Fuxe et al, 1970; Freedman et al, 1975], the hippocampus [Lindvall and Bjorklund, 1974; Pickel et al, 1974; Segal et al, 1973], and cingulate gyrus [Pickel et al, 1974]. There appears to be a loose topographic organization within the LC [Mason and Fibiger, 1979; Guyenet, 1980; Loughlin et al, 1979]. For example, neurons projecting to the hippocampus are clustered in the dorsal LC, whereas cells projecting to the spinal cord lie in the caudal portion of the LC. Cells projecting to the other terminal fields exhibit a more complex pattern of distribution within the LC.

B. Postsynaptic Neurotransmitter Effects

In keeping with the existence of diffuse anatomical projections from the LC and other brain NE systems, iontophoretically applied NE affects neurons in virtually all parts of the central nervous system [Bloom 1975; Szabadi, 1979; Krnjevic, 1974; Amaral and Sinnamon, 1977]. Initially, it was thought that the postsynaptic action of NE was exclusively inhibitory and β receptor-mediated, and that reported NE-mediated excitations were artifacts due to variation in ionotophoretic techniques or anesthesia [Bloom,

1975; Szabadi, 1979]. This view was elaborated by Bloom and his associates in their studies of the cerebellum [Hoffer et al, 1971; Siggins et al, 1971] and hippocampus [Segal and Bloom, 1974a, b; see also reviews by Bloom, 1975, and Moore and Bloom, 1979]. In these studies, the effects of iontophoretically applied NE on the spontaneous activity of Purkinje cells in the cerebellum and pyramidal cells in the hippocampus were compared with the effects of stimulation of the endogenous NE input pathway which originates in the LC. LC stimulation and NE caused a similar inhibition of spontaneous firing. This inhibition was characterized by a relatively slow onset (> 50 msec) and prolonged duration (350 msec). Furthermore, this effect was believed to be mediated by β receptors coupled to adenylate cyclase. Intracellular recordings in cerebellar Purkinje cells revealed that the inhibition induced by NE was associated with hyperpolarization and with a decrease in membrane conductance. This type of inhibition is unlike classical postsynaptic potentials, which are associated with increases in membrane conductance.

It has now become increasingly evident that α receptors mediate some postsynaptic effects of NE and the LC in the brain, and that these effects are excitatory. Binding studies have established that both α and β receptor sites are present in the brain [U'Prichard et al, 1977, 1981; Alexander et al, 1975]. The two receptor types have been found to coexist in the cerebral cortex and hippocampus [Greenberg et al, 1976; Skolnick et al, 1978; Crutcher and Davis, 1980]. A portion of these central α receptors are located postsynaptically to NE neurons since they do not disappear after 6-OHDA-induced degeneration of NE terminals [U'Prichard et al, 1980; Skolnick et al, 1978]. In a detailed study of the effects of NE on the lateral geniculate nucleus (LGN), iontophoretic NE activated neurons through α receptors [Rogawski and Aghajanian, 1980a]. The relative potency of a number of adrenergic agonists (E > NE > phenylephrine > = α-methylnorepinephrine > dopamine > isoproterenol) resembled that for peripheral α-1 receptors. Furthermore, the response to NE was blocked by the α antagonists phentolamine, piperoxane, and WB-4101. This fact is consistent with the view of Szabadi [1979] that, as in the sympathetic nervous system, α receptors mediate excitatory responses to NE in the brain, whereas β receptors mediate predominantly inhibitory responses.

Recent studies, however, have reminded us that neither spontaneous neuronal activity nor the characterization of a receptor as α or β can be used to determine functional effects of brain NE originating from the locus coeruleus. Iontophoresis of NE or LC stimulation appears to modulate the response of neurons to inputs from other sources. Segal and Bloom [1976a] observed this phenomenon in their studies of single units from the hippocampus of awake, unrestrained rats, in which LC stimulation restored a previously habituated inhibitory response to a tone. Furthermore, a conditioned response to a tone previously paired with food was enhanced by LC stimulation. Neither of these effects would be predicted from the inhibitory action of LC stimulation or of NE application on spontaneous activity in the hippocampus [Segal and Bloom, 1974a, b; 1976a]. Similar facilitatory effects have since been investigated in a number of other areas. In the cerebellum the excitatory response of Purkinje cells to climbing fiber stimulation and the inhibitory response to stimulation of mossy fibers and cerebellar interneurons were enhanced by LC stimulation and NE [Freedman et al, 1977; Woodward et al, 1979]. The facilitation was not just a consequence of a reduction in the level of spontaneous neuronal activity since iontophoresis of GABA, which also decreased the level of spontaneous activity, did not facilitate afferent input. These findings have been extended to include facilitation of glutamate excitation and GABA-mediated inhibition by LC stimulation and iontophoresis of NE [Moises et al, 1979; Moises and Woodward, 1980]. Activation of nonadrenergic cerebellar inputs, however, did not facilitate the response to amino acid transmitters. Like the effects of NE on spontaneous neuronal activity, the NE-mediated facilitation was slow in onset, prolonged in duration, and, contrary to the generalization previously stated, was blocked by a β rather than an α antagonist.

Neurons in the cerebral cortex also show facilitation of inputs by NE. In the auditory cortex of the squirrel monkey, iontophoresis of NE increased acoustically evoked responses as compared with spontaneous levels of activity [Foote et al, 1975]. A recent preliminary report described how NE facilitated the responses of neurons in the rat somatosensory cortex to both the excitation produced by acetylcholine (ACh) and the inhibition produced by GABA [Moises and Woodward, 1980]. In addition, responses to stimulation of efferent inputs to the cortex were facilitated by NE [Waterhouse and Woodward, 1980]. The facilitation of ACh appeared to be mediated by an α receptor, whereas the facilitation of GABA was mediated by a receptor not easily characterized as either α or β [Waterhouse et al, 1980].

In the lateral geniculate nucleus (LGN), LC stimulation and iontophoresis of NE facilitate the firing of spontaneously active neurons [Rogawski and Aghajanian, 1980a]. However, LC stimulation and iontophoresis of NE do not activate LGN neurons if their spontaneous activity is abolished after suppression of the excitatory input from the retina by enucleation of the eyes [Rogawski and Aghajanian, 1980b]. This suggests that NE does not directly excite LGN neurons but may enhance existing excitation. LC stimulation or iontophoresis of NE also facilitates the excitation of LGN neurons produced by glutamate, optic chiasm stimulation, or photic stimulation. Like the NE excitation of spontaneous neuronal activity, this facilitation is blocked by α antagonists. These studies suggest that a major function of the brain NE system may be the gating or enhancement of synaptic activity temporally correlated with the activation of NE neurons by enhancing the effectiveness of incoming signals. There are also indications that NE-mediated changes in synaptic efficiency may persist for extended periods [Pettigrew, 1979; Pettigrew and Kasamatsu, 1978].

IV. SUMMARY

Several points are particularly relevant to an understanding of the effects of clonidine in the brain: Clonidine appears to act preferentially at α-2 adrenergic receptors and, in systemic doses of less than 50–100 μg/kg, to exert its effects at autoreceptors, which initially decrease noradrenergic neuronal firing rates, NE release, and NE turnover. This action results in functional decreases of the usual effects of these neurons at their post-synaptic α-1 and β-adrenergic receptor-mediated projections, which are widely distributed throughout the limbic system, cerebrum, cerebellum, and spinal cord. Higher doses of clonidine appear to produce agonist effects at α-1 adrenergic receptors, counteracting the effects of decreases in firing rates and turnover. However, decreased function at β receptors would continue after these higher doses owing to continued inhibition of neuronal activity and the lack of direct effects of clonidine on β receptors. Receptors for GABA, endorphins, substance P, and ACh on LC neurons provide an anatomical and physiological basis for interactions among systems utilizing these substances as neurotransmitters in that they act on a common final noradrenergic pathway.

These noradrenergic pathways, in turn, also project to and mediate functional changes in areas utilizing other neurotransmitters. Although these changes affect numerous types of behavior and responses that are measurable by psychopharmacologists, it is the neurons of the locus coeruleus and other noradrenergic neurons with similar receptor combinations that provide the entry point to this NE system. Studies of the LC, therefore, may help to determine the nature of these specific effects and to characterize the effects of clonidine and other α-2 agonists on the brain.

V. ACKNOWLEDGMENTS

This work was supported by grants from the National Institute of Mental Health, Nos. MH 25642, MH 31176; National Institute of Drug Abuse, No. DA 02321; and the State of Connecticut. S.J.G. is a Behavioral Science Training Program Fellow (MH 14276). D.E.R. is supported by Research Scientist Development Award (KOZ-DA00075). We thank G.K. Aghajanian, M. Rogawski, J.D. Elsworth, and A. Grace for helpful comments and advice, and B.G. Erb and L. Rubino for editorial assistance.

VI. REFERENCES

Aghajanian GK: Tolerance of locus coeruleus neurons to morphine and suppression of withdrawal response by clonidine. Nature (Lond) 276(5684):186–188, 1978.

Aghajanian GK, Cedarbaum JM, Wang RY: Evidence for norepinephrine-mediated collateral inhibition of locus coeruleus neurons. Brain Res 136:570–577, 1977.

Alexander RW, Davis JN, Lefkowitz RJ: Direct identification and characterization of beta-adrenergic receptors in rat brain. Nature 258:437–440, 1975.

Amaral DG, Sinnamon HM: The locus coeruleus: Neurobiology of a central noradrenergic nucleus. Prog Neurobiol 9:147–196, 1977.

Anden NE, Corrodi H, Fuxe K, Hokfelt B, Hokfelt T, Rydin C, Svensson T: Evidence for a central noradrenaline receptor. Stimulation by clonidine. Life Sci 9:513–523, 1970.

Anden NE, Dahlström A, Fuxe K, Larsson K, Olson L, Ungerstedt U: Ascending monoamine neurons to the telencephalon and diencephalon. Acta Physiol Scand 6(7):313–326, 1966.

Anden NE, Strombom U: Different alpha-adrenoreceptors in the central nervous system mediating biochemical and functional effects of clonidine and receptor blocking agents. Naunyn-Schmiedeberg's Arch Pharmacol 292:43–52, 1976.

Battista A, Fuxe K, Goldstein M, Ogawa M: Mapping central monoamine neurons in the monkey. Experientia 288:688–690, 1972.

Bauman PA, Koella WP: Feedback control of noradrenaline release as a function of noradrenaline concentration in the synaptic cleft in cortical slices of the rat. Brain Res 189:437–448, 1980.

Bird SJ, Kuhar MJ: Iontophoretic applications of opiates to the locus coeruleus. Brain Res 122:523–533, 1977.

Bjorklund A, Lindvall O: Regeneration of normal terminal innervation patterns by central noradrenergic neurons after 5,7-dihydroxytryptamine-induced axotomy in the adult rat. Brain Res 171:271–293, 1979.

Bjorklund A, Segal M, Stenevi U: Functional reinnervation of rat hippocampus by locus coeruleus implants. Brain Res 170:409–426, 1979.

Bloom FE: Amine receptors in the CNS. I. Norepinephrine. In Iversen LL, Iversen SD, Snyder SH (eds): "Handbook of Psychopharmacology." New York: Plenum Press, 1975, pp 1–22.

Bloom FE, Battenberg ELF: A rapid, simple and more sensitive method for the demonstration of central catecholamine-containing neurons and axons by glyoxylic acid induced fluorescence. II. A detailed description of methodology. J Histochem Cytochem 24:561–571, 1976.

Bloom FE, Rossier J, Battenberg EL, Bayon A, French E, Henrikson SJ, Siggens GR, Segal D, Browne R, Ling N, Guillemin R: Beta-endorphin: Cellular localization, electrophysiological, and behavioral effects. Adv Biochem Pharm 18:89–109, 1978.

Bolme P, Fuxe K, Lidbrink P: On the function of central catecholamine neurons — Their role in cardiovascular and arousal mechanisms. Res Commun Chem Pathol Pharmacol 4(3):657–697, 1972.

Cedarbaum JM, Aghajanian GK: Activation of locus coeruleus neurons by peripheral stimuli: Modulation by a collateral inhibitory mechanism. Life Sci 23:1383–1392, 1978a.

Cedarbaum JM, Aghajanian GK: Afferent projections to the rat locus coeruleus as determined by a retrograde tracing technique. J Comp Neurol 178:1–16, 1978b.

Cedarbaum JM, Aghajanian GK: Catecholamine receptors on locus coeruleus neurons: Pharmacological characterization. Eur J Pharmacol 44:375–385, 1977.

Cedarbaum JM, Aghajanian GK: Noradrenergic neurons of the locus coeruleus: Inhibition by epinephrine and activation by the alpha-antagonist piperoxane. Brain Res 112:413-419, 1976.

Chu NS, Bloom FE: The catecholamine-containing neurons in the cat dorso-lateral pontine tegmentum: Distribution of the cell bodies and some axonal projections. Brain Res 66:1-21, 1974.

Chu NS, Bloom FE: Norepinephrine-containing neurons: Changes in spontaneous discharge patterns during sleep and waking. Science 179:908-910, 1973.

Conrad LCA, Leonard CM, Pfaff DW: Connections of the median and dorsal raphe nuclei in the rat: An autoradiographic and degeneration study. J Comp Neurol 156:179-206, 1974.

Conrad LCA, Pfaff DW: Efferents from medial basal forebrain and hypothalamus in the rat. I. An autoradiographic study of the medial pre-optic area. J Comp Neurol 167:185-220, 1976a.

Conrad LCA, Pfaff DW: Efferents from medial basal forebrain and hypothalamus in the rat. II. An autoradiographic study of the anterior hypothalamus. J Comp Neurol 167:221-262, 1976b.

Costa E, Guidotti A: Molecular mechanisms of the receptor action of benzodiazepines. Ann Rev Pharm Toxicol 19:531-545, 1979.

Crutcher KA, Davis JN: Hippocampal alpha- and beta- adrenergic receptors: Comparison of H3-dihydroalprenolol and WB4101 binding with noradrenergic innervation in the rat. Brain Res 182:107-118, 1980.

Dahlström A, Fuxe K: Evidence for the existence of monoamine-containing neurons in the central nervous system. I. Demonstration of monoamines in the cell bodies of brain stem neurons. Acta Physiol (Scand) 62 (Suppl 232):1-55, 1964.

DeLangen C, Hagenboom F, Mulder AH: Pre-synaptic noradrenergic alpha-receptors and modulation of 3H-noradrenaline release from rat brain synaptosomes. Eur J Pharm 60:79-89, 1979.

Demirjian C, Grossman R, Meyer R, Katzman R: The catecholamine pontine cellular groups locus coeruleus, A4, subcoeruleus in the primate cebus apella. Brain Res 115:395-411, 1976.

Descarries L, Droz B: Intraneural distribution of exogenous norepinephrine in the central nervous system. J Cell Biol 49:385-399, 1970.

Descarries L, Lapierre Y: Noradrenergic axon terminals in the cerebral cortex of the rat. I. Radiographic visualization after topical application of d,1 3H-norepinephrine. Brain Res 51:141-160, 1973.

Descarries L, Watkins KC, Lapierre Y: Noradrenergic axon terminals in the cerebral cortex of the rat. III. Topometric ultrastructural analysis. Brain Res 133:197-222, 1977.

Engberg G, Svensson TH: Amphetamine-induced inhibition of central noradrenergic neurons: A pharmacological analysis. Life Sci 24:2245-2254, 1979.

Faiers AA, Mogenson GJ: Electrophysiological identification of neurons in locus coeruleus. Exp Neurol 53:254-266, 1976.

Fallon JH, Koziell D, Moore RY: Catecholamine innervation of the basal forebrain. II. Amygdala, suprarhinal cortex and autorhinal cortex. J Comp Neurol 180:509-532, 1978.

Fallon JH, Moore RY: Catecholamine innervation of the basal forebrain. III. Olfactory bulb, anterior olfactory nuclei, olfactory tubercle, and piriform cortex. J Comp Neurol 180:533-544, 1978.

Felten DL, Crutcher KA: Neuronal-vascular relationships in the raphe nucleus, locus coeruleus, and substantia nigra in primates. Am J Anat 155:467-482, 1979.

Finely KH, Cobb S: The capillary bed of the locus coeruleus. J Comp Neurol 73: 49-58, 1940.

Foote SL, Aston-Jones G, Bloom FE: Impulse activity of locus coeruleus in awake rats and monkeys is a function of sensory stimulation and arousal. Pnas 77:3033-3037, 1980.

Foote SL, Freedman R, Oliver AP: Effects of putative neurotransmitters on neuronal activity in monkey auditory cortex. Brain Res 86:229-242, 1975.

Freedman R, Foote SL, Bloom, FE: Histochemical characterization of neocortical projection of the nucleus locus coeruleus in the squirrel monkey. J Comp Neurol 164:209-232, 1975.

Freedman R, Hoffer BJ, Woodward DJ, Puro D: Interaction of norepinephrine with cerebellar activity evoked by mossy and climbing fibers. Exp Neurol 55:269-288, 1977.

Fuxe K, Hokfelt T, Ungerstedt U: Morphological and functional aspects of central monoamine neurons. Int Rev Neurobiol 13:93-126, 1970.

Fuxe K, Hokfelt T, Agnati LF, Johansson M, Goldstein M, Perez de la Mora M, Passanti L, Tapia R, Teran L, Palacio J: Mapping out central catecholamine neurons: Immunohisto-chemical studies on catecholamine-synthesizing enzymes. In Lipton MA, DiMascio A, Killam KF (eds): "Psychopharmacology: A Generation of Progress." New York: Raven Press, 1978, pp 67-95.

Garver DL, Sladek JR Jr: Monoamine distribution in primate brain: I. Catecholamine-containing parikarya in the brain stem of Macaca speciosa. J Comp Neurol 159:289-304, 1975.

German DC, Bowden DM: Locus ceruleus in rhesus monkey (Macaca mulatta): A combined histochemical fluorescence, Nissl and silver study. J Comp Neurol 161:19-29, 1975.

German DC, Sungher MK, Kiser RS, McMillan BA: Electrophysiological and biochemical responses of noradrenergic neurons to a non-amphetamine CNS stimulant. Brain Res 166:331-339, 1979.

German DC, Fetz EE: Responses of primate locus coeruleus and subcoeruleus neurons to stimulation at reinforcing brain sites and to natural reinforcers. Brain Res 109:497-514, 1976.

Gold MS, Donabedian RK, Redmond DE Jr: Prolactin response to piperoxane suggests antipsychotic activity. Lancet 8028:96-97, 1977.

Gold MS, Redmond DE Jr, Kleber HD: Clonidine in opiate withdrawal. Lancet 8070:929-930, 1978.

Graham AW, Aghajanian GK: Effects of amphetamine on single cell activity in a catecholamine nucleus, the locus coeruleus. Nature 234:100-103, 1971.

Grant SJ, Huang YH, Redmond DE Jr: Benzodiazepines attenuate single unit activity in the locus coeruleus. Life Sciences 27:2231-2237, 1980.

Greenberg, DA, U'Prichard DC, Snyder, SH: Alpha-noradrenergic receptor binding in mammalian brain: Differential labeling of agonist and antagonist states. Life Sci 19:69-76, 1976.

Grzanna R, Mollevier ME: The locus coeruleus in the rat: An immunohistochemical delineation. Neuroscience 5:21-40, 1980.

Guyenet PG: The coeruleospinal noradrenergic neurons: Anatomical and electrophysiological studies in the rat. Brain Res 189:121-133, 1980.

Guyenet P, Aghajanian GK: ACh, substance-P and met-enkephalin in the locus coeruleus: Pharmacological evidence for independent sites of action. Eur J Pharm 53:319-328, 1979.

Guyenet PG, Aghajanian GK: Excitation of neurons in the nucleus locus coeruleus by substance P and related peptides. Brain Res 136:178-184, 1977.

Hobson JA, McCarley RW, Wyzinski PW: Sleep cycle oscillation: Reciprocal discharge by two brainstem neuronal groups. Science 189:55-58, 1975.

Hoffer BJ, Siggins GR, Bloom FE: Studies on norepinephrine containing afferents to Purkinje cells of rat cerebellum. II. Sensitivity of purkinje cells to norepinephrine and related substances administered by microiontophoresis. Brain Res 25:523-534, 1971.

Hokfelt T: On the ultrastructural localization of noradrenaline in the central nervous system of the rat. Z Zellforsch 79:110-117, 1967.

Hokfelt T, Fuxe K, Goldstein M, Johansson O: Immunohistochemical evidence for the existence of adrenaline neurons in the rat brain. Brain Res 66:235–251, 1974.

Huang YH, Redmond DE Jr, Snyder DR, Maas JW: In vivo location and destruction of the locus coeruleus in the stumptail macaque (Macaca arctoides). Brain Res 100:157–162, 1975.

Hubbard JE, DiCarlo V: Fluorescence histochemistry of monoamine-containing cell bodies in the brain stem of the squirrel monkey. I. The locus coeruleus. J Comp Neurol 147:553–556, 1973.

Igarashi S, Sasa M, Takaori S: Feedback loop between locus coeruleus and spinal trigeminal nucleus neurons responding to tooth pulp stimulation in the rat. Brain Res Bull 4:75–83, 1979.

Iversen LL, Schon F: The use of autoradiographic techniques for the identification and mapping of transmitter specific neurons in CNS. In Mandell A, Segal D (eds): "New Concepts of Transmitter Regulation." New York; Plenum Press, 1973, pp 153–193.

Jones BE, Moore RY: Catecholamine-containing neurons of the nucleus locus coeruleus in the cat. J Comp Neurol 157:43–51, 1974.

Kafka MS, Wirz-Justice A, Naber L, Lewy AJ: Circadian rhythms in alpha- and beta-adrenergic receptor binding in rat brain. Brain Res 207:409–419, 1981.

Kobayashi RM, Palkovits M, Jacobowitz DM, Kopin I: Biochemical mapping of the noradrenergic projection from the locus coeruleus. Neurology 25:223–233, 1975.

Koda LY, Bloom FE: A light and electron microscopic study of noradrenergic terminals in the rat dentate gyrus. Brain Res 120:327–335, 1977.

Korf J, Bunney BS, Aghajanian GK: Noradrenergic neurons: Morphine inhibition of spontaneous activity. Eur J Pharmacol 25:165–169, 1974.

Krnjevic K: Chemical nature of synaptic transmission in vertebrates. Physiol Rev 54: 418–504, 1974.

Kuypers HGJ, Maisky VA: Retrograde axonal transport of horseradish peroxidase from spinal cord to brain stem cell groups in the cat. Neurosci Lett 1:9–14, 1975.

Lapierre Y, Beaudet A, Demianczuk N, Descarries L: Noradrenergic axon terminals in the cerebral cortex of the rat. II. Quantitative data revealed by light and electron microscopic radioautography of the frontal cortex. Brain Res 63: 175–182, 1973.

Levitt P, Moore RY: Origin and organization of brainstem catecholamine innervation in the rat. J Comp Neurol 186:505–528, 1979.

Levitt P, Moore RY: Organization of brain stem noradrenaline hyperinnervation following neonatal 6-hydroxydopamine treatment in rat. Annal Embryol 158:133–150, 1980.

Lindvall O, Bjorklund A: The organization of the ascending catecholamine neuron systems in the rat brain as revealed by the glyoxylic acid fluorescence method. Acta Physiol Scand Suppl 412:1–48, 1974.

Loisou LA: Projections of the nucleus locus coeruleus in the albino rat. Brain Res 15:563–566, 1969.

Loughlin SE, Foote SL, Bloom FE: Topographic organization of locus coeruleus: Efferent projections of constituent neurons. Neurosci Abstr 5:342, 1979.

Maas JW, Hattox SE, Landis DH, Roth RH: A direct method for studying 3-methoxy-4-hydroxyphenethyleneglycol (MHPG) production by brain in awake animals. Eur J Pharmacol 46:221–228, 1977.

Mason ST, Fibiger HC: Regional topography within noradrenergic locus coeruleus as revealed by retrograde transport of horseradish peroxidase. J Comp Neurol 187:703–724, 1979.

Medina MA, Giachetta A, Shore PA: On the physiological disposition and possible mechanism of the antihypertensive action of debrisoquin. Biochem Pharmacol 18:891–901, 1969.

Moises HC, Woodward DJ: Potentiation of GABA inhibitory action in cerebellum by locus coeruleus stimulation. Brain Res 182:327–344, 1980.

Moises HC, Woodward DJ, Hoffer BJ, Freedman R: Interactions of norepinephrine with purkinje cell responses to putative amino acid neurotransmitters applied by microiontophoresis. Exp Neurol 64:493-515, 1979.

Moore RY, Bloom FE: Central catecholamine neuron system: Anatomy and physiology of the norepinephrine and epinephrine system. Ann Rev Neurosci 2:113-168, 1979.

Moore RY, Bjorklund A, Stenevi U: Plastic changes in the adrenergic innervation of the rat septal area in response to denervation. Brain Res 33:13-35, 1971.

Nakamura S: Some electrophysiological properties of rat locus coeruleus neurons. J Physiol 267:641-658, 1977.

Nyback H, Walters JR, Aghajanian GK, Roth RH: Tricyclic antidepressants: Effects on the firing rate of brain noradrenergic neurons. Eur J Pharmacol 32:302-312, 1975.

Nygren LG, Olsen L: A new major projection from locus coeruleus: The main source of noradrenergic terminals in the ventral and dorsal columns of the spinal cord. Brain Res 132:85-94, 1977.

Olsen L, Fuxe K: On the projections from the locus coeruleus noradrenaline neurons: The cerebellar innervation. Brain Res 28:165-171, 1971.

Olsen L, Fuxe K: Further mapping out of the central noradrenaline neuron systems: Projections of the subcoeruleus area. Brain Res 43:289-295, 1972.

Pasquier DA, Kemper TL, Forbes WB, Morgane PJ: Dorsal raphe, substantia nigra, and locus coeruleus: Interconnections with each other and the neostriatum. Brain Res Bull 2:323-339, 1977.

Peroutka SJ, U'Prichard DC, Greenber DA, Snyder SH: Neuroleptic drug interactions with norepinephrine alpha receptor bindng sites in rat brain. Neuropharm 16:549-556, 1977.

Pert CB, Kuhar MJ, Snyder SH: Autoradiographic localization of the opiate receptor in rat brain. Life Sci 16:1849-1854, 1975.

Pettigrew JD: The locus coeruleus and cortical plasticity. Trends Neurosci 1:73-74, 1979.

Pettigrew JD, Kasamatsu T: Local perfusion of noradrenaline maintains visual cortical plasticity. Nature 271:761-763, 1978.

Pickel VM, Segal M, Bloom FE: A radioautographic study of the afferent pathways of the nucleus coeruleus. J Comp Neurol 155:15-42, 1974.

Pickel VM, Joh TH, Reis DJ: A serotonergic innervation of noradrenergic neurons in nucleus locus coeruleus: Demonstration by immunocytochemical localization of the transmitter specific enzymes tryrosine and tryptophan hydroxylase. Brain Res 131:197-214, 1977.

Pickel VM, Joh TH, Reis DJ, Leeman SE, Miller RJ: Electron microscopic localization of substance P and enkephalin in axon terminals related to dendrites of catecholaminergic neurons. Brain Res 160:387-400, 1979.

Pohorecky LA, Brick J: Activity of neurons in the locus coeruleus of the rat: Inhibition by ethanol. Brain Res 3:174-179, 1977.

Redmond DE, Jr: New and old evidence for the involvement of a brain norepinephrine system in anxiety. In Fann WE (ed): "The Phenomenology and Treatment of Anxiety." New York: Spectrum, 1979, pp 153-203.

Redmond DE Jr, Huang YH: New evidence for a locus coeruleus-norepinephrine connection with anxiety. Life Sci 25:2149-2162, 1979.

Redmond DE Jr, Huang YH, Snyder DR, Maas JW: Behavioral effects of stimulation of the locus coeruleus in the stumptail monkey (Macaca arctoides). Brain Res 116:502-510, 1976.

Redmond DE Jr: Alterations in the function of the nucleus locus coeruleus: A possible model for studies of anxiety. In Usdin E, Hanin I (eds): "Animal Models in Psychiatry and Neurology. Oxford and New York: Pergamon Press, 1977, pp 293-305.

Redmond DE Jr, Gold MS, Huang YH: Enkephalin acts to inhibit locus coeruleus mediated behaviors. Neurosci Abstr 4:413, 1978.

Reil JC: Das verlangerte Ruckenmark, die hinteren, seitlichen and vorderen Schenkels des Kleinen gehirns und die theils strangformig, theils als ganglienkette in der axe dex ruckenmarks und des gehirns forlanfende graue substanz. Archiv Physiol (Holle) 9:511, 1809.

Rogawski MA, Aghajanian GK: Activation of lateral geniculate neurons by norepinephrine: Mediation by an alpha-adrenergic receptor. Brain Res 182:345–359, 1980a.

Rogawski MA, Aghajanian GK: Modulation of lateral geniculate neuron excitability by noradrenaline microiontophoresis or locus coeruleus stimulation. Nature 287:731–734, 1980b.

Rogawski MA, Aghajanian GK: Norepinephrine and serotonin: Opposite effects on the activity of lateral geniculate neurons evoked by optic pathway stimulation. Exp Neurol 69:678–694, 1980c.

Russell GV: The nucleus locus coeruleus (dorsolateralis tegmenti). Tex Rep Biol Med 13:939–988, 1955.

Sakai K, Touret M, Salvert D, Leger L, Jouvet M: Afferent projections to the cat locus coeruleus as visualized by the horseradish peroxidase technique. Brain Res 119:21–41, 1977.

Saper CB, Swanson LW, Cowan WM: The efferent connections of the ventro-medial nucleus of the hypothalamus in the rat. J Comp Neurol 167:409–442, 1976.

Satoh K, Tohyama M, Yamamoto K, Sakwanoto T, Shimzu N: Noradrenaline innervation of the spinal cord studied by the horseradish peroxidase method combined with monoamine oxidase staining. Exp Brain Res 30:175–186, 1977.

Segal M: Serotonergic innervation of the locus coeruleus from the dorsal raphe and its action on responses to noxious stimuli. J Physiol 286:401–405, 1979.

Segal M, Bloom FE: The action of norepinephrine in the rat hippocampus. III. Hippocampal cellular responses to the locus coeruleus stimulation in the awake rat. Brain Res 107:499–511, 1976a.

Segal M, Bloom FE: The action of norepinephrine in the rat hippocampus. IV. The effects of locus coeruleus stimulation on evoked hippocampal unit activity. Brain Res 197:513–525, 1976b.

Segal M, Bloom FE: The action of norepinephrine in the rat hippocampus. I. Iontophoretic studies. Brain Res 72:79–97, 1974a.

Segal M, Bloom FE: The action of norepinephrine in the rat hippocampus. II. Activation of the input pathway. Brain Res 72:99–114, 1974b.

Segal M, Pickel V, Bloom FE: The projections of the nucleus locus coeruleus: An autoradiographic study. Life Sci 13:817–821, 1973.

Shimizu N, Imamoto K: Fine structure of the locus coeruleus in the rat. Arch Histol Jpn. 31:329–346, 1970.

Shimizu N, Ohnishi S, Tohyami M, Maeda T: Demonstration by degeneration silver method of the ascending projection from the locus coeruleus. Exp Brain Res 20:181–192, 1974.

Siggins GR, Hoffer BJ, Oliver AP, Bloom FE: Activation of a central noradrenergic projection to cerebellum. Nature 233:481–483, 1971.

Skolnick P, Stalvey LP, Daly JW, Hoyler E, Davis JN: Binding of alpha and beta adrenergic ligands to cerebral cortical membranes: Effect of 6-hydroxydopamine treatment and relationship to the responsiveness of cylic-AMP generating systems in two rat strains. Eur J Pharm 47:201–210, 1978.

Sladek JR, Walker P: Serotonin-containing neuronal perikarya in the primate locus coeruleus and sub-coeruleus. Brain Res 134:359–366, 1977.

Snider RS: A cerebellar-coeruleus pathway. Brain Res 88:59–67, 1975.

Stjarne L: Basic mechanism and local feedback control of secretion of adrenergic and cholinergic neurotransmitters. In Iversen LL, Iversen SD, Synder SH (eds): "Handbook of Psychopharmacology." New York: Plenum Press, 1975, pp 179–234.

Strahlendorf HK, Strahlendorf JC, Barnes CD: Endorphin-mediated inhibition of locus coeruleus neurons. Brain Res 191:284–288, 1980.

Svensson TH, Bunney BS, Aghajanian GK: Inhibition of both noradrenergic and serotonergic neurons in brain by the alpha-adrenergic antagonist clonidine. Brain Res 92:291–306, 1975.

Swanson LW, Connelly MA, Hartman BK: Ultrastructural evidence for central monoaminergic innervation of blood vessels in the paraventricular nucleus of the hypothalamus. Brain Res 136:166–173, 1977.

Swanson LW, Hartman BK: The central adrenergic system: An immunofluorescent study of the location of cell bodies and their efferent connections in the rat using dopamine B-hydroxlylases as a marker. J Comp Neurol 163:467–506, 1975.

Swanson LW: The locus coeruleus: A cytoarchitectonic, Golgi and immunohistochemical study in the albino rat. Brain Res 110:39–56, 1976.

Szabadi E: Adrenoceptors on cortical neurons: Microelectrophoretic studies. Neuropharm 18:831–845, 1980.

Takigawa M, Morgenson GJ: A study of inputs to antidromically identified neurons of the locus coeruleus. Brain Res 135:217–230, 1977.

Tallman JF, Paul SM, Skolnick P, Gallager DW: Receptors for the age of anxiety: Pharmacology of the benzodiazepines. Science 207:274–281, 1980.

Ungerstedt U: Stereotaxic mapping of the manoamine pathways in the rat brain. Acta Physiol Scand (Suppl) 367:1–48, 1971.

U'Prichard DC, Greenberg DA, Snyder SH: Binding characteristics of radiolabeled agonists and antagonists at central nervous system alpha noradrenergic receptors. Mol Phar 13:445–473, 1977.

U'Prichard DC, Reissine TD, Mason ST, Fibiger HC: Modulation of rat brain alpha and beta adrenergic receptor populations by lesions of the dorsal noradrenergic bundle. Brain Res 187:143–154, 1980.

Watabe K, Satoh T: Mechanism underlying prolonged inhibition of rat locus coeruleus neurons following anti- and orthodromic activation. Brain Res 165:343–348, 1979.

Waterhouse BD, Moises HC, Woodward DJ: Noradrenergic modulation of somatosensory cortical neuronal responses to iontophoretically applied putative neurotransmitters. Exp Neurol 69:30–49, 1980.

Waterhouse BD, Woodward DJ: Interaction of cerebrocortical activity evoked by stimulation of somatosensory afferent pathways in the rat. Exp Neurol 67:11–34, 1980.

Wemer J, Vanderlogt JC, DeLangen CDJ, Mulder AH: Capacity of pre-synaptic alpha-receptors to modulate norepinephrine release from slices of rat neocortex and the affinity of some agonists and antagonists for these receptors. J Pharm Exp Ther 211:445–451, 1979.

Westlund KN, Coulter JD: Descending projections of the locus coeruleus and sub-coeruleus/medial parabrachial nuclei in monkey. Brain Res Rev 2:235–264, 1980.

Woodward DJ, Moises HC, Waterhouse BD, Hoffer BJ, Freedman R: Modulatory actions of norepinephrine in the central nervous system. Fed Proc 38:2109–2116, 1979.

Young WS, Kuhar MJ: Noradrenergic α_1 and α_2 receptors: Autoradiographic visualization. Eur J Pharm 59:317–319, 1979.

Psychopharmacology of Clonidine, pages 29–39

Brain Sites for the Antihypertensive Action of Clonidine

Lawrence Isaac

I. INTRODUCTION

The major objective of this presentation is to examine the pharmacologic actions of clonidine in the central nervous system, primarily focusing on the vasomotor center in the medulla oblongata. I have intentionally omitted much of the literature, confining many remarks instead to that which investigated the actions of clonidine utilizing the most direct approach. These data demonstrate that clonidine is both an α-adrenergic agonist and antagonist in the central nervous system. In addition, these results demonstrate that clonidine interacts with the catecholaminergic neuronal systems, which modulate reflex blood pressure regulation.

Clonidine (2-(2,6-dichlorophenylamino)-2-imidazoline hydrochloride) is reported to decrease arterial pressure and heart rate by an action in the central nervous system (CNS) [Kobinger and Walland, 1967; Sattler and van Zweiten, 1967; Sherman et al, 1968; Rand and Wilson, 1968; Schmitt et al, 1968; Constantine and McShane, 1968]. It has a direct α-adrenergic agonistic action on the peripheral smooth muscle [Kobinger and Walland, 1967; Boissier et al, 1968], and it is suggested that the reduction of central sympathetic outflow is due to stimulation by clonidine of α-adrenergic receptors in the brain [Bolme and Fuxe, 1971; Schmitt and Schmitt, 1970; Schmitt et al, 1973; Haeusler, 1973].

Clonidine also possesses α-adrenergic antagonistic activity in the peripheral sympathetic nervous system [Boissier et al, 1968; Bentley and Li, 1968; Davis et al, 1977; Doxey and Everitt, 1977; Davis and Maury, 1978]. In addition, clonidine stimulates the presynaptic α-adrenoceptors that regulate transmitter release in sympathetic nerves [Doxey and Everitt, 1977]. Stimulation of these presynaptic receptors (autoreceptors) reduces the release of norepinephrine from nerve endings both peripherally [Arbilla and Langer, 1978] and centrally [Starke and Endo, 1976; Svenson and Usdin, 1978].

When clonidine is injected intravenously in animals, it causes an initial transient rise in arterial blood pressure followed by a sustained hypotension [Constantine and McShane, 1968; Kobinger and Walland, 1967]. When injected intracisternally [Kobinger, 1967; Schmitt and Schmitt, 1969], intraventricularly [Schmitt and Schmitt, 1969; Sherman et al, 1968], or into the vertebral artery [Constantine and McShane, 1968; Sattler and van Zwieten, 1967], it produces only a long-lasting hypotensive effect and bradycardia. These data suggest that clonidine produces its hypotensive effect at sites within the central nervous system; however, these routes of administration make it difficult to localize the site of action. Consequently, more recent investigations into the site and mechanism of action of clonidine have employed more direct methods. Sharma et al [1978] used microiontophoresis, applying clonidine to specific cardiovascular neurons. Tadepalli and Mills [1978] injected the drug intraventricularly and confined it to brain structures above the midcollicular level.

II. CLONIDINE AS AN α-ADRENERGIC RECEPTOR ANTAGONIST

In an effort to localize the site and mechanism of action of clonidine induced hypotension, Sharma et al [1978] applied the drug by the technique of microiontophoresis directly to neurons of the bulbar cardiovascular center in decerebrate cats. This technique permits simultaneous electrophysiological recording and drug application in the vicinity of a single cardiovascular neuron in bulbar sympathetic centers. Initially, excitatory cardiovascular neurons (CVN) were identified by a reduction in firing rate following an increase in systemic blood pressure. Inhibitory cardiovascular neurons (ICVN) were identified by an increase in firing rate following an increase in systemic blood pressure. Clonidine applied by microiontophoresis in a low dose (30 nA) reduced the spontaneous firing rate of CVN but had no effect on ICVN. It also had no effect on neurons from the same area whose firing rate was not affected by changes in systemic blood pressure (noncardiovascular neurons). Thus clonidine (in this dosage) depresses neuronal firing rate somewhat selectively. Norepinephrine applied by iontophoresis (25 nA) increased the spontaneous firing rate of CVN. When norepinephrine (25 nA) was applied to an excitatory cardiovascular neuron (CVN) while clonidine was also being applied at a dose of 10 nA, the excitatory response (increased firing rate) of norepinephrine was completely inhibited, although full recovery of the norepinephrine response occurred after termination of clonidine application. These data demonstrate that clonidine blocks norepinephrine excitation of cardiovascular neurons presumably by acting on α-adrenergic receptors. These receptors have been located postsynaptically [U'Prichard and Snyder, 1979]. Also, one can postulate that norepinephrine is the transmitter at the synapse between the tonic excitatory synapse from higher brain centers and the vasomotor center (Fig. 1).

This conclusion is consistent with the findings of Chalmers and Reid [1972] and Doba and Reis [1974]. These authors sectioned afferent baroreceptor nerves, which produced hypertension and tachycardia. Injection of 6-hydroxydopamine (a catecholaminergic neurotoxin) into the cisternal

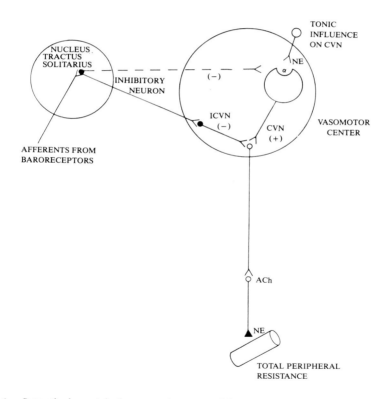

Fig. 1. Synaptic elements in the vasomotor center of the medulla demonstrating excitatory (+) and inhibitory (−) neural pathways. CVN = excitatory cardiovascular neuron; ICVN = inhibitory cardiovascular neuron. The firing rate of the CVN is reduced as blood pressure is increased and increased as norepinephrine (NE) is applied microiontophoretically. ACh = acetylcholine. [From Issac, 1980.]

space prevented the development of hypertension. Chalmers and Reid [1972] concluded that norepinephrine neurons (tonic influence on CVN in Fig. 1) exist at the level of bulbospinal pathways, which form connections with the baroreceptor reflex pathway. Doba and Reis [1974] reached similar conclusions following hypertension in rats by lesions in the nucleus tractus solitarius.

Additionally, electrical stimulation of the cerebellar fastigial nucleus of dogs results in a hypertensive response with tachycardia [Dormer and Stone, 1978]; this response is believed to be exerted through the parasolitary portion of the nucleus tractus solitarius [Batton et al, 1977]. During clonidine administration, the fastigial nucleus hypertensive response was reduced. Based on the combined work of Dormer and Stone [1978] and Sharma et al [1978], it appears that this antagonism is further evidence that the fastigial nucleus is exerting its influence in medullary regions associated with sympathetic efferent pathways and incoming baroreceptor reflex information, and that the site of the clonidine suppression of the fastigial nucleus response may be at the α-adrenergic receptor on the excitatory cardiovascular neuron (Fig. 1).

In contrast to clonidine, when norepinephrine was applied to an excitatory cardiovascular neuron while propranolol was also being applied, the excitatory response of norepinephrine was not inhibited [Sharma et al, 1979]. Propranolol alone, however, did reduce the spontaneous firing rate of excitatory cardiovascular neurons when applied by microiontophoresis (25 nA). This response was shown to be due to its β-adrenergic receptor blocking action and not to a nonspecific local anesthetic effect. These data demonstrate that β-adrenoceptors may play a role in bulbar cardiovascular neuron systems. It is clear that the actions of clonidine and propranolol differ greatly with respect to mechanism, although they both produce the same effect (suppression of CVN firing rate). Clonidine blocks α receptors (postsynaptically) to inhibit the actions of applied norepinephrine, whereas propranolol blocks β receptors. Blockade of β receptors presynaptically presumably can lead to a reduction in the release of norepinephrine from the adrenergic nerve ending [Adler-Graschinsky and Langer, 1975]. It is conceivable that propranolol reduces neuronal firing rate by inhibition of norepinephrine release.

Another recent characterization of the mechanism of action of clonidine in the central nervous system was conducted by Tadepalli et al [1976] and Tadepalli and Mills [1978]. Their objective was to determine whether clonidine can produce cardiovascular effects opposite to those of α-adrenergic receptor blocking agents under similar experimental conditions. They determined the actions of clonidine, phentolamine, and hydergine following intraventricular injection in vagotomized cats with the brain intact and with the brain transected at the midcollicular level. More importantly, however, they limited drug access to neural structures above the midcollicular level following injection into the third ventricle using a drainage cannula from the cerebral aqueduct. These data are summarized in Table I.

When clonidine was injected into the fourth ventricle of vagotomized cats with brain intact, it decreased arterial pressure, heart rate, and preganglionic sympathetic nerve activity. These data suggest that clonidine acts centrally to decrease sympathetic activity to peripheral vasculature and heart, a fact repeatedly demonstrated (see above). In addition, clonidine depressed both the rise in blood pressure and the increase in preganglionic sympathetic nerve activity in response to bilateral carotid occlusion (BCO), whereas it failed to reduce the BCO response in decerebrate cats and failed to reduce the response to BCO in cats when the drug was confined to sites above the colliculus (third ventricular injection). These data indicate that the decrease in BCO response is due to a central action of clonidine, and that the drug does not affect primary baroreceptor efferent pathways. This latter point is in harmony with the fact that clonidine reduced arterial pressure in the three preparations but did not reduce the BCO response in decerebrate and third ventricular injection preparations. That clonidine reduced the BCO response following injection into the fourth ventricle with brain intact, but not when the brain was lesioned at the midcollicular level, indicates that the actions of the drug are on sites in the caudal brain stem that are part of the pathways connecting with supracollicular brain structures. It also appears (see Table I) that depression of the baroreceptor pressor response is mediated by sites different from those through which clonidine acts to reduce arterial pressure, because this latter variable decreased in all three preparations but BCO did not. Finally, these data clearly indicate that the hypotensive effect is the net result of drug action on sub- and supracollicular areas of the brain.

A comparison of the effects (see Table I) of clonidine with those of the α-adrenergic receptor antagonists shows that both drugs have the same cardiovascular actions below the midcollicular level, whereas they have different actions above this level. These comparisons would suggest that clonidine is acting as an α-adrenergic antagonist below the midcolliculus and as an α-adrenergic agonist above this site. These data are consistent with the fact that clonidine blocks the norepinephrine-induced excitation of medullary cardiovascular neurons [Sharma et al, 1978] and excitation of medullary cardiovascular neurons induced by stimulation of cerebellar fastigial nucleus (Dormer and Stone, 1978).

This site and mechanism of action of clonidine explains how, in humans, this drug lacks severe orthostatic hypotensive side effects [Schwartz et al, 1973; Onesti, 1978] compared with reserpine or guanethidine. Clonidine decreases the resting tone of the sympathetic nervous system by interfering with tonic influences on the excitatory cardiovascular neuron (Fig. 1), but still permits the passage of reflex information over the inhibitory cardiovas-

TABLE I. Cardiovascular Effects of Drugs Administered Intraventricularly and Confined to Brain Areas Above and Below the Midcolliculus

Treatment	Above			Below					
	Third ventricular injection intact brain			Fourth ventricular injection					
				decerebrate			intact brain		
	AP	HR	BCO	AP	HR	BCO	AP	HR	BCO
Clonidine	−	−	0	−	−	0	−	−	−
Alpha antagonists[a]	0	0,+	+	−	0,−	0	−	0,−	−

[a]phentolamine, hydergine

AP = arterial pressure; HR = heart rate; BCO = response to bilateral carotid occlusion (rise in blood pressure and increase in preganglionic sympathetic nerve activity).

All cats were vagotomized, and those that were decerebrate had their brains transected dorsally at the midcollicular level and ventrally at the rostral termination of the pontine grey.

+ = increase; − = decrease; 0 = no change.

cular neurons without influencing the final efferent sympathetic vasomotor neurons of the medulla. Reserpine and guanethidine interfere with these latter neurons by decreasing norepinephrine content at the adrenergic nerve ending, which interrupts neurotransmission, and by producing adrenergic neuron blockade, which interrupts neurotransmission at the final effector junction (arteriole). In this respect, reserpine and guanethidine (which block adrenergic neurons at peripheral sites) interfere with pressor reflexes, whereas clonidine (which blocks adrenergic neurons at central sites) does not.

III. CLONIDINE AS AN α-ADRENERGIC RECEPTOR AGONIST

As early as 1936, physiologists sought sites in the brain that could explain the actions of chemical stimulants that could produce either a pressor response or a depressor when applied directly to brain tissue. According to Price et al [1965], the anatomical distribution of independent sites in the bulbar cardiovascular region mediating either a rise in arterial blood pressure or a fall are not predictable stereotaxically. A generally accepted belief is that "pressor" and "depressor" centers may exist anatomically at higher brain levels than the bulbar region [Palkovits and Zaborszky, 1977]. It is the hypothalamus that has been implicated as a possible site of the higher brain structures modulating cardiovascular control mechanisms at the medullary level [McAllen, 1976] (Fig. 2).

Electrical stimulation of the posterior hypothalamus elicits tachycardia and hypertension [Philippu et al, 1973]. This response is antagonized by local application of the α-adrenergic antagonist tolazoline [Philippu et al, 1973] and by local application of clonidine (10^{-3} M), whereas lower doses of clonidine (10^{-5} M) enhance the response [Philippu et al, 1974]. In the anesthetized rat, 3–10 μg of clonidine lowers blood pressure and heart rate for up to 2 hours following microinjection to the posterior area [Struyker Boudier and van Rossum, 1972]. In addition, clonidine applied topically to the ventral face of the brain stem (medullary region) decreases the blood pressure response to posterior hypothalamic stimulation [Bloch et al, 1977]. Finally, Przuntek et al [1971] have shown that the rise in blood pressure evoked by electrical stimulation of this area is reduced by bretylium (an adrenergic neuron blocking agent) and enhanced by desipramine (norepinephrine reuptake blocker), which elevates the local concentration of norepinephrine.

Electrical stimulation of the anterior hypothalamus elicits bradycardia and hypotension [Hilton and Spyer, 1971]. Injection of norepinephrine into this area induces a fall in blood pressure and heart rate. These effects are probably due to stimulation of α-adrenergic receptors by norepinephrine because both the hypotension and bradycardia could be induced by phenylephrine (a pure α agonist) but not by isoproterenol (a pure β agonist) or

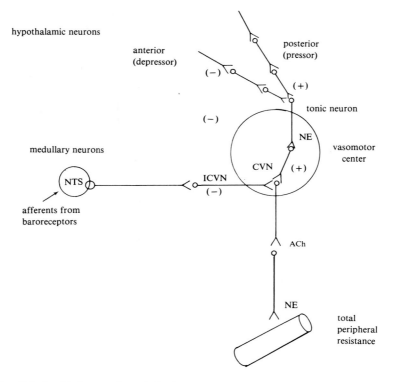

Fig. 2. Relationship between hypothalamic areas and bulbar cardiovascular neurons. Stimulation of the anterior hypothalamus inhibits ($-$) activity of the excitatory cardiovascular neuron (CVN); stimulation of the posterior area enhances ($+$) activity of the CVN. NTS = nucleus tractus solitarius; ICVN = inhibitory cardiovascular neuron; ACh = acetylcholine; NE = norepinephrine. [From Isaac, 1980.]

dopamine, and could be prevented by phentolamine (an α antagonist) [Struyker Boudier et al, 1974].

These data suggest that α receptors that mediate hypertension and tachycardia can be located in fiber tracts of the posterior hypothalamus, and that α receptors that mediate hypotension and bradycardia can be detected in fiber tracts of the anterior hypothalamus. This oversimplification defines the posterior hypothalamus as the cardiovascular "pressor" center, and the anterior hypothalamus as the cardiovascular "depressor" center. Neural pathways from these sites may be multisynaptic or directly descend to the medulla and to the spinal cord [Palkovits and Zaborszky, 1977]. In any case, it is possible that the fibers from the posterior and anterior hypothalamus ultimately make synaptic connections with fibers modulating the tonic influence on the excitatory cardiovascular neuron (CVN) (Fig. 1). Stimulation of the anterior hypothalamic pathway would tend to suppress activity of the excitatory cardiovascular neuron, leaving inhibitory influences from the nucleus tractus solitarii unopposed in reducing sympathetic nervous system outflow from the vasomotor center. It is interesting that the pattern of response elicited from stimulation of the depressor area is indistinguishable from that to baroreceptor afferent stimulation [Hilton and Spyer, 1971]. Conversely, stimulation of the posterior hypothalamic pathway would tend to increase activity of the excitatory cardiovascular neuron, making inhibitory influences from the nucleus tractus solitarii less effective in reducing sympathetic activity.

These data, in conjunction with the facts that clonidine is both an α-adrenergic agonist and antagonist, would imply that clonidine is acting as an α agonist in the anterior hypothalamic tract to increase inhibition on the excitatory cardiovascular neuron and thus effectively increase sympathetic inhibition by the NTS, and that clonidine is acting as an α antagonist in the posterior hypothalamic tract to decrease excitation on the excitatory cardiovascular neuron and thus effectively increase sympathetic inhibition by the NTS to lower blood pressure. These implications are consistent with the data of Tadepalli and Mills [1978] that clonidine acts as an α antagonist below the midcollicular level of the brain and as an α agonist above this level. In addition, these implications will explain how clonidine induces hypotension in midbrain-transected animals; that is, having sites of action (one above the transection and one below) that are complementary in reducing sympathetic activity [Table 1; Tadepalli and Mills, 1978; Schmitt and Schmitt, 1969; Kobinger and Pichler, 1975].

IV. SUMMARY

In conclusion, I reviewed recent literature that directly investigated the site and mechanism of action of clonidine in the central nervous system. One can interpret these data in the following manner. In the medulla, clonidine is acting as an α-adrenergic receptor antagonist that inhibits excitatory input to the sympathetic nervous system. In the anterior hypothalamus, clonidine is acting as an α-adrenergic receptor agonist that excites an inhibitory pathway which inhibits excitatory input to the sympathetic nervous system. Both actions produce the same final response; that is, diminished sympathetic outflow from the central nervous system.

V. REFERENCES

Adler-Graschinsky E, Langer SZ: Possible role of a beta-adrenoceptor in the regulation of noradrenaline release by nerve stimulation through a positive feedback mechanism. J Pharmacol 53:43–50, 1975.

Arbilla S, Langer SZ: Differences between presynaptic and postsynaptic alpha-adrenoceptors in the isolated nictitating membrane of the cat: Effects of metanephrine and tolazoline. Br J Pharmacol 64:259–264, 1978.

Batton RR, Jayaraman A, Ruggiero D, Carpenter MB: Fastigial efferent projections in the monkey: An autoradiographic study. J Comp Neurol 174:281–306, 1977.

Bentley GA, Li DMF: Studies of the new hypotensive drug ST 155. Eur J Pharmacol 4:124–134, 1968.

Bloch R, Feldman J, Bousquet P, Schwartz J: Relationship between the ventromedullary clonidine-sensitive area and the posterior hypothalamus. Eur J Pharmacol 45:55–60, 1977.

Boissier JR, Guidicelli JF, Fichelle J, Schmitt H, Schmitt H: Cardiovascular effects of 2-(2,6-dichlorophenylamino)-2-imidazoline hydrochloride (ST 155): Peripheral sympathetic system. Eur J Pharmacol 2:333–339, 1968.

Bolme P, Fuxe K: Pharmacological studies on the hypotensive effects of clonidine. Eur J Pharmacol 13:168–174, 1971.

Chalmers JP, Reid JL: Participation of central noradrenergic neurons in arterial baroreceptor reflexes in the rabbit. A study with intracisternally administered 6-hydroxydopamine. Circ Res 31:789–804, 1972.

Constantine JW, McShane WK: Analysis of the cardiovascular effects of 2-(2,6-dichlorophenylamino)-2-imidazoline hydrochloride (Catapres). Eur J Pharmacol 4:109–123, 1968.

Davis JM, Maury W: Clonidine and related imidazolines are postsynaptic alpha adrenergic antagonists in dispersed rat parotid cells. J Pharmacol Exp Ther 207:425–430, 1978.

Davis JM, Maury W, Hoyler E: Clonidine is a postsynaptic and adrenergic antagonist in the rat parotid; Correlation of (^{3}H) DHE binding and K$^+$ release. Soc Neurosci Abstr 3:454, 1977.

Doba N, Reis D: Role of central and peripheral adrenergic mechanisms in neurogenic hypertension produced by brainstem lesions in rat. Circ Res 34:293–301, 1974.

Dormer KJ, Stone HL: The effect of clonidine on the fastigial pressor response in dogs. J Pharmacol Exp Ther 205:212–220, 1978.

Doxey JC, Everitt J: Inhibitory effects of clonidine on responses to sympathetic nerve stimulation in the pithed rat. Br J Pharmacol 61:559–566, 1977.

Haeusler G: Activation of the central pathway of the baroreceptor reflex, a possible mechanism of the hypotensive action of clonidine. N-S Arch Pharmacol 278:231–246, 1973.

Hilton SM, Spyer KM: Participation of the anterior hypothalamus in the baroreceptor reflex. J Physiol 218:271–293, 1971.

Isaac L: Clonidine in the central nervous system: Site and mechanism of hypotensive action. J Cardiovasc Pharmacol 2 (Suppl 1): S5–S19, 1980.

Kobinger W: Uber den Wirkungsmechanismus einer neuen antihypertensiven Substanz mit Imidazolin-Struktur. Arch Pharmak Exp Pathol 258:48–58, 1967.

Kobinger W, Pichler L: Localization in the CNS of adrenoceptors which facilitate a cardioinhibitory reflex. N-S Arch Pharmacol 286:371–377, 1975.

Kobinger W, Walland A: Investigations into the mechanism of the hypotensive effect of 2-(2,6-dichlorophenylamino)-2-imidazoline-HCl. Eur J Pharmacol 2:155–162, 1967.

McAllen RM: Inhibition of the baroreceptor input to the medulla by stimulation of the hypothalamic defence area. J Physiol (Lond) 257:45P–46P, 1976.

Onesti G: Antihypertensives and their modes of action. Drug Ther Bull 8(2):35–48, 1978.

Palkovits M, Zaborszky L: Neuroanatomy of central cardiovascular control. Nucleus tractus solitarii: Afferent and efferent neuronal connections in relation to the baroreceptor reflex arc. In DeJong W, Provoost AP, Shapiro AP (eds): "Hypertension and Brain Mechanisms," Vol. 47. Amsterdam–Oxford–New York: Elsevier Scientific Publishing Co., 1977, pp 9–34.

Philippu A, Demmeler R, Roensberg G: Effects of centrally applied drugs on pressure responses to hypothalamic stimulation. N-S Arch Pharmacol 287:389–400, 1974.

Philippu A, Rosenberg W, Przuntek H: Effects of adrenergic drugs on pressure responses to hypothalamic stimulation. N-S Arch Pharmacol 278:373–386, 1973.

Price HL, Price ML, Morse HT: Effects of cyclopropane, halothane, and procaine on the vasomotor "center" of the dog. Anesthesiology 26:55–60, 1965.

Przuntek H, Guimaraes S, Philippu A: Importance of adrenergic neurons of the brain for the rise of blood pressure evoked by hypothalamic stimulation. N-S Arch Pharmacol 271:311–319, 1971.

Rand MJ, Wilson J: Mechanisms of the pressor and depressor actions of ST 155 (2-(2,6-dichlorophenylamino)-2-imidazoline hydrochloride) (Catapres). Eur J Pharmacol 3:27–33, 1968.

Sattler PW, van Zwieten PA: Acute hypotensive action of 2-(2,6-dichlorophenylamino)-2-imidazoline hydrochloride (ST 155) after infusion into the cat's vertebral artery. Eur J Pharmacol 2:9–13, 1967.

Schmitt H, Schmitt H: Localization of the hypotensive effect of 2-(2,6-dichlorophenylamino)-2-imidazoline hydrochloride. Eur J Pharmacol 6:8–12, 1969.

Schmitt H, Schmitt H: Interactions between 2-(2,6-dichlorophenylamino)-2-imidazoline hydrochloride (ST 155, Catapres) and alpha-adrenergic blocking drugs. Eur J Pharmacol 9:7–13, 1970.

Schmitt H, Schmitt H, Boissier JR, Giudicelli JF, Fichelle J: Cardiovascular effects of 2-(2,6-dichlorophenylamino)-2-imidazoline hydrochloride (ST 155): II. Central sympathetic structures. Eur J Pharmacol 2:340–346, 1968.

Schmitt H, Schmitt H, Fenard S: Action of alpha-adrenergic blocking drugs on the sympathetic centres and their interactions with the central sympatho-inhibitory effect of clonidine. Arzneimittel-Forschung 23:40–45, 1973.

Schwartz A, Banach S, Smith JS, Kim KE, Onesti G, Swartz C: Clinical efficacy of clonidine in hypertension. In Onesti G, Kim KE, Moyer JH (eds): "Hypertension: Mechanisms and Management." New York: Grune and Stratton, 1973, pp 389–403.

Sharma JN, Sandrew BB, Wang SC: CNS site of clonidine-induced hypotension: A microiontophoretic study of bulbar cardiovascular neurons. Brain Res 151:127–133, 1978.

Sharma JN, Sandrew BB, Wang SC: CNS site of beta-adrenergic blocker-induced hypotension in the cat: A microiontophoretic study of bulbar cardiovascular neurons. Neuropharmacology 18:1–5, 1979.

Sherman GP, Grega GJ, Woods PJ, Buckley JP: Evidence for a central hypotensive mechanism of 2-(2,6-dichlorophenylamino)-2-imidazoline (Catapresan, ST 155). Eur J Pharmacol 2:326–328, 1968.

Starke K, Endo T: Presynaptic alpha-adrenoceptors. Gen Pharmacol 7:307–312, 1976.

Struyker Boudier HAJ, Smeets GWM, Brouwer GM, van Rossum JM: Hypothalamic alpha-adrenergic receptors in cardiovascular regulation. Neuropharmacology 13:837–846, 1974.

Struyker Boudier H, van Rossum JM: Clonidine-induced cardiovascular effects after stereotaxic application in the hypothalamus of rats. J Pharm Pharmacol 24:410–411, 1972.

Svensson TH, Usdin T: Feedback inhibition of brain noradrenalin neurons by tricyclic antidepressants: Alpha-receptor mediation. Science 202:1089–1091, 1978.

Tadepalli AS, Mills E: Contribution of supracollicular structures of the brain to the central depression of cardiovascular function by clonidine. J Pharmacol Exp Ther 205:693–701, 1978.

Tadepalli AS, Mills E, Schanberg SM: Depression and enhancement of baroreceptor pressor response in cats after intracerebroventricular injection of noradrenergic blocking agents. Dependence on supracollicular areas of the brain. Circ Res 39:724–730, 1976.

U'Prichard DC, Snyder SH: Distinct alpha-noradrenergic receptors differentiated by binding and physiological relationships. Life Sci 24:79–88, 1979.

Psychopharmacology of Clonidine, pages 41–52

Anatomical Mapping of Clonidine (α-2 Noradrenergic) Receptors in Rat Brain: Relationship to Function

W. Scott Young III and Michael J. Kuhar

I. INTRODUCTION

Langer [1974] and others [Berthelsen and Pettinger, 1977] have proposed two distinct α-adrenergic receptor populations, designated as α-1 and α-2. This distinction has pharmacological importance since centrally acting antihypertensive agents fall into the category of α-2 agents, whereas α-1 agents have no comparable pharmacological effects. Like many other receptor sites, noradrenergic α receptors can be identified by binding methods. Suitable ligands for selectively identifying α-1 and α-2 receptors are WB-4101 and p-aminoclonidine (PAC), respectively [U'Prichard and Snyder, 1979; Rouot and Snyder, 1979]. We have localized distinct populations of α-1 and α-2 binding sites in intact tissue sections of rat brain by means of a generally applicable light-microscopic autoradiographic method for localizing receptors [Young and Kuhar, 1979]. These studies have provided insights into the distribution and action of α-adrenergic drugs. In this communication, we summarize some of our studies on α-2 receptors, for which clonidine is a clinically important agonist.

II. METHODS

The overall autoradiographic procedure involves labeling receptors in slide-mounted tissue sections with a high degree of specificity and generating autoradiograms by the subsequent apposition of emulsion-coated coverslips [Young and Kuhar, 1979a].

After extensive preliminary biochemical studies on the binding of PAC to the slide-mounted tissue sections, we were able to show that the properties of the receptors were unaltered by our tissue preparation procedure. The binding of PAC was characterized by high affinity, saturability, and the appropriate pharmacology associated with α-2 receptors. ^{3}H-PAC dissociated from the receptors in slide-mounted tissue sections at a half-time of 44 minutes at 0°C (Fig. 1) and reached equilibrium by approximately 60 minutes (Fig. 2). Figure 3 shows a typical binding curve for ^{3}H-PAC. Specific binding saturation is attained and a Scatchard curve (Fig. 3, inset) reveals a K_d of 0.92 nM and a B_{max} of 3.47 fmoles/mg tissue wet weight for this experiment. Figure 4 shows that clonidine and $(-)-$ norepinephrine displace ^{3}H-PAC with high affinity, whereas $(+)-$ norepinephrine and prazosin, an α-1 adrenergic agent, do not.

The following procedure was used for routine autoradiographic studies as it provided optimal labeling of receptors with good specific to nonspecific ratios: Sections (6 microns) of rat brain were thaw-mounted onto microscope slides. The mounted tissue sections were incubated with 2.5 nM

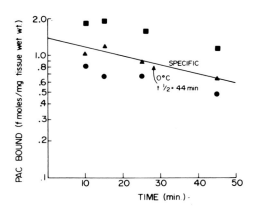

Fig. 1. Dissociation of ^{3}H-PAC from rat tissue sections. Ten-micron sections were incubated in 1.1 nM ^{3}H-PAC for 60 minutes, washed for various lengths of time, and then wiped from the slides and measured for radioactivity. Nonspecific binding was measured in the presence of 10^{-4} M norepinephrine. Symbols: ■ = total; ▲ = specific; ● = nonspecific binding.

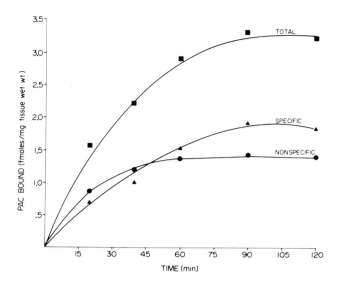

Fig. 2. Association of ³H-PAC with rat tissue sections. Sections were incubated for various lengths of time, washed twice for 5 and 10 minutes, and processed as in Figure 1. For symbols, see legend to Figure 1.

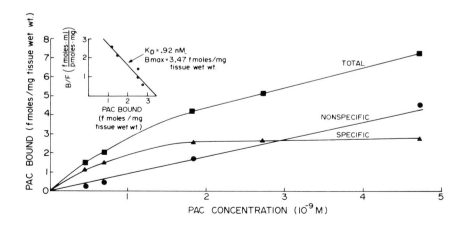

Fig. 3. Saturation curve of ³H-PAC binding to rat tissue sections. Sections were incubated in various concentrations of ³H-PAC for 60 minutes and washed and processed as in Figure 2.

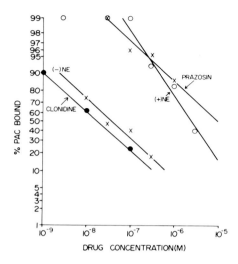

Fig. 4. Pharmacological specificity of ³H-PAC binding in mounted tissue sections. ● = clonidine; X = (−)−norepinephrine; ○ = (+)−norepinephrine; ⊕ = prazosin.

³H-PAC (47.5 Ci/mM) for 60 minutes. After being washed twice for 5 and 10 minutes, the mounted tissue sections were dried in a stream of cold, dry air. Controls were generated by adding 10^{-4} M norepinephrine to separate incubations. In some experiments, adjacent sections were incubated with 1.1 nM ³H-WB4101, an α-1 adrenergic antagonist, instead. The sections were then processed similarly as for ³H-PAC [Young and Kuhar, 1979b, 1980]. Autoradiograms were exposed for four months and developed, fixed and stained as previously described [Young and Kuhar, 1979a, 1980]. The slides were viewed by both brightfield and darkfield microscopy. Under these conditions the autoradiographic technique provides quantitative data because autoradiographic grain densities are proportional to time of exposure and tissue content of radioactivity. All of the observations reported here were readily reproducible and were made in several sections from the same and three different animals.

III. RESULTS

Alpha-2 receptors were found in several different regions of the rat brain. White matter areas in general always showed a low level of autoradiographic grains comparable to the background level observed in controls.

In the olfactory bulb, PAC binding was very high in the external plexiform layer of the olfactory nucleus. In the cerebral cortex moderate to low levels were widely distributed. However, in general, PAC binding was higher in the more superficial layers. The anterior pyriform cortex showed high levels of α-2 receptors, as did a medial portion of the very anterior part of the cerebral cortex. There was low to moderate binding in the caudateputamen, whereas the lateral septum showed a high level of PAC binding. High levels of PAC binding were also found in the basal forebrain anterior to the optic chiasm. Another area showing high levels of α-2 receptors was the interstitial nucleus of the stria terminalis, especially in its dorsal parts.

In the thalamus and hypothalamus, levels of α-2 receptors were elevated in the supraoptic nucleus, the arcuate nucleus, the dorsal medial nucleus of the hypothalamus, and in some periventricular areas (Fig. 3). There was an almost complementary disposition of α-1 and α-2 receptors about the third ventricle, with α-1 receptors located more laterally. In the thalamus, the periventricular nucleus (pars rotundocellularis) also had elevated levels of clonidine receptors (Fig. 5). Binding was generally low in the hippocampus and most midbrain areas, but somewhat elevated in the superior colliculus (Fig. 6).

In the hindbrain, we observed high densities of α-2 receptors in the locus ceruleus (Fig. 7), nucleus tractus solitarii (Fig. 8), nucleus commissuralis, and nucleus raphe pallidus. Other areas that had lower levels that were still considerably above background included the cochlear nuclei, parts of the floor of the fourth ventricle, and the substantiae gelatinosae of the spinal trigeminal nucleus and the spinal cord.

IV. DISCUSSION

Radiohistochemical studies of the distribution of α-2 adrenergic receptors in brain have several potential uses. These studies provide a fairly detailed map of the action of clonidine in the brain. They are also valuable complements to other histochemical studies involving norepinephrine and its synthesizing enzymes for purposes of mapping functional catecholaminergic pathways. Yet another value of these studies is that they provide some insight into the mechanism of the multiple actions of clonidine (Table 1). This aspect will be discussed in more detail.

An important therapeutic property of clonidine is its antihypertensive activity. It has been shown that the antihypertensive effect is due to a central action of the drug. Many experiments have suggested that a primary site of its action is the lower medulla and possibly the hypothalamus [Kobinger, 1978; Schmitt et al, 1971]. In agreement with this, we observed high densities of receptors in the nucleus tractus solitarii and in the medial hypothalamus. The nucleus tractus solitarii is clearly involved in blood pressure control as lesions of this structure cause fulminating hypertension [Doba and Reis, 1974; Talman et al, 1979].

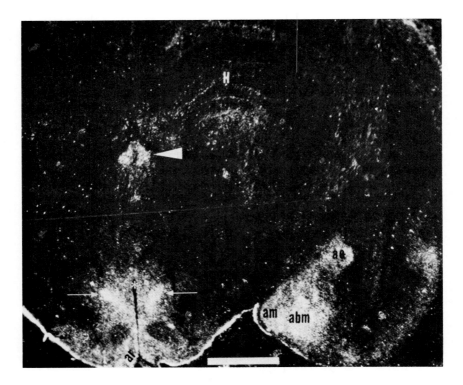

Fig. 5. Darkfield micrographs showing α-2-receptor distribution in a coronal section of rat brain. The level shown is approximately the same as A 3990 μ of König and Klippel [1963]. The bar equals 1,000 μM. In darkfield photomicrographs, the receptors are represented by the white silver grain accumulations. Note the high densities of α-2 receptors in the medial hypothalamus, the amygdala, and the periventricular nucleus (pars rotundocellularis) in the dorsomedial thalamus (large arrowhead). The bilateral smaller arrows touch the dorsomedial nucleus of the hypothalamus, pars dorsalis. An adjacent control section did not have any of these grain accumulations. Adjacent sections incubated in 10⁻⁴ M norepinephrine had very low levels comparable to that shown below the large arrowhead. Abbreviations: ar = nucleus arcuatus; am = nucleus amygdaloideus medialis; abm = nucleus amygdaloideus basalis, pars medialis; ac = nucleus amygdaloideus centralis; H = hippocampal formation.

Another interesting use of clonidine is the blocking of opiate withdrawal symptoms. It has been shown that administration of clonidine blocks onset of the withdrawal syndrome in animals [Fielding et al, 1978; Spaulding et al, 1979] as well as humans [Gold et al, 1978]. In this connection, we found high densities of α-2 receptors in several areas previously shown to have high densities of opiate receptors [Atweh and Kuhar, 1977a, b, c]. These areas

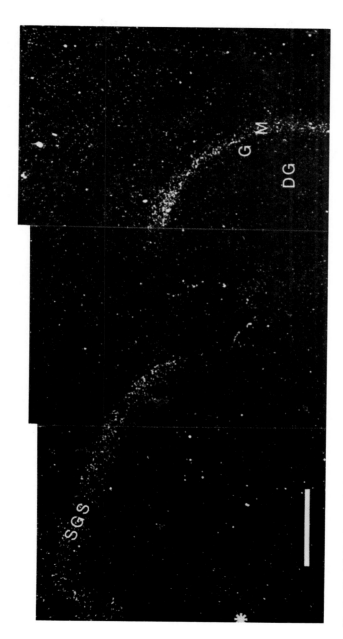

Fig. 6. Darkfield micrograph showing α-2-receptor distribution at level A1610 μ of König and Klippel [1963]. The bar equals 1,000 μ. There is very little binding except over the superficial layer of the superior colliculus (SGS) and the molecular layer (M) of the dentate gyrus (DG). The positions of the granule cells (G) in DG and the cerebral aqueduct (*) in the central gray are shown.

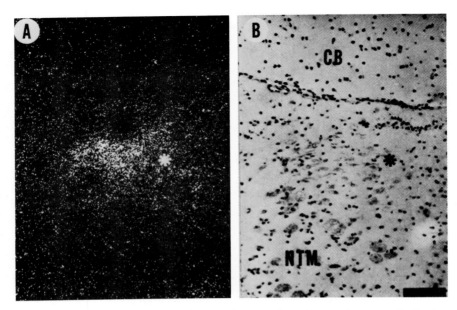

Fig. 7. Distribution of α-2 receptors in area of locus ceruleus. A) The α-2 receptor distribution is shown. Note the strikingly high level of α-2 receptors in the locus ceruleus. B) Brightfield micrograph shows the cerebellum (CB), the mesencephalic nucleus of the trigeminal nerve (NTM), and the locus ceruleus (asterisk is placed immediately to its right). Bar = 100 μ.

TABLE I. Tentative Correlations Between Anatomical Areas, Receptors, and Drug Actions

Drug action	Region
Antihypertensive	Nucleus tractus solitarius
	Hypothalamus
Opiate-like (antinociceptive action and blockade of opiate withdrawal)	Substantiae gelatinosae (spinal cord and trigeminal)
	Raphe pallidus
	Locus ceruleus
	Periventricular nucleus (thalamus)
Anxiolytic	Locus ceruleus
	Limbic areas (amygdala, septum)
Endocrine	Arcuate nucleus
	Median eminence

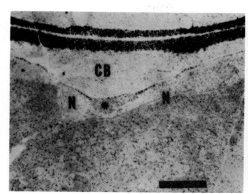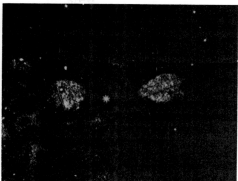

Fig. 8.   Brightfield (left) and darkfield (right) photomicrographs of the same area of a slide showing the bilateral nucleus tractus solitarius (N) situated in the floor of the fourth ventricle immediately below the cerebellum (CB). The area postrema is identified with an asterisk. Note the striking concentration of α-2 receptors in the nucleus tractus solitarius, which is much higher than in any of the other areas in this section. The bar equals 500 microns.

include the substantiae gelatinosae of the spinal cord and spinal trigeminal nucleus, the vagal nuclei, the locus ceruleus and adjacent areas of the fourth ventricle, the dorsomedial thalamus, and parts of the amygdala and olfactory nucleus. Thus, administration of clonidine would affect many of the same brain areas as opiates. Aghajanian [1978] has found that clonidine inhibits the firing of locus ceruleus neurons, and we have found that opioids have a similar effect on this nucleus [Young et al, 1977]. Thus, when systemic opiate levels fall to low values, as in withdrawal, administration of clonidine is likely to result in a morphine-like action on a number of areas normally affected by opiates. Interestingly, there is evidence that naloxone, an opiate antagonist, can reverse clonidine-induced hypotensive effects [Farsang and Kunos, 1979; Resnick et al, 1980].

There have been some reports indicating that clonidine has an antianxiety effect [Redmond, 1977; Redmond and Huang, 1979]. We have in fact found high densities of clonidine receptors in a number of brain areas normally associated with anxiety [Papez, 1937; Zeman and Innes, 1963]. Perhaps the most striking would be the limbic areas. We observed high densities in parts of the amygdala and in the lateral septum. The locus ceruleus also has been connected to the syndrome of anxiety [Redmond, 1977; Redmond and Huang, 1979], and we found high densities of α-2 receptors in this area as well.

Administration of clonidine has certain endocrine effects [Brown et al, 1978; Weiner and Ganong, 1978]. For example, clonidine administration results in an increase of the plasma level of growth hormone, and we also found high densities of α-2 adrenergic receptors in areas intimately involved in hormonal regulation, such as the median eminence and the arcuate nucleus in the hypothalamus.

Using similar techniques, we further examined the distribution of α-1 receptors and β-adrenergic receptors in the rat brain [Palacios and Kuhar, 1980; Young and Kuhar, 1979, 1980]. The distributions of these receptors were different from each other and different from that of the α-2 receptors. In general, α-1 receptors were more widely distributed throughout the brain. They did not show high concentrations in areas in which α-2 receptor levels were found to be elevated. Alpha-1 adrenergic receptors were found in increased amounts in the external plexiform layer of the olfactory bulb, whereas α-2 receptors were found in the external plexiform layer of the olfactory nucleus.

Alpha-1 receptors were also found in the hypothalamus but more lateral in location than α-2 receptors. In the hippocampal formation, the molecular layer of the dentate gyrus had higher levels of α-1 receptors than did the remainder of the structure, but the overall levels were moderate to low. Caudally, however, the dentate gyrus showed fairly high levels. ^{3}H-PAC binding was low in these areas. ^{3}H-WB 4101 was bound to a greater extent in the central gray than ^{3}H-PAC, and the reverse was true for the superior colliculus. Finally, whereas α-2 receptors were prominent in several brain stem areas, α-1 receptor levels were consistently lower.

Similarly, preliminary studies have shown β-adrenergic receptors to have their own unique pattern of distribution [Palacios and Kuhar, 1980]. For example, β receptors are found in the molecular layer of the cerebellum but not in the hypothalamus, in contrast to the α receptors. Another area, the cerebral cortex, shows a greater variation in the density of β receptors in its laminae than of α receptors.

Original experiments designed to identify α-2 adrenergic receptors in the periphery suggested a presynaptic localization of these receptors, whereas α-1 receptors were thought to be predominantly postsynaptic [Langer, 1974; Berthelsen and Pettinger, 1977]. In the brain, some of the α-2 receptors may be located presynaptically as well. For example, several workers have found that α-2 receptors appear to block norepinephrine release in brain slices [Farnebo and Hamberger, 1971; Starke, 1977]. However, lesion experiments suggest that perhaps not all α-2 receptors are located presynaptically. For example, administration of 6-hydroxydopamine to deplete noradrenergic nerve terminals in the forebrain resulted in only a slight decrease of α-2 receptors in the septum and amygdala, whereas the remainder of the brain showed an increase in receptors [U'Prichard et al, 1979]. The resolution necessary to settle this issue was lacking in our light-microscopic studies. In the brain, however, the localization of α-2 adrenergic receptors is likely to be both presynaptic and postsynaptic.

V. ACKNOWLEDGMENTS

We wish to thank Ms. Mary Conrad and Mrs. Naomi Taylor for excellent technical assistance and Ms. Darlene Weimer for clerical assistance. This work was supported by PHS grants MH 25951, DA 00266, and MH 00053, and by PHS postdoctoral fellowship MS 07624 to Dr. Young.

VI. REFERENCES

Aghajanian GK: Tolerance of locus ceruleus neurons to morphine and suppression of withdrawal response by clonidine. Nature 276:186–188, 1978.

Atweh S, Kuhar MJ: Autoradiographic localization of opiate receptors in rat brain. I. Spinal cord and lower medulla. Brain Res 124:53–67, 1977a.

Atweh S, Kuhar MJ: Autoradiographic localization of opiate receptors in rat brain. II. The brain stem. Brain Res 129:1–12, 1977b.

Atweh S, Kuhar MJ: Autoradiographic localization of opiate receptors in rat brain. III. The telencephalon. Brain Res 134:393–405, 1977c.

Berthelsen S, Pettinger WA: A functional basis for classification of alpha-adrenergic receptors. Life Sci 21:595–606, 1977.

Brown GM, Friend WC, Chambers JW: Neuropharmacology of hypothalamic pituitary regulation. In Tolis G, Labrie F, Martin J, Naftolin F (eds): "Clinical Neuroendocrinology." New York: Raven Press, 1978, pp 47–81.

Doba N, Reiss D: Role of central and peripheral adrenergic mechanisms in neurogenic hypertension produced by brainstem lesions in rat. Circulation Res 34:293–301, 1974.

Farnebo LO, Hamberger B: Drug-induced changes in the release of ^{3}H-monoamines from field stimulated rat brain slices. Acta Physiol Scand Suppl 371:35–44, 1971.

Farsang C, Kunos G: Naloxone reverses the antihypertensive effect of clonidine. Br J Pharmacol 67:161–164, 1979.

Fielding SJ, Walker MH, Szewczak M, Novick WJ Jr, Lal H: A comparison of clonidine with morphine for antinociceptive and antiwithdrawal actions. J Pharmacol Exp Ther 207:899–905, 1978.

Gold MS, Redmond DE Jr, Kleber HD: Clonidine blocks acute opiate withdrawal symptoms. Lancet 2:599–602, 1978.

Kobinger W: Central alpha-adrenergic systems as targets for hypotensive drugs. Rev Physiol Biochem Pharmacol 81:39–100, 1978.

König JR, Klippel RA: "A Stereotoxic Atlas of the Forebrain and Lower Parts of the Brain Stem." New York: Robert E. Krieger Publishing Co., 1963.

Langer SZ: Presynaptic regulation of catecholamine release. Biochem Pharmacol 23:1793–1800, 1974.

Palacios JM, Kuhar MJ: Beta-adrenergic receptor localization by light microscopic autoradiography. Science, 1980.

Papez JW: A proposed mechanism of emotion. Arch Neurol Psychiatr 38:725–743, 1937.

Redmond DE Jr: Alterations in the function of the nucleus locus ceruleus: A possible model for studies of anxiety. In Hanin I, Usdin E (eds): "Animal Models in Psychiatry and Neurology." New York: Pergamon Press, 1977, pp 293–304.

Redmond DE Jr, Huang YH: New evidence for a locus coeruleus–norepinephrine connection with anxiety. Life Sci 25:2149–2162, 1979.

Resnick RB, Washton AM, Lal H: Reversal of clonidine-induced hypotension by opioid antagonists in man. In Way EL (ed): "Endogenous and Exogenous Opiate Agonists and Antagonists." New York: Pergamon Press, 1980, pp 565–566.

Rouot BR, Snyder SH: (^{3}H)Para-amino-clonidine: A novel ligand which binds with high affinity to alpha-adrenergic receptors. Life Sci 25:769–774, 1979.

Schmitt H, Schmitt H, Fernard S: Evidence for α-sympathomimetic component in the effects of catapresan on vasomotor centers: Antagonism by piperoxane. Eur J Pharmacol 14:90–100, 1971.

Spaulding TC, Fielding S, Venafro JJ, Lal H: Antinociceptive activity of clonidine and its potentiation of morphine analgesia. Eur J Pharmacol 58:19–25, 1979.

Starke K: Regulation of noradrenaline release by presynaptic receptor systems. Rev Physiol Biochem Pharmacol 77:1–124, 1977.

Talman W, Perrone MH, Doba N, Reis DJ: Fulminating hypertension produced by local injection of kainic acid into the nucleus tractus solitarii in the rat. Proc Soc Neurosci 9:176 (Abstract), 1979.

U'Prichard DC, Snyder SH: Distinct alpha-noradrenergic receptors differentiated by binding and physiological relationships. Life Sci 24:79–88, 1979.

U'Prichard DC, Yamamura HI, Reisine TD: Characterization and differential in vivo regulation of brain adrenergic receptor subtypes. In Pepeu G, Kuhar MJ, Enna S (eds): "Neurotransmitter and Hormone Receptors." New York: Raven Press, 1979.

Weiner RI, Gonong WF: Role of brain monoamines and histamine in regulation of anterior pituitary secretion. Physiol Rev 58:905–976, 1978.

Young WS III, Bird SJ, Kuhar MJ: Iontophoresis of methionine-enkephalin in the locus coeruleus area. Brain Res 129:366–370, 1977.

Young WS III, Kuhar MJ: A new method for receptor autoradiography: ^{3}H-opioid receptors in rat brain. Brain Res 179:255–270, 1979a.

Young WS III, Kuhar MJ: Noradrenergic alpha-1 and alpha-2 receptors: Autoradiographic visualization. Eur J Pharmacol 59:317–319, 1979b.

Young WS III, Kuhar MJ: Noradrenergic alpha-1 and alpha-2 receptors: Light microscopic autoradiographic localization. Proc Natl Acad Sci USA, 77, 1980.

Zeman W, Innes JRM: "Craigie's Neuroanatomy of the Rat." New York: Academic Press, 1963.

Psychopharmacology of Clonidine, pages 53–74

^{3}H-Clonidine and ^{3}H-p-Aminoclonidine Interactions In Vitro With Central and Peripheral α_2-Adrenergic Receptors

David C. U'Prichard

I. INTRODUCTION

The use of in vitro radioligand binding techniques to label selectively different adrenergic receptor types has yielded much information in the past 5 years about the molecular characteristics of adrenergic receptors and the manner in which these receptors are coupled to cellular effector mechanisms [Williams and Lefkowitz, 1978]. This has been true especially for β-adrenergic receptors ever since the introduction of specific, high-affinity antagonist radioligands [Aurbach et al, 1974; Lefkowitz et al, 1974]. Corresponding studies on α receptors and their associated mechanisms have until now proceeded at a somewhat slower pace, owing initially to the lack of a clear distinction between α_1 and α_2 receptor binding sites and to the relative ignorance about α-receptor-effector coupling, in contrast to the array of knowledge concerning β-receptor-adenylate cyclase interactions in many homogeneous cell systems [Maguire et al, 1977]. Recently, however, the availability of ^{3}H-clonidine and a substituted derivative, ^{3}H-p-aminoclonidine, possessing high specific radioactivity, has led to the successful use of these ligands as probes to examine the molecular characteristics of an α receptor type in the brain known as the α_2 receptor that modulates the release of norepinephrine (NE).

Clonidine, which is used clinically as an antihypertensive agent, has profound centrally mediated hypotensive and sedative activity. Although it also shows some histamine-like activity, the major pharmacological characteristic of clonidine is its potent interaction with classic postjunctional α receptors (α_1 receptors) and α_2 receptors. In the brain and at the periphery, clonidine is more potent at α_2 than at α_1 receptors [Langer, 1979; Starke et al, 1975], but it acts as a partial rather than a full agonist at both types of α receptor [Starke et al, 1974; Medgett et al, 1978]. p-Aminoclonidine is a vasopressor agent with extraordinarily high potency at vascular α receptors [Ronot and Snyder, 1979], but it is of limited therapeutic usefulness because it does not readily enter the brain. However, since it is more potent than clonidine at α_2 receptor sites, it is useful as an α_2 receptor probe in tissues in which tissue yield or receptor density is a limiting factor.

The aims of the present paper are: 1) to describe recent studies demonstrating the interaction of ^{3}H-clonidine and ^{3}H-p-aminoclonidine with brain and peripheral tissue α_2 receptors, and 2) to outline evidence that a population of the α_2 receptors labeled by these ligands which is postsynaptic at central NE synapses may be coupled to adenylate cyclase in an inhibitory manner or, in other words, "inversely coupled." More direct evidence for this hypothesis is presented on the basis of experiments from our laboratory on the interactions of ^{3}H-p-aminoclonidine with α_2 receptors on human platelets and neuroblastoma × glioma (NG108-15) hybrid cell line membranes. The characteristics of the ^{3}H-clonidine and ^{3}H-p-aminoclonidine binding to α-receptors in bovine vascular tissues are also described, as is evidence that brain β- and α_2-receptors are functionally linked in such a way that procedures that cause a desensitization of β-receptors lead to an increase in the number of α_2-receptors.

II. BASIC CHARACTERISTICS OF ^{3}H-CLONIDINE AND ^{3}H-p-AMINOCLONIDINE BINDING TO RAT BRAIN MEMBRANES

In initial studies [Greenberg et al, 1976; U'Prichard et al, 1977b], the NE-displaceable binding of ^{3}H-clonidine (^{3}H-CLO) at 1.6 Ci/mM was found to be saturable and appeared to have single site characteristics. Binding was rapidly and linearly dissociable, and had the inhibitor potency spectrum of an

α receptor. The ranking order of catecholamines was the same as at the site labeled by a benzodioxane α antagonist, ³H-WB-4101, except that at the ³H-CLO site α-methyl-NE was more potent than NE. Imidazolines were generally as potent as or more potent than (-)-epinephrine (EPI)($K_i = 2 - 11$ nM) (Table I). Compared with brain ³H-WB sites, antagonists such as ergot alkaloids and phentolamine were as potent in inhibiting ³H-CLO binding, whereas yohimbine and tolazoline were more potent, and phenoxybenzamine and WB-4101 were less potent (Table II). Methoxamine, a selective α_1 agonist, was a weak inhibitor of ³H-CLO binding [U'Prichard et al, 1977b].

In general, at K_i values of 6 nM for (-)-EPI and 17 nM for (-)-NE, agonists were much more potent inhibitors of ³H-CLO binding, than of ³H-WB binding. The finding that many antagonists were more potent inhibitors of ³H-WB binding, however, led Snyder and collaborators to suggest that ³H-CLO labels an agonist-preferring conformation, whereas ³H-WB labels an antagonist-preferring conformation, of the same postsynaptic α receptor in the brain; they had observed initially that ³H-CLO binding did not decrease in 6-OHDA-treated animals [Greenberg et al, 1976, U'Prichard et al, 1977b]. However, different regional distributions of the two binding sites in rat and bovine brain [U'Prichard et al, 1977a, b], along with inconsistencies in this hypothesis with regard to the affinities of some antagonists, culminating in the later discovery that prazosin is 10,000 times more potent in inhibiting ³H-WB than ³H-CLO binding [U'Prichard et al, 1978], led to the revised suggestion that ³H-CLO labels a population of predominantly postsynaptic α_2 receptors in the brain, whereas ³H-WB labels α_1 receptors [U'Prichard et al, 1978; U'Prichard and Snyder, 1979]. The much higher potency of yohimbine than of prazosin at ³H-CLO sites [U'Prichard et al, 1979a] and the reverse situation at ³H-WB sites [U'Prichard et al, 1977b, 1978] confirmed this classification. ³H-CLO sites in the brain show a significant correlation of drug potency with α_2 receptor-mediated effects on transmitter release in the rabbit duodenum, cat cardioaccelerator nerves, and brain slices [Titeler et al, 1978; U'Prichard and Snyder, 1979]. The catecholamine radioligands ³H-NE and ³H-EPI label the same α_2 receptor site in the brain as ³H-CLO [U'Prichard and Snyder, 1978a].

In the rat cortex, binding of the ergot alkaloid ³H-dihydroergocryptine (³H-DHEC) under the appropriate conditions is α receptor-specific. The affinity constants of agonist and antagonist inhibitors of ³H-DHEC binding are the logarithmic means of constants at the ³H-CLO and ³H-WB sites (Tables I and II) [Greenberg and Snyder, 1978]. This evidence, together with the observations: a) that drugs selective at either the ³H-CLO or the ³H-WB sites had shallow ³H-DHEC inhibition curves (n_H about 0.6 [Greenberg and Snyder, 1978]); b) that in bovine cerebellum, which contains many more ³H-catecholamine than ³H-WB sites [U'Prichard et al, 1977a], kinetic con-

TABLE I. Apparent Dissociation Constants of Some Agonist and Partial Agonist Inhibitors of Binding to Putative α-Adrenergic Receptor Sites in Rat Brain

Drug	α_2 Sites		α_1 Sites		$\alpha_1 + \alpha_2$	
	^{3}H-EPI	^{3}H-CLO	^{3}H-PAC	^{3}H-WB	^{3}H-PRAZ	^{3}H-DHEC
			K_i app (nM)			
(−) − Epinephrine	5.2	2.1	2.9	590	600	46
(+) − Epinephrine	92	65	−	28,000	−	2,700
(−) − α-Methylnorepine- phrine	11.5	3.4	−	2,800	−	160
(−) − Norepinephrine	20	6.1	10.5	1,000	900	120
(+) − Norepinephrine	2,200	170	363	67,000	43,000	3,000
Dopamine	200	250	−	44,000	−	720
(−) − Phenylephrine	580	115	−	2,600	1,400	1,200
(−) − Isoproterenol	2,800	5,600	2,900	70,000	−	18,000
p-Aminoclonidine	−	0.63	0.91	130	−	−
Clonidine	3.0	2.0	2.8	430	340	52
Tramazoline	−	2.0	−	110	290	−
Oxymetazoline	3.0	1.2	1.7	24	23	15
Naphazoline	−	1.5	−	110	43	−
Methoxamine	−	940	−	11,000	−	−

Inhibition of the binding of epinephrine (EPI), clonidine (CLO), p-aminoclonidine (PAC), WB-4101 (WB), prazosin (PRAZ) and dihydroergocryptine (DHEC) was determined under equilibrium (sodium- and nucleotide-free) conditions at 25°C, using ^{3}H-ligand concentrations equal to the K_D value or less. The formula of Cheng and Prusoff was applied to obtain K_i values. Data taken from Greenberg and Snyder, 1978; Greengrass and Bremner, 1979; Rouot and Snyder, 1979; U'Prichard et al, 1977b, 1978, 1979a.

TABLE II. Apparent Dissociation Constants of Some Antagonist Inhibitors of Binding to Putative α-Adrenergic Receptor Sites in Rat Brain

Drug	α_2 Sites		α_1 Sites		$\alpha_1 + \alpha_2$	
	^{3}H-EPI	^{3}H-CLO	^{3}H-PAC	^{3}H-WB	^{3}H-PRAZ	^{3}H-DHEC
			K_i app (nM)			
Phentolamine	19	2.0	3.1	3.6	−	6.2
Tolazoline	−	80	−	2,100	2,000	−
Phenoxybenzamine[a]	490	20	17.2	4.0	0.9	31
Dibenamine[a]	−	270	−	83	−	260
Ergotamine	6.3	2.4	−	12	−	2.2
Dihydroergotamine	−	3.0	−	3.5	−	1.6
Dihydroergocryptine	7.1	7.0	−	2.4	−	1.7
Ergonovine	1,400	1,400	−	1,800	−	150
Yohimbine	−	47	57	480	1,000	62
Piperoxan	−	36	−	180	360	110
WB-4101	340	108	138	0.6	1.0	29
Prazosin	−	5,000	−	0.49	0.1	39
Indoramin	36,000	26,000	−	5.9	5.0	240

See footnote to Table I.

[a]Noncompetitive inhibition.

stants of ³H-DHEC and ³H-catecholamine binding site inhibitors were identical [Peroutka et al, 1978]; c) that the number of cortical ³H-DHEC sites was equal to the sum of ³H-WB sites and sites labeled with ³H-CLO, ³H-EPI, or ³H-NE [U'Prichard et al, 1979b; U'Prichard and Snyder, 1979], and that cortical ³H-DHEC binding in the presence of 300 nM indoramin (sufficient to occupy selectively all α_1 receptors) assumed the pharmacological and site number characteristics of ³H-EPI or ³H-CLO binding [Peroutka et al, 1978]; and d) that inhibition of ³H-DHEC binding by prazosin was markedly biphasic [U'Prichard et al, 1979b], all led to the general conclusion that in the brain ³H-DHEC labels α_1 receptors (selectively labeled by ³H-WB) and α_2 receptors (selectively labeled by ³H-CLO, ³H-EPI, and ³H-NE [U'Prichard et al, 1978]) with equal affinity. Other data suggest that this finding also applies to many peripheral tissues [U'Prichard and Snyder, 1979]. The hypothesis concerning ³H-DHEC interactions in rat cortex was confirmed by Miach and co-workers [1978]. More recently there is evidence in some peripheral tissues that ³H-WB can label α_2-receptors [Daiguji et al, 1981].

Preliminary studies at our laboratory indicate that ³H-DHEC binding to bovine cortex membranes in the presence of 100 nM prazosin indeed has α_2 receptor characteristics, and that the affinity constants of yohimbine and piperoxan (α_2 antagonists) are the same as at the ³H-EPI or ³H-CLO site [U'Prichard, 1979]. However, catecholamine agonists are 6–20 times weaker inhibitors of ³H-DHEC binding to α_2 receptors than of ³H-EPI or ³H-CLO α_2 receptor binding (Table III), suggesting that central α_2 receptors, like β receptors in general [Maguire et al, 1977], can exist in both high and low agonist affinity states, the former state being selectively labeled by ³H-catecholamines and ³H-CLO. It is interesting to note that although ³H-CLO and ³H-catecholamine α_2 receptor sites are very similar, the affinity of clonidine for inhibiting ³H-DHEC α_2 receptor binding is as high as at the ³H-EPI site (Table III). This may mean that clonidine is a partial rather than a full agonist at the central α_2 receptors labeled in binding studies.

The selective labeling of brain α_2 receptors by ³H-CLO has been demonstrated in another way. Lefkowitz and co-workers have shown that, as in the brain, prazosin and yohimbine inhibit ³H-DHEC α-receptor binding in the rabbit uterus in a shallow, biphasic manner. These investigators utilized computer-modeled curve fitting procedures to determine the number of uterine α_1 sites and α_2 sites with high affinity for prazosin and yohimbine, respectively, and the affinity constants of these inhibitors for each α receptor population [Hoffman et al, 1979]. α_2-Receptors constituted 55% of the total number of ³H-DHEC sites, at which the K_i values of prazosin and yohimbine were 7600 and 14 nM [Hoffman et al, 1979]. These affinity constants correspond well to the values for prazosin and yohimbine as inhibitors of α_2 sites in the brain labeled by the specific ligand ³H-CLO.

TABLE III. Inhibition of Binding α Receptor Sites in Bovine Cortex Labeled by an Agonist, ^{3}H-Epinephrine, and an Antagonist, ^{3}H-Dihydroergocryptine: Effects on Drug Affinities of 100 μM GTP and 100 mM NaCl

Drug	^{3}H-EPI	^{3}H-DHEC Control	GTP	NaCl
		IC$_{50}$ (nM)		
$(-)$ – Epinephrine	2.5	50	380	1,000
$(-)$ – Norepinephrine	24	150	400	5,000
Clonidine	3.3	3.6	10	250
Dihydroergocryptine	8.3	4.6	5.6	4.5
Dihydroergotamine	3.2	2.2	1.8	5.7
Yohimbine	60	46		75
Piperoxan	24	20		34

Cortex membranes were incubated for 60 min at 25°C with 0.3 nM ^{3}H-DHEC in the presence of 100 nM prazosin to eliminate α_1 receptor binding. IC$_{50}$ concentrations were determined by log probit analysis.

Sites in the rat cerebral cortex labeled by the analog ^{3}H-p-aminoclonidine (^{3}H-PAC) (40–50 Ci/mM) have the same α_2 receptor characteristics as ^{3}H-CLO sites [Rouot and Snyder, 1979]. ^{3}H-PAC is about three times more potent than clonidine itself at both the α_2 receptor labeled by ^{3}H-CLO (K$_D$ 0.87 nM vs 2.0 nM) and at the α_1 receptor labeled by ^{3}H-WB. Therefore, clonidine and p-aminoclonidine have similar selectivity for the α_2 receptor. The increased affinity of ^{3}H-PAC for brain α_2 receptor sites is due both to increased rates of association and to decreased rates of dissociation as compared to ^{3}H-CLO. ^{3}H-PAC is also 2–3 times more potent than ^{3}H-CLO in the bovine cortex and in some peripheral tissues such as rat kidney and spleen [Rouot and Snyder, 1979]. Although p-aminoclonidine is a potent vasopressor agent [Rouot and Snyder, 1979], not enough is known about its in vitro pharmacology to decide whether it, like clonidine, is a partial agonist rather than a full agonist at both α_1 and α_2 receptors.

The differences in pharmacological potencies at brain α_2 receptor sites labeled by ^{3}H-imidazolines or ^{3}H-catecholamines, and at α_1 receptor sites labeled by ^{3}H-WB or ^{3}H-prazosin, compared to the non-receptor-specific labeling of ^{3}H-DHEC, are illustrated in Tables I and II for agonists and antagonists.

Other laboratories have examined structure–activity relationships at brain ^{3}H-CLO sites in more detail. Many imidazoline components and the hypotensive agent guanabenz and analogs have potencies similar to that of clonidine, but clonidine metabolites are one-tenth to one-fiftieth as potent as the parent compound [Jarrot et al, 1979a]. Tanaka and Starke [1980] have observed that among the diastereoisomers of yohimbine, rauwolscine (α-yohimbine) is as potent as yohimbine in inhibiting ^{3}H-CLO binding, but rauwolscine is much more α_2-selective, ie, much less potent at the ³H-WB site, which is in keeping with the pharmacological specificity of rauwolscine. Corynanthine, α_1-selective yohimbine isomer, is more potent at the ³H-WB site. Bovine cortex have recently been labeled in our laboratory in a very selective manner with ³H-rauwolscine (80 Ci/mmole). As with ³H-DHEC (Table III), both high and low affinity states are labeled [Perry and U'Prichard, 1981].

III. MULTIPLE RAT BRAIN α₂-RECEPTOR SITES LABELED BY ³H-CLONIDINE

Before the initial experiments with ³H-CLO, it was expected that this ligand would preferentially label α_2 receptors on NE-presynaptic terminal membranes, since this is the hypothetical location of the NE release-modulating receptor. Recent studies with ³H-CLO (27 Ci/mM) have shown two components of α_2 receptor binding sites in rat cerebral cortex that differ in affinity for ³H-CLO (K_D values 0.4 nM and 2 nM) and other agonists [U'Prichard et al, 1979a]. Both the equilibrium binding isotherms and the dissociation of ³H-CLO were nonlinear, and by selectively dissociating the low-affinity component of the specific binding sites, U'Prichard et al were able to isolate the high-affinity component [1979a]. The distribution of the high-affinity component of ³H-CLO binding sites differed from that of the low-affinity component; distribution of the latter was much more uniform and widespread, whereas the high-affinity component was prevalent in forebrain areas, especially the cerebral cortex, but not in the corpus striatum. Even in the cortex, however, the binding capacity of the high-affinity component was much lower than that of the low-affinity component. It seemed possible that the low-capacity, high-affinity component represents receptors on NE terminals. However, after i.c.v. 6-OHDA, neither component of ³H-CLO binding was reduced significantly in any brain region, and the number of high-affinity sites was in fact increased 100% in the cerebral cortex [U'Prichard et al, 1979a]. This led to speculation that ³H-CLO binds to different types of central α_2 receptor, and that the α_2 receptor species with higher affinity for agonists might be located postsynaptically at central NE synapses and therefore subject to "denervation supersensitivity." At neither binding site did terminal receptors predominate. However, the data could also be interpreted as pointing to two states or conformations of the α_2 receptor with different agonist affinities, as had been suggested for the β receptor [Maguire et al, 1977]. In addition to these two receptor states ("super-high" and "high" affinity), there is also a third state ("low" affinity) which is undetectable with ³H-CLO or other ³H-agonists, but may be observed with ³H-antagonists (see Table III). Equally important, the absence of a reduction in ³H-CLO binding after NE terminal destruction does not prove the nonexistence of α_2 receptors on central NE terminal membranes if one accepts the coexistence of pharmacologically identical postsynaptic α_2 receptors. In the presence of a more specific lesion of the dorsal noradrenergic bundle, ^{3}H-CLO binding is increased the rat cortex, and the increase is preferentially associated with the high-affinity component [U'Prichard et al, 1980]. In this study, ^{3}H-CLO binding was decreased in lesioned amygdala and septum, suggesting that in these areas there is a greater prevalence of true presynaptic α_2 receptors.

IV. IN VITRO ALLOSTERIC EFFECTS ON α_2-RECEPTOR BINDING OF ^{3}H-CLONIDINE IN BRAIN

Extensive investigation of two hormone receptor systems that are "positively" coupled to adenylate cyclase in plasma membranes (ie, interaction of the hormone or other agonists with the receptor stimulates adenylate cyclase activity) has shown that the guanine nucleotide GTP acts as a "coupling" agent for the receptor and cyclase moieties. At cyclase-coupled glucagon receptors in hepatocytes [Rodbell et al, 1971] and β receptors in frog erythrocytes [Lefkowitz, 1974] and other cells [Maguire et al, 1977], GTP is required for full agonist-mediated stimulation of the enzyme. At the glucagon and β receptors, GTP has the additional observed effect of decreasing the affinity of agonist ligands specifically by accelerating dissociation [Lin et al, 1977; Williams and Lefkowitz, 1977]. It has been suggested that the GTP-induced conversion of the receptor from a high-affinity to a low-affinity state for agonist is an integral step in the coupling of the receptor to adenylate cyclase that results in stimulation of the enzyme [Williams and Lefkowitz, 1977].

Alpha receptors in mammalian brain have been indirectly associated with increased adenylate cyclase activity [Skolnick and Daly, 1975]. Soon after the identification of brain α receptors by ^{3}H-CLO and ^{3}H-catecholamines, it was observed that the guanine nucleotides GTP and GDP and the phosphohydrolase-resistant analog guanylyl-5'-imidodiphosphate (Gpp(NH)p) potently decrease ^{3}H-EPI and ^{3}H-NE-specific binding to bovine cortex α receptors [U'Prichard and Snyder, 1978b]. These nucleotides were approximately equipotent (ED_{50} 1–5 μM) and were several orders of magnitude more effective than adenine nucleotide analogs. The nucleotide-induced reduction in agonist affinities at ^{3}H-catecholamine α receptor sites in brain membranes is closely similar to nucleotide effects on ^{3}H-glucagon or ^{3}H-hydroxybenzylisoproterenol binding to glucagon and β receptors, respectively [Lin et al, 1977; Williams and Lefkowitz, 1977], suggesting that the brain α receptor site is associated with the components of an adenylate cyclase system. Not until later was it realized that the brain ^{3}H-catecholamine sites represent α_2 receptors [U'Prichard et al, 1978].

After these studies it became apparent that the α_2 receptors in several tissues — eg, platelets and NG 108-15 cells — are coupled to adenylate cyclase in an "inverse" manner. Tsai and Lefkowitz [1979] observed that GTP and

Gpp(NH)p were equally effective (ED_{50} 4 μM) in decreasing the affinities of agonists, but not antagonists, at ^{3}H-DHEC sites in human platelet membranes. Furthermore, in these studies, the extent to which GTP altered the affinity of an agonist was directly correlated to its intrinsic activity in inhibiting adenylate cyclase. In our laboratory, we have shown that GTP and Gpp(NH)p will directly reduce the high-affinity binding of the α_2 agonist ligands ^{3}H-PAC and $(-) - ^3$H-EPI to human platelet and NG 108-15 membranes, with ED_{50}s in the 0.1-1.0 μM range. The above studies lead to two conclusions: a) that a receptor like the α_2 receptor, which is "inversely" linked to adenylate cyclase activity, is coupled to the enzyme via a regulatory protein with a GTP site, similarly to "positively" coupled receptors; and b) that the α receptors labeled in mammalian brain may also be "inversely" coupled to adenylate cyclase. Another "inversely" coupled receptor, the opiate receptor, has been shown to be very similarly influenced by guanine nucleotides in brain and NG 108-15 membranes [Blume, 1978].

The effect of guanine nucleotides on frog erythrocyte β receptors is dependent on the presence of magnesium to induce a high agonist affinity state, which is then influenced by the nucleotide [Williams and Lefkowitz 1977]. A similar relationship between GTP and Mg^{2+} exists at the platelet α_2 receptor in that Mg^{2+} greatly facilitates the ability of GTP to decrease agonist affinities at ^{3}H-DHEC sites [Tsai and Lefkowitz, 1979], and guanine nucleotides decrease the specific binding of the agonists ^{3}H-PAC and ^{3}H-EPI much better in the presence of at least 1.0 mM Mg^{2+} (Mitrius and U'Prichard, in preparation). However, in bovine and rat brain membranes, Mg^{2+} and other divalent cations, especially Mn^{2+}, antagonize rather than facilitate the reduction of α_2 agonist ligand binding by GTP and GDP [U'Prichard and Snyder, 1978c, 1980]. The significance of this difference between platelet and neural α_2 receptors, and its relation to possible differences in modes of cyclase coupling, is at present unclear, but it is noteworthy that Mg^{2+} and other divalent cations did not affect the ability of the nonhydrolyzable analog Gpp(NH)p to inhibit brain α_2 agonist binding, from which the inference may be drawn that in brain membranes the nucleotide–cation interactions could be associated with GTPase activity or membrane protein phosphorylation [U'Prichard and Snyder, 1980]. Similar cation–nucleotide interactions at ^{3}H-clonidine binding sites in the brain were observed by Glossman and Presek [1979].

In rat cortex membranes, where two α_2 receptor sites with differential affinities for ^{3}H-CLO and other agonists can be discerned [U'Prichard et al, 1979a], only the high-affinity site is sensitive to GTP and divalent cations. Kinetic and equilibrium analyses of binding indicated that GTP decreases the number of high-affinity ^{3}H-CLO sites, with no change in the number of low-affinity sites and no change in the observed K_D for ^{3}H-CLO at either site [Rouot et al, 1980]. It has been suggested that GTP converts the majority of the high-affinity receptors to a state with sufficiently low affinity for ^{3}H-CLO to make them undetectable in the binding assay. An alternative explanation to a partial GTP sensitivity of ^{3}H-CLO binding in rat brain is that clonidine is a partial agonist at rat brain α_2 receptors, as it is in platelets and NG 108-15 cells. However, the binding of ^{3}H-EPI was much less susceptible to GTP in rat cortex than in bovine cortex, from which we may infer that either fewer α_2 receptors are cyclase-coupled or all α_2 receptors are less efficiently coupled in rat cortex [Rouot et al, 1980].

Another similarity between opiate and α_2 receptor sites is the effect of small monovalent cations on agonist binding. Previously Na$^+$ had been found to decrease ^{3}H-agonist binding to central opiate receptors [Pert and Synder, 1974]. Opiate binding of ^{3}H-antagonists was increased by Na$^+$ [Pert and Snyder, 1974], probably on account of accelerated dissociation of endogenous opioid peptides. It has been suggested that at "inversely" coupled receptors Na$^+$ and GTP regulate the receptor conformation and receptor-cyclase coupling in the same manner, whereas Na$^+$ influences may be absent from "positively" coupled receptors [Blume et al, 1979].

Both Na$^+$ and Li$^+$ are potent in reducing the specific binding to brain α_2 receptors of the agonist ligands ^{3}H-CLO, ^{3}EPI, and ^{3}H-NE (ED$_{50}$ 10–20 mM) [Greenberg et al, 1978]. Monovalent cations with a larger, hydrated radius, such as K$^+$ and Cs$^+$, are much less effective. At submaximal Na$^+$ and GTP concentrations, the actions of these allosteric agents on brain α_2 agonist binding are strictly additive [U'Prichard and Snyder, 1978b], whereas Na$^+$ has a significant permissive effect on the ability of GTP to reduce the agonist affinities of opiate receptors [Childers and Snyder, 1978]. Divalent cations, especially Mn^{2+}, antagonize Na$^+$ influences at central α_2 receptors with the same potency as they antagonize GTP effects [U'Prichard and Snyder, 1978c, 1980], suggesting that a common mechanism is responsible for the regulation of α agonist affinities by nucleotides and monovalent cations. It should be noted, however, that in the rat cortex both high- and low-affinity components of ^{3}H-CLO α_2 receptor binding sites were Na$^+$-sensitive, whereas only the high-affinity component proved GTP-sensitive [Rouot et al, 1980]. At bovine cortex α_2 receptor sites specifically labeled by the antagonist ^{3}H-DHEC (in the presence of 100 nM prazosin), the potencies of agonists, not antagonists, where reduced by both Na$^+$ and GTP, but the "Na$^+$ shift" was much more extensive [U'Prichard, 1979] (Table III). The receptor binding of ^{3}H-DHEC on rabbit platelet membranes has been found to be subject to similar ionic influences [Tsai and Lefkowitz, 1978b].

V. REGULATION OF α_2-RECEPTORS LABELED BY ^{3}H-CLONIDINE

In contrast to the great number of investigations of the mechanisms of β receptor desensitization in various tissues, relatively few studies have been done to date concerning the regulation of either α_1 or α_2 receptors. The study of desensitization mechanisms in peripheral tissues containing α_2 receptors such as platelets [Cooper et al, 1978], NG 108-15 cells [Sabol and Nirenberg, 1979], or rat salivary glands [Strittmatter et al, 1977], either did not involve receptor–ligand binding measurements or utilized the nonselective ligand ³H-DHEC. In brain slices, down regulation of β receptors (a decrease in β receptor sites and β-mediated cAMP accumulation) occurs very rapidly and is easily reversible [Dibner and Molinoff, 1979; U'Prichard and Enna, 1979; Wagner and Davis, 1979]. Incubation of brain slices with 100 μM clonidine will also rapidly reduce the number of α receptor sites labeled by ³H-PAC (U'Prichard and Enna, unpublished observations).

An intriguing observation is that several in vivo and in vitro procedures which down regulate β receptors cause a parallel increase in the number of α_2 receptors in the brain. Thus, incubation of rat cortical slices with 100 μM isoproterenol causes a rapid decrease in the number of β receptor sites, but an even more rapid increase in the number of cortical α_2 receptor sites labeled by ³H-PAC [Maggi et al, 1980] (Fig. 1). Both events are readily reversible by washing out the isoproterenol (Fig. 1), and the increase in the number of α_2 receptors is prevented by concurrent incubation with the β antagonist sotalol. Similarly, chronic immobilization stress decreases the number of cortical β receptors, whereas acute stress (one 150-minute period) does not. However, both acute and chronic stress increase the number of cortical α_2 receptor sites labeled by ³H-CLO [U'Prichard and Kvetnansky, 1980]. Rats treated with a combination of amphetamine and iprindole (which retards the metabolism of amphetamine) for 3 days show a loss of cortical β receptors, whereas each drug given separately for the same time has no effect on β receptors. However, a 3-day treatment with the drugs given either separately or together causes an increase in the number of cortical α_2 receptor sites labeled by ³H-PAC [Reisine et al, 1980]. The increase is limited to the high-affinity component of the ³H-PAC binding sites, which, according to denervation studies, have a postsynaptic cortical localization. Similar findings have been made after chronic desipramine treatment [Johnson et al, 1980]. These data are summarized in Table IV.

A possible explanation for data showing reciprocal modulation of β and α_2 receptors in the brain is that: a) the α_2-receptor population involved is postsynaptic at NE synapses and may occur on the same plasma membranes as cortical postsynaptic β receptors; b) in rat cortex, α_2 receptors and β receptors are "inversely" and "positively" coupled to the same pool of adenylate cyclase, possibly via the same pool of guanine nucleotide regulatory sites; c) the opposite changes in the receptor binding sites are reflected in parallel changes in catecholamine-mediated cyclic AMP accumulation, ie, changes in the direction of "desensitization." The regulation of cortical α_2 receptors appears to be dependent on initial β receptor activation, but perhaps not on β receptor "desensitization." In the cortex, the postsynaptic α_2 receptor may be allosterically linked to β receptors. This hypothesis is supported at a func-

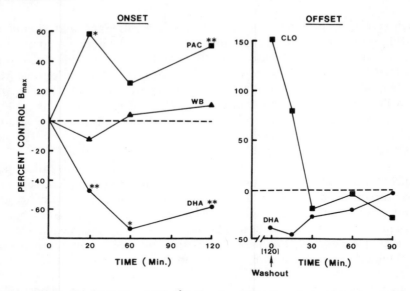

Fig. 1. Time course of onset and offset of alterations in number of adrenergic receptors in rat cerebral cortex induced by preincubation of cortical slices with 100 μM $(-)$ – isoproterenol. At each time point the numbers of α_1 receptors, α_2 receptors, and β receptors were determined from saturation isotherms of ^{3}H-WB-4101 (WB) binding, ^{3}H-p-aminoclonidine (PAC), or ^{3}H-clonidine (CLO) binding, and ^{3}H-dihydroalprenolol (DHA) binding, respectively, in slices from 2–10 rats. To determine the reversibility of receptor alterations (B), slices were preincubated with isoproterenol for 120 min, then washed and transferred to isoproterenol-free medium.

tional level by the finding of Skolnick and Daly [1975] that clonidine potentiates the isoproterenol-induced increase in the concentration of cyclic AMP in cortical slices, an effect that is blocked by phentolamine.

VI. ALPHA-RECEPTOR BINDING IN HOMOGENEOUS CELL POPULATIONS

Platelets present a useful, homogeneous model system for studying the biochemical pharmacology of α_2 receptor function and regulation. Two α receptor-mediated responses, inhibition of adenylate cyclase activity [Robison et al, 1969] and platelet aggregation [Barthel and Markwardt, 1974], can be determined and correlated with receptor binding studies. The aggregation response has been shown to have α_2 receptor characteristics [Grant and Scrutton, 1979].

TABLE IV. Reciprocal Effects on Numbers of β- and α_2-Adrenergic Receptors in Rat Cortex In Vitro and In Vivo

Treatment	β Receptor (³H-DHA B_{max})	α Receptor (³H-PAC or ³H-CLO B_{max})
	fmoles/mg protein	
A) Incubation of cortex slices with isoproterenol		
Control	550 ± 50	$1{,}200 \pm 150$
100 μM Isoproterenol	230 ± 30**	$1{,}800 \pm 200$*
B) Chronic immobilization stress		
Control	67 ± 6	58 ± 8
Stressed (14 days)	41 ± 2*	78 ± 4*
C) Treatment with amphetamine plus iprindole		
Control	113 ± 7	140 ± 15
Treated (3 days)	81 ± 3*	185 ± 15*

In saturation experiments, β receptor binding was determined in each case with ³H-dihydroalprenolol (DHA), and α_2 receptor binding with ³H-p-aminoclonidine (PAC), except in the stress experiments, in which ³H-clonidine (CLO) was used. In treatment (A), slices were incubated for 120 min at 37°C; in treatment (B), rats were immobilized for a 150-min period every day, and sacrificed immediately after the last period; in treatment (C), rats were treated twice daily with amphetamine (10 mg/kg) and once daily with iprindole (25 mg/kg), and sacrificed 16 hrs after the last amphetamine treatment.
*P < 0.05.
**P < 0.01.

In our laboratory we have labeled human platelet membranes with $(-)-$³H-EPI, a full agonist for the cyclase and aggregating response, and ³H-PAC, at platelet α receptors a partial agonist. Both ligands specifically label platelet α receptors with high affinity. The interaction of these ligands, unlike their binding in the brain, is to some extent magnesium-dependent (with 1.0 mM magnesium, ³H-PAC $K_D = 1.9$ nM; ³H-EPI $K_D = 8.3$ nM). The pharmacological characteristics of the sites are closely similar to the brain α_2 receptor sites labeled by the same ligands (Table V). No specific platelet binding of ³H-prazosin was found, indicating that platelets have a pure α_2 receptor population. Although antagonists such as yohimbine and phentolamine exhibited similar affinities for inhibiting ³H-EPI, ³H-PAC, or ³H-DHEC binding to platelets, catecholamines and other agonists proved to be much more potent inhibitors of ³H-EPI and ³H-PAC binding than of ³H-DHEC binding (Table V). The data suggest that ³H-EPI and ³H-PAC label conformations of the α_2 receptor having a high agonist affinity, even though PAC, like clonidine, may be only a partial agonist. Similar results have been obtained with ³H-CLO [Shattil et al, 1981]. We have recently confirmed this in an examination of the interactions of the po-

TABLE V. Alpha Receptor Binding of [3]H Ligands on Human Platelet Membranes: Comparison of Drug Potencies With α Receptor-Mediated Effects on Platelet Adenylate Cyclase

Drug	^{3}H-EPI	^{3}H-PAC	^{3}H-DHEC	Adenylate cyclase
		K_i or K_D (nM)		
Agonists				
(−) − Epinephrine	−	2.6	260	1,500
(−) − Norepinephrine	7.7	6.2	850	10,000
(+) − Norepinephrine	380	230	17,000	100,000
(−) − Isoproterenol	400	650	142,000	100,000
(−) − Phenylephrine[a]	−	135	860	−
Clonidine[a]	1.6	1.7	17	−
Antagonists				
Phentolamine	3.2	5.6	6.9	200
Yohimbine	7.7	6.4	2.0	60
Prazosin	10,000	15,000	−	−

Platelet membranes were incubated at 25°C with 0.6 nM ^{3}H-p-aminoclonidine (PAC) or with 1-2 nM (−)-^{3}H-epinephrine (EPI) in the presence of 1.0 mM pyrocatechol. Binding was defined as specific if it was displaceable by 1.0 μM phentolamine (PAC), or 1.0 μM oxymetazoline (EPI). K_i values were determined by the Cheng-Prusoff equation. ^{3}H-Dihydroergocryptine (DHEC) binding and adenylate cyclase data have been taken from Newman et al [1978].
[a]Partial agonist in inhibiting adenylate cyclase.

tent, selective antagonist ^{3}H-yohimbine with platelet α_2 receptors [Daiguji et al, 1981]. Agonists are 10–100 times weaker in inhibiting ^{3}H-yohimbine than in inhibiting ^{3}H-PAC binding, and they give "shallow" inhibition curves vs ^{3}H-yohimbine in the absence of guanine nucleotides.

The study of the properties of α receptors in neural tissue is hampered by the lack of clearly devined α receptor-mediated responses at the cellular level. For this reason, it is significant that a neuroblastoma × glioma hybrid cell line NG108-15 (108CC15) [Hamprecht, 1977] was recently shown to possess an α receptor, stimulation of which, as in platelets, reduces basal and PGE-stimulated adenylate cyclase activity [Sabol and Nirenberg, 1979]. These cells also possess opiate [Klee and Nirenberg, 1974] and muscarinic [Matsuzawa and Nirenberg, 1975] receptors, which inhibit adenylate cyclase activity, and the inversely coupled receptors appear to be functionally coupled to the same pool of catalytic cyclase — or regulatory — molecules [Sabol and Nirenberg, 1979]. We have shown that the NG108-15 α receptors are, as in platelets, of the α_2 type, since there is no specific binding of ^{3}H-WB-4101 or ^{3}H-prazosin.

The α_2 ligands ^{3}H-PAC and (−) − ^{3}H-EPI bind with high affinity to about 10,000–20,000 receptors per cell, which is somewhat less than the number of opiate receptors on these cells. While ³H-PAC, which is, like clonidine, a weak partial agonist at the NG108-15 α_2 receptor [Kahn et al, 1982], and binds to a single class of sites with K_D of about 4 nM, the binding of $(-)-³H$-EPI is nonlinear, a high affinity component of about 4–5 nM accounting for somewhat more sites per cell than labeled by ³H-PAC. The relation between affinity constants at the sites labeled by these ligands and the adenylate cyclase response is very similar to that in human platelets (Table VI); antagonists are equipotent in inhibiting the ³H-PAC binding and in antagonizing catecholamine-induced inhibition of adenylate cyclase, but agonists are in general two orders of magnitude more potent at the α_2 receptor binding site. This seems to mean that ³H-PAC (and ³H-EPI) label a high-agonist affinity conformation of the receptor, just as they do in the brain. ³H-Yohimbine labels about 30,000 sites per cell, and, as in platelets, binds to both high and low affinity forms of the receptor [Kahn et al, 1982]. One difference between platelet and NG108-15 receptors is that high-affinity interactions of ³H-PAC and ³H-EPI at the NG108-15 α_2 receptor are not dependent on the presence of magnesium. The lack of magnesium dependence is also seen in brain α_2 receptor–agonist interactions and may reflect a fundamental difference between the properties of neural and nonneural α_2 receptors.

TABLE VI. Drug Inhibition of ³H-p-Aminoclonidine Binding to α Receptors in Neuroblastoma $\times$ Glioma (NG 108-15) Cells: Comparison With α Receptor-Mediated Effects on Adenylate Cyclase

Drug	³H-PAC	Adenylate cyclase
	K_i (nM)	IC_{50}/K_D (nM)
Agonists		
$(-)$ – Norepinephrine	1.6	510
$(+)$ – Norepinephrine	62.0	380,000
$(-)$ – Epinephrine	1.9	250
$(-)$ – Phenylephrine[a]	30.0	4,500
$(-)$ – Isoproterenol	41.0	24,000
Clonidine[a]	3.3	470
Oxymetazoline[a]	3.6	575
Antagonists		
Dihydroergocryptine	2.6	10
Phentolamine	9.3	10
Yohimbine	11.8	40
WB-4101	100	200

³H-PAC assays were performed on washed cell membranes as in Table V. Assays of basal adenylate cyclase activity at 37°C were performed according to Kahn et al [1982].
[a]Partial agonists in inhibiting adenylate cyclase.

VII. ³H-CLONIDINE AND ³H-p-AMINOCLONIDINE BINDING IN PERIPHERAL TISSUES

³H-PAC and ³H-CLO binding to α_2 receptors has been reported in a few peripheral rat tissues, such as kidney, spleen, and salivary glands, as well as in rabbit duodenum [U'Prichard and Snyder, 1979]. Alpha receptor-mediated responses in the salivary glands (K⁺ release) and kidney (renin release) have α_2 receptor characteristics [Arnett and Davis, 1979; Berthelson and Pettinger, 1977], and α_2 sites in these tissues labeled by ³H-CLO or ³H-DHEC are not reduced in number by peripheral chemical sympathectomy, a fact suggesting a postjunctional location [Arnett and Davis, 1979; U'Prichard and Snyder, 1979]. In tissues such as the heart, however, where α_2 receptor-mediated regulation of NE release from cardioaccelerator neurons is well established, and especially in the vas deferens, where sympathetic innervation is of great density, ³H-CLO α_2 receptor binding is, surprisingly, not readily demonstrable. These negative findings suggest that the concentration of α_2 receptors on sympathetic terminals is generally very low. In extensive characterizations of ³H-CLO binding in guinea pig kidney, Jarrott and co-workers [1979b] found that kidney and brain sites were pharmacologically very similar, and that binding occurred primarily in the renal cortex [Jarrott et al, 1980].

A receptor system of great physiological and therapeutic importance is the postjunctional α receptor located on vascular smooth muscle, stimulation of which causes vasoconstriction. The identification and characterization of vascular α receptors in binding studies is of prime importance but vascular tissue has proved more refractory to this kind of in vitro analysis than other organs, the chief problem in small mammals being the low yield of membranes. One published report [Tsai and Lefkowitz, 1978a] has described the binding of ³H-DHEC to semipurified membranes from dog aorta. Recent experiments in our laboratory have demonstrated a specific binding of ³H-WB and ³H-prazosin to α_1 receptors, and of ³H-CLO, ³H-PAC and ³H-rauwolscine to α_2 receptors, in a purified preparation of smooth muscle membranes from the tunica media of bovine aorta [U'Prichard and Rosendorff, submitted].

Both ³H-WB and ³H-prazosin bound with high affinity to a single class of sites in the bovine aortic media membranes; the number of sites labeled by these ligands were similar, as were the α_1 characteristics of the specific binding (Table VII). ³H-CLO and ³H-PAC labeled a site in the same membranes having a lower density and showing α_2 receptor characteristics since yohimbine proved a considerably more potent displacer than prazosin (Table VII). The interactions of ³H-CLO with the aortic α_2 receptor showed significant positive cooperativity (Fig. 2), unique among ³H-CLO interactions in various

TABLE VII. Drug Inhibition of α Receptor Binding of Radioligands in Tunica Media Membranes of Bovine Aorta

	³H-WB-4101	³H-Prazosin	³H-Clonidine	³H-PAC
		K_i (nM)		
Agonists				
(−) – Epinephrine	470	3,900	4.3	2.8
(−) – Norepinephrine	3,100	3,500	300	27
(+) – Norepinephrine	72,800	—	3,200	—
(±) – Isoproterenol	45,500	—	1,000	—
Clonidine	1,070	1,320	2.4	13.8
Antagonists				
Prazosin	5.2	1.7	1,200	265
Phentolamine	7.3	23	6.3	0.6
Yohimbine	730	190	20	15.6
Piperoxan	1,080	—	—	—

Membranes from a low-speed supernatant fraction were sonicated and washed, and incubated to equilibrium at 25°C with ³H ligand. Binding in each case was defined as specific if displaced by 10 μM phentolamine.

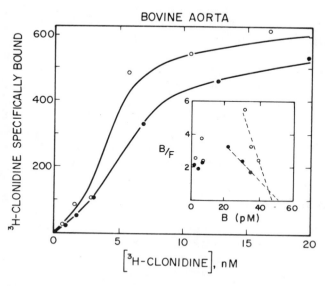

Fig. 2.   Saturation isotherms of ³H-clonidine-specific binding (10 μM phentolamine blank) to α_2 receptors in tunica media membranes of bovine aorta. Points are from two different experiments. Inset: Scatchard plots of ³H-clonidine saturation.

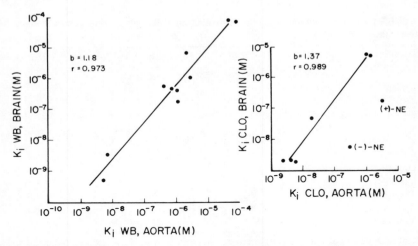

Fig. 3. Correlations between potencies of α receptor agonists and antagonists at rat brain and tunica media α_1 receptor sites in bovine aorta labeled by ^{3}H-WB-4101 (WB), and α_2 receptor sites labeled by ^{3}H-clonidine (CLO).

tissues, but similar to α_2 receptor interactions of ^{3}H-DHEC reported in the rat heart [Guicheney et al, 1978]. In general, the α_1 and α_2 receptor sites in the bovine aorta were similar to those in the brain (Fig. 3), but the NE isomers were considerably less potent at the aortic than at the brain α_2 receptor. The tissue distribution of aortic binding differed for the two receptor types, α_1 binding being slightly higher in the media than in the adventitia and α_2 binding much higher in the adventitia. It is not clear from these studies whether the aortic α_2 receptor sites are pre- or postjunctional, but the techniques used in this study are applicable to vascular tissue from other large species in which denervation is possible. We have recently shown that ^{3}H-rauwolscine labels high and low affinity forms of the α_2 receptor in media membranes with a K_D of 1.0 nM [U'Prichard and Rosendorf, submitted].

VIII. CONCLUSIONS

Since the initial identification of α receptors by radioligand binding methods in 1976, ^{3}H-CLO and ^{3}H-PAC have become extremely useful probes for the identification and characterization of α_1 and α_2 receptor subtypes. It is becoming more and more likely that correlation of functional studies with the binding of ^{3}H-CLO and other α_2 ligands will soon allow the mechanisms of α_2 receptor coupling to adenylate cyclase and of α_2 receptor regulation to be clarified in some cellular systems, at least to the extent of our present knowledge about β receptors.

Still to be accomplished is a conclusive demonstration of the existence of true NE "autoreceptors," ie, α_2 receptors located on sympathetic or central noradrenergic terminal membranes. However, binding studies have indicated that postjunctional or postsynaptic α_2 receptors are more prevalent than previously suspected, and there is strong evidence from both binding and functional studies that these α_2 receptors are in general "inversely" coupled to adenylate cyclase. However, the physiological role of postjunctional α_2 receptors is very unclear in most instances. These questions are critical for the precise localization of the action of clonidine at central synapses.

IX. ACKNOWLEDGMENTS

This research was supported by USPHS grant NS 15595 and a grant-in-aid from the American Heart Association. The author is indebted to Joan Mitrius and Deborah Kahn for their assistance.

X. REFERENCES

Arnett CD, Davis JH: Denervation-induced changes in alpha and beta adrenergic receptors of the rat submandibular gland. J Pharmacol Exp Ther 211:394–400,1979.

Aurbach GD, Fedak SA, Woodard CJ, Palmer JS, Hauser D, Troxler F: β-Adrenergic receptor: Stereospecific interaction of iodinated β-blocking agent with high affinity site. Science 186:1223–1224, 1974.

Barthel W, Markwardt F: Aggregation of blood platelets by biogenic amines and its inhibition by antiadrenergic and antiserotinergic agents. Biochem Pharmacol 24:37–46, 1974.

Berthelsen S, Pettinger WA: A functional basis for classification of α-adrenergic receptors. Life Sci 21:595–606, 1977.

Blume AJ: Opiate binding to membrane preparation of neuroblastoma × glioma hybrid cells NG108-15: Effects of ions and nucleotides. Life Sci 22:1845–1852, 1978.

Blume AJ, Lichtshtein D, Boone G: Coupling of opiate receptor to adenylate cyclase: Requirement for Na⁺ and GTP. Proc Natl Acad Sci USA 76:5626–5630, 1979.

Childers SR, Snyder SH: Guanine nucleotides differentiate agonist and antagonist interactions with opiate receptors. Life Sci 23:759–762, 1978.

Cooper B, Handin RI, Young LH, Alexander RW: Agonist regulation of the human platelet α-adrenergic receptor. Nature (Lond) 274:703–706, 1978.

Daiguji M, Meltzer HY, U'Prichard DC: Human platelet α_2-adrenergic receptors: labeling with ³H-yohimbine, a selective antagonist ligand. Life Sci 28:2705–2717, 1981.

Dibner MD, Molinoff PB: Agonist-induced changes in β-adrenergic receptor density and receptor-mediated responsiveness in slices of rat cerebral cortex. J Pharmacol Exp Ther 210:433–439, 1979.

Glossman H, Presek P: Alpha noradrenergic receptors in brain membranes: Sodium, magnesium and guanyl nucleotides modulate agonist binding. Naunyn-Schmied Arch Pharmacol 306:67–73, 1979.

Grant JA, Scrutton MC: Noval α_2-adrenoreceptors primarily responsible for platelet aggregation. Nature (Lond) 277:659–661, 1979.

Greenberg DA, Snyder SH: Pharmacological properties of ³H-dihydroergocryptine binding sites associated with alpha noradrenergic receptors in rat brain membranes. Mol Pharmacol 14:38–49, 1978.

Greenberg DA, U'Prichard DC, Snyder SH: Alpha noradrenergic receptor binding in mammalian brain: Differential labeling of agonist and antagonist states. Life Sci 19:69–76, 1976.

Greenberg DA, U'Prichard DC, Sheehan P, Snyder SH: Alpha-noradrenergic receptors in the brain: Differential effects of sodium on binding of [3H] agonists and [3H] antagonists. Brain Res 140:378–384, 1978.

Greengrass P, Bremner R: Binding characteristics of ^{3}H-prazosin to rat brain α-adrenergic receptors. Eur J Pharmacol 55:323–326, 1979.

Guicheney P, Garay RP, Levy-Marchal C, Meyer P: Biochemical evidence for presynaptic and postsynaptic α-adrenoceptors in rat heart membranes: Positive homotropic cooperativity of presynaptic binding. Proc Natl Acad Sci USA 75:6285–6289, 1978.

Hamprecht B: Structural, electrophysiological, biochemical and pharmacological properties of neuroblastoma–glioma cell hybrids in cell culture. Int Rev Cytol 49:99–169, 1977.

Hoffman B, DeLean A, Wood CL, Schocken DD, Lefkowitz RJ: Alpha-adrenergic receptor subtypes: Quantitative assessment by ligand binding. Life Sci 24:1739–1746, 1979.

Jarrott B, Louis WJ, Summers RJ: The effect of a series of clonidine analogues on ^{3}H-clonidine binding in rat cerebral cortex. Biochem Pharmacol 28:141–144, 1979a.

Jarrott B, Louis WJ, Summers RJ: The characteristics of ^{3}H-clonidine binding to an α-adrenoceptor in membranes from guinea-pig kidney. Br J Pharmacol 65:663–670, 1979b.

Jarrott B, Culvenor AJ, Louis WJ, Summers RJ: Localization of ^{3}H-clonidine binding in guinea-pig kidney. Circ Res 46:I15–I21, 1980.

Johnson RW, Reisine TD, Spotnitz S, Wiech N, Ursillo R, Yamamura HI: Eur J Pharmacol 67:23–27, 1980.

Kafka MS, Tallman JF, Smith CC: Alpha-adrenergic receptors on human platelets. Life Sci 21:1429–1438, 1977.

Kahn DJ, Mitrius JC, U'Prichard DC: α_2-Adrenergic receptors in neuroblastoma × glioma hybrid cells: Characterization with agonist and antagonist radioligands and relationship to adenylate cyclase. Mol Pharmacol, in press, 1982.

Klee WA, Nirenberg M: A neuroblastoma × glioma hybrid cell line with morphine receptors. Proc Natl Acad Sci USA 71:3474–3477, 1974.

Langer SZ: Presynaptic adrenoceptors and regulation of release. In Paton DM (ed): "The Release of Catecholamines from Adrenergic Neurons." Oxford: Pergamon Press, 1979, pp 59–85.

Lefkowitz RJ: Stimulation of catecholamine-sensitive adenylate cyclase by 5′-guanyl-imido-phosphate. J Biol Chem 249:6119–6125, 1974.

Lefkowitz RJ, Mukherjee C, Coverstone M, Caron MG: Stereospecific ^{3}H-(-)-alprenolol binding sites, β-adrenergic receptors and adenylate cyclase. Biochem Biophys Res Commun 60:703–709, 1974.

Lin MC, Nicosia S, Lad PM, Rodbell M: Effects of GTP on binding of ^{3}H-glucagon to receptors in rat hepatic plasma membranes. J Biol Chem 252:2790–2792, 1977.

Maggi A, U'Prichard DC, Enna SJ: Beta-adrenergic regulation of α_2-adrenergic receptors in the central nervous system. Science 207:645–647, 1980.

Maguire ME, Ross EM, Gilman AG: β-Adrenergic receptor: Ligand binding properties and the interaction with adenylyl cyclase. Adv Cyclic Nucleotide Res 8:1–83, 1977.

Matsuzawa H, Nirenberg M: Receptor-mediated shifts in cAMP and cGMP levels in neuroblastoma cells. Proc Natl Acad Sci USA 72:3472–3476, 1975.

Medgett C, McCulloch MW, Rand MJ: Partial agonist action of clonidine on prejunctional and postjunctional α-adrenoceptors. Naunyn-Schmied Arch Pharmacol 304:215–221, 1978.

Miach PJ, Dausse JP, Meyer P: Direct biochemical demonstration of two types of α-adrenoceptor in rat brain. Nature (Lond) 274:492–494, 1978.

Newman KD, Williams LT, Bishopric NH, Lefkowitz RJ: Identification of α-adrenergic receptors in human platelets by ^{3}H-dihydroergocryptine binding. J Clin Invest 61:395–402, 1978.

Peroutka SJ, Greenberg DA, U'Prichard DC, Snyder SH: Regional variations in α-noradrenergic receptor interactions of [³H] dihydroergokryptine in calf brain: Implications for a two-site model of α-receptor function. Mol Pharmacol 14:403–412, 1978.

Perry BD, U'Prichard DC: ³H-Rauwolscine (α-yohimbine): A specific antagonist radioligand for brain α_2-adrenergic receptors. Eur J Pharmacol, in press, 1981.

Pert CB, Snyder SH: Opiate receptor binding of agonists and antagonists affected differentially by sodium. Mol Pharmacol 10:868–879, 1974.

Reisine TD, U'Prichard DC, Wiech NL, Ursillo RC, Yamamura HI: Effects of combined administration of amphetamine and iprindole on brain adrenergic receptors. Brain Res 188:587–592, 1980.

Robison GA, Arnold A, Hartmann RC: Divergent effects of epinephrine and prostaglandin E1 on level of cyclic AMP in human blood platelets. Pharmacol Res Commun 1:325–334, 1969.

Rodbell M, Birnbaumer L, Pohl SL, Krans HMJ: The glucagon-sensitive adenyl cyclase system in plasma membranes of rat liver. V. An obligatory role of guanyl nucleotides in glucagon action. J Biol Chem 246:1877–1882, 1971.

Rouot BR, Snyder SH: 3H-Para-amino-clonidine: A novel ligand which binds with high affinity to α-adrenergic receptors. Life Sci 25:769–774, 1979.

Rouot BR, U'Prichard DC, Snyder SH: Multiple α-noradrenergic receptor sites in rat brain: Selective regulation of high-affinity [³H] clonidine binding by guanine nucleotides and divalent cations. J Neurochem 34:374–384, 1980.

Sabol SL, Nirenberg M: Regulation of adenylate cyclase of neuroblastoma × glioma hybrid cells by α-adrenergic receptors. I. Inhibition of adenylate cyclase mediated by α-receptors. J Biol Chem 254:1913–1920, 1979.

Sabol SL, Nirenberg M: Regulation of adenylate cyclase of neuroblastoma × glioma hybrid cells by alpha-adrenergic receptors. II. Long lived increase of adenylate cyclase activity mediated by α-receptors. J Biol Chem 254:1921–1926, 1979.

Shattil SJ, McDonough M, Turnbull J, Insel PA: Characterization of alpha-adrenergic receptors in human platelets using ³H-clonidine. Mol Pharmacol 19:179–183, 1981.

Skolnick P, Daly JW: Stimulation of adenosine 3',5'-mono-phosphate formation by α- and β-adrenergic agonists in rat cerebral cortical slices: Effects of clonidine. Mol Pharmacol 11:545–551,1975.

Starke K, Endo T, Taube HD: Relative pre- and postsynaptic potencies of α-adrenergic agonists in the rabbit pulmonary artery. Naunyn-Schmied Arch Pharmacol 291:55–78, 1975.

Starke K, Montel H, Gayk W, Merker R: Comparison of the effects of clonidine on pre- and postsynaptic adrenoceptors in the rabbit pulmonary artery. Naunyn-Schmied Arch Pharmacol 285:133–150,1974.

Strittmater WJ, Davis JN, Lefkowitz RJ: α-Adrenergic receptors in rat parotid cells. II. Desensitization of receptor binding sites and potassium release. J Biol Chem 252:5478–5482, 1977.

Tanaka T, Starke K: Antagonist/agonist-preferring α-adrenoceptors or α_1-/α_2-adrenoceptors? Eur J Pharmacol 63:191–195, 1980.

Titeler M, Tedesco JL, Seeman P: Selective labeling of presynaptic receptors by 3H-dopamine, 3H-apomorphine and 3H-clonidine; labeling of postsynaptic sites by 3H-neuroleptics. Life Sci 23:587–592, 1978.

Tsai BS, Lefkowitz RJ: 3H-Dihydroergocryptine binding to alpha adrenergic receptors in canine aortic membranes. J Pharmacol Exp Ther 204:606–614, 1978a.

Tsai BS, Lefkowitz RJ: Agonist-specific effects of monovalent and divalent cations on adenylate cyclase-coupled alpha adrenergic receptors in rabbit platelets. Mol Pharmacol 14:540–548, 1978b.

Tsai BS, Lefkowitz RJ: Agonist-specific effects of guanine nucleotides on alpha-adrenergic receptors in human platelets. Mol Pharmacol 16:61–68, 1979.

U'Prichard DC: Multiple CNS receptor interactions of ergot aklaloids: Affinity and intrinsic activity analysis in in-vitro binding systems. In Goldstein M(ed): "Ergot Compounds and Brain Function: Neuroendocrine and Neuropsychiatric Aspects." New York: Raven Press, 1979, pp 103–115.

U'Prichard DC, Bechtel WD, Rouot B, Snyder SH: Multiple α-noradrenergic receptor binding sites in rat brain: Effect of 6-hydroxydopamine. Mol Pharmacol 16:47–60, 1979a.

U'Prichard DC, Charness ME, Robertson D, Snyder SH: Prazosin: Differential affinities for two populations of α-noradrenergic receptor binding sites. Eur J. Pharmacol 50:87–89, 1978.

U'Prichard DC, Enna SJ: In vitro modulation of CNS β-receptor number by antidepressants and β-agonists. Eur J Pharmacol 59:297–301, 1979.

U'Prichard DC, Greenberg DA, Sheehan P, Snyder SH: Regional distribution of α-noradrenergic receptor binding in calf brain. Brain Res 138:151–158, 1977a.

U'Prichard DC, Greenberg DA, Snyder SH: Binding characteristics of a radiolabeled agonist and antagonist at central nervous system alpha noradrenergic receptors. Mol Pharmacol 13:454–473, 1977b.

U'Prichard DC, Greenberg DA, Snyder SH: CNS α-adrenergic receptor binding: Studies with normotensive and spontaneously hypertensive rats. In Meyer P, Schmitt H (eds): "Nervous System and Hypertension." New York: Wiley-Flammarion, 1979b, pp 38–48.

U'Prichard DC, Kvetnansky R: Central and peripheral adrenergic receptors in acute and repeated immobilization stress. In Usdin E, Kvetnansky R, Kopin IJ (eds): "Catecholamines and Stress." Amsterdam: Elsevier, 1980, pp 299–308.

U'Prichard DC, Reisine TD, Mason ST, Fibiger HC, Yamamura HI: Modulation of rat brain α-and β-adrenergic receptor populations by lesion of the dorsal noradrenergic bundle. Brain Res 187:143–154, 1980.

U'Prichard DC, Rosendorff C: Direct identification of α_1- and α_2-adrenergic receptor subtypes in bovine aorta membranes. Brit J Pharmacol (submitted).

U'Prichard DC, Snyder SH: Catecholamine binding to CNS adrenergic receptors. J Supramol Struct 9:189–206, 1978a.

U'Prichard DC, Snyder SH: Influences of guanyl nucleotides upon 3H-ligand binding to alpha-noradrenergic receptors in calf brain membranes. J Biol Chem 253:3444–3452, 1978b.

U'Prichard DC, Snyder SH: Nucleotide and ion regulation of CNS adrenergic receptors. In Szabadi E, Bradshaw CM, Bevan P (eds): "Recent Advances in The Pharmacology of Adrenoceptors." Amsterdam: Elsevier, 1978c, pp 153–162.

U'Prichard DC, Snyder SH: Distinct α-noradrenergic receptors identified by binding and physiological relationships. Life Sci 24:79–88, 1979.

U'Prichard DC, Snyder SH: Interactions of divalent cations and guanine nucleotides at α_2-noradrenergic receptor binding sites in bovine brain membranes. J Neurochem 34:385–394, 1980.

Wagner HR, Davis JN: β-Adrenergic receptor regulation by agonists and membrane depolarization in slices. Proc Natl Acad Sci USA 76:2057–2061, 1979.

Williams LT, Lefkowitz RJ: Slowly reversible binding of catecholamine to a nucleotide-sensitive state of the β-adrenergic receptor. J Biol Chem 252:7207–7213, 1977.

Williams LT, Lefkowitz RJ: "Receptor Binding Studies in Adrenergic Pharmacology." New York: Raven Press, 1978.

Psychopharmacology of Clonidine, pages 75–97

Mechanisms of Antihypertensive Action of Clonidine in Relation to Its Psychotropic Effects

W. Hoefke and H.M. Jennewein

I. INTRODUCTION

As investigators who had the opportunity to work with clonidine from the beginning, we would like to recall some older experiments to elucidate the mechanisms of the antihypertensive action of clonidine.

Clonidine exerts a complex influence on the circulation of anesthetized dogs (Fig. 1). A transient rise in blood pressure is followed by a lasting fall. Increasing the dose causes a more distinct rise in blood pressure, which may even conceal the hypotensive activity. Hypertensive and hypotensive actions are accompanied by bradycardia. The nictitating membrane is contracted to a degree depending on the dose. The carotid occlusion reflex—clamping both common carotid arteries—is inhibited by clonidine in dose-dependent measure. This increase in blood pressure and contraction of the nictitating membrane can be explained by action of clonidine on peripheral adrenergic α receptors, whereas hypotension, bradycardia, and inhibition of carotid sinus reflex are centrally mediated. The initial blood pressure increase secondary to vasoconstriction is due to direct activation of α adrenoceptors since clonidine is effective after pretreatment with reserpine [Hoefke and Kobinger, 1967], guanethidine [Robson and Kaplan, 1969], and bretylium [Nayler et al, 1968]. This α-adrenergic effect can be blocked by α adrenoceptor antagonists such as phentolamine and phenoxybenzamine [Hoefke and Kobinger, 1967; Schmitt and Schmitt, 1969].

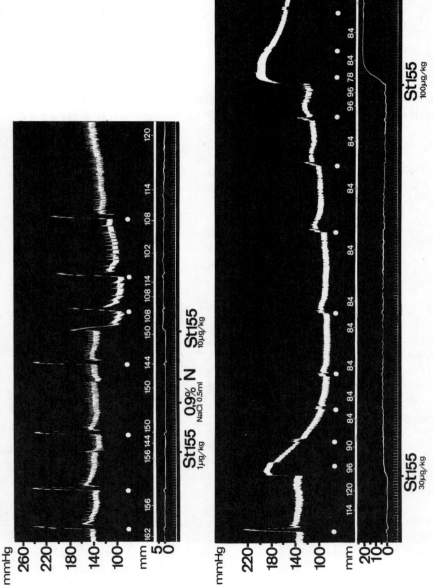

Fig. 1. Cardiovascular effects of clonidine (St 155) in an anesthetized dog. Upper curve: Blood pressure, heart rate values; lower curve: nictitating membrane. At the dots the carotid sinus occlusion reflex was elicited. (Hoefke and Kobinger [1966].)

The vasoconstriction has been seen in the rabbit ear artery, isolated rabbit aortic strips, isolated dog veins, and perfused hind limbs of cats and dogs [Constantine and McShane, 1968; Hoefke and Kobinger, 1966; Haeusler, 1976]. Most of these effects can also be blocked by α adrenoceptor antagonists. High doses of clonidine reduce or reverse the pressor effects of epinephrine as well as those of norepinephrine [Boissier et al, 1966; Hoefke and Kobinger, 1967]. Constantine and McShane [1968] found that clonidine had lower intrinsic activity than epinephrine on the isolated rabbit aorta. The maximum effect of clonidine on rabbit aorta and rat tail artery was also smaller than that of norepinephrine [Hodge and Robinson, 1972; Starke et al, 1974]. Clonidine thus seems to be a partial agonist. Cocaine fails to potentiate vasoconstriction induced by clonidine. Clonidine does not block the uptake of norepinephrine into postganglionic terminals of sympathetic nerves (uptake I) [Autret et al, 1971; Salt, 1972].

II. CENTRAL ACTION

The hypotensive effect of clonidine could not be explained satisfactorily by action on the peripheral circulation. The possibility of a direct vasodilating action, a peripheral inhibitory action on the heart, and ganglionic blocking activity could also be ruled out for all practical purposes [Hoefke and Kobinger, 1966].

Numerous studies have therefore been performed to explore the possibility of action on the central nervous system. Investigations in spinalized animals provided the answer (Fig. 2). In this cat experiment, the action of clonidine on blood pressure and heart rate before and after spinalization could be visualized. If the site of action is in the brain, neither a fall in blood pressure nor bradycardia would occur after spinalization, and this is actually what was observed after the administration of clonidine. Clonidine in fact caused an even sharper rise in blood pressure in the peripheral circulation after pithing.

Administration of clonidine, 1 μg/kg, into the cisterna cerebellomedullaris of a cat caused a lasting fall in blood pressure and bradycardia, whereas intravenous injection of the same dose was largely ineffective [Kobinger, 1967] (Fig. 3). It is assumed that compounds injected into the cisterna reach the fourth ventricle via the foramina of Magendie and Luschka and then pass on to the medulla oblongata. Low concentrations of clonidine infused into one of the vertebral arteries cause a fall in blood pressure and bradycardia, whereas hardly any effect can be observed after infusion of the same doses into a peripheral vein [Sattler and van Zwieten, 1967]. Clonidine injected intracerebroventricularly also decreases the blood pressure [Schmitt and Schmitt, 1969].

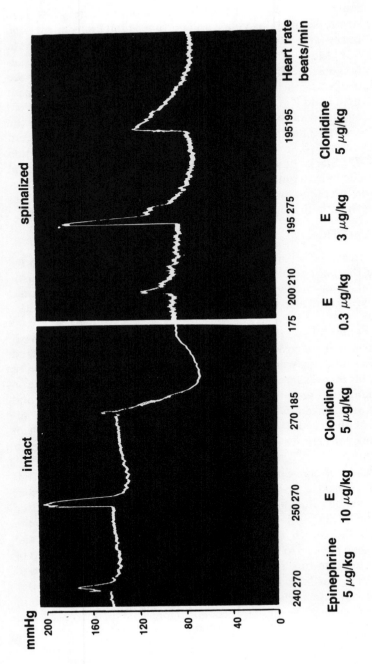

Fig. 2.   Blood pressure and heart rate under the action of clonidine before and after pithing in a cat. Pithing was performed between the two parts of the figure. Epinephrine and clonidine were given IV. (Hoefke [1976].)

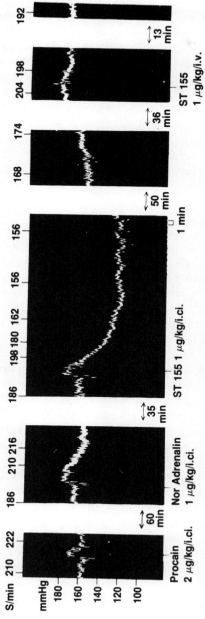

Fig. 3. Blood pressure and heart rate in an anesthetized cat with sectioned vagi, pretreated with atropine (1 mg/kg). Decrease of blood pressure and heart rate, in beats/min (S/min), after intracisternal (i.ci) and intravenous (IV) injection of clonidine. (Kobinger [1967].)

Additional proof for a central site of the hypotensive action was provided in experiments involving crossed circulation [Sherman et al, 1968]. Schmitt and co-workers [1969; Sinha et al, 1973] made further attempts to identify the site of the hypotensive action of clonidine. In cats and dogs in which the brainstem was cut rostrally to the medulla oblongata, the effect of clonidine was retained. However, if the brainstem was cut below the medulla oblongta, neither a decrease in blood pressure nor bradycardia was produced by clonidine.

To investigate the effect of clonidine on sympathetic tone, the electrical activity of sympathetic preganglionic nerves was recorded in anesthetized animals. After intravenous as well as intracerebroventricular administration of clonidine—eg, in dogs and cats—a decrease in the frequency of action potentials was observed in the preganglionic splanchnic nerve [Schmitt and Schmitt, 1969].

III. PRE- AND POST-SYNAPTIC ACTION

A great deal of recent research has been concerned with possible pre- and postsynaptic actions of clonidine. Effects of clonidine on peripheral postsynaptic α adrenoceptors leading to the initial blood pressure increase have been mentioned. We have seen initial indications of a presynaptic action in isolated pieces of rabbit ileum. Electrical stimulation of the nerves supplying the plain muscle as well as administration of norepinephrine reduced the contractility of the gut. In a relatively high range of concentrations, $10^{-7} - 10^{-6}$ g/ml, clonidine inhibited the effect of electrical stimulation but not that of norepinephrine [Hoefke, 1964, unpublished].Tachycardia induced by low-frequency stimulation of the accelerator nerve in cats and dogs was also reduced [Kobinger, 1967; Scriabine et al, 1968, 1970]. Werner et al [1972] were the first to show that clonidine significantly reduces the norepinephrine outflow elicited by electrical stimulation of the accelerator nerve from isolated rabbit hearts, which again points to an action on presynaptic adrenergic receptors.

Starke et al [1974] estimated the affinity of clonidine for pre- and postsynaptic α adrenoceptors in isolated pulmonary arteries of rabbits and calculated EC_{20} values. According to their results, clonidine is approximately six times more potent on presynaptic than on postsynaptic receptors. Drew [1976] demonstrated that clonidine in pithed rats was equipotent on both types of receptors. He investigated the inhibition of tachycardia induced by stimulation of the thoracic sypathetic nerves and the pressor effect. Similar results were reported by Doxey and Everitt [1977]. Effects of clonidine have also been observed on presynaptic α-adrenergic receptors in the rat vas deferens [Drew, 1977]. In studies of the differential activity of clonidine in isolated rabbit aorta strips and in isolated spontaneously beating guinea pig atria, Medgett et al [1978] confirmed the results of Starke and found clonidine to be a partial agonist having a much higher potency at presynaptic than at postsynaptic sites. Differences in the species and tissues used may account for the seemingly large differences in the observed levels of pre- and postsynaptic activity of clonidine. The significance of peripheral presynaptic action for the antihypertensive effect of clonidine remains to be determined. Haeusler [1976] could not demonstrate its functional role in stimulation-induced pressor responses of auto-perfused hindquarters of cats, except at a rather high dose of clonidine, 100 μg/kg iv.

The differences in the ability of different α agonists to act on pre- or postsynaptic adrenergic receptors reflects fundamental differences in the structural requirements of the two receptors. Berthelsen and Pettinger [1977] classified adrenergic receptors that behave like postsynaptic ones as α_1 receptors and those behaving like presynaptic ones as α_2 receptors. They mentioned, however, that "there is evidence for postsynaptic location on other organs for this α_2 receptor."

Alpha-adrenergic antagonists have likewise displayed different effects on pre- and postsynaptic α-adrenergic receptors. In the pithed rat, Drew [1976] tested several α adrenoceptor antagonists antagonizing the bradycardiac effect of clonidine. Phentolamine, yohimbine, and piperoxan were the most active compounds inhibiting the effect of clonidine, which indicates that a presynaptic α_2 receptor is being acted upon. Prazosin, however, inhibited the contractile response of the rabbit pulmonary artery to stimulation without affecting the simultaneously occurring overflow of norepinephrine [Cambridge et al, 1978], and this finding points to action on a postsynaptic α_1 receptor. In view of these findings Timmermans [1980] looked for both types of receptors at postsynaptic sites in the circulatory system of the pithed rat. The increase of diastolic blood pressure induced by clonidine was moderately inhibited by yohimbine, whereas the pressor effect of phenylephrine was not influenced. Prazosin, however, blocked the effects of phenylephrine strongly and those of clonidine moderately. Clonidine behaved as a nonselective agonist (α_1 and α_2), whereas phenylephrine seemed to be an α_1 agonist. According to these and other results, prazosin may be viewed as an α_1-adrenoceptor antagonist and yohimbine as an α_2-adrenoceptor antagonist. Figure 4 gives an overview of these data.

Alpha-noradrenergic receptor sites in brain and peripheral tissues can be labeled by a variety of ligands, such as the agonists H^3-clonidine, H^3-norepinephrine, and H^3-epinephrine, and the antagonist H^3-WB 1401. The H^3-clonidine site has been postulated as the α_2 receptor. According to Starke [1980], yohimbine had nine and rauwolscine 54 times higher affinities for the H^3-clonidine than for the H^3-WB 1401 site in rat brain

	α_1	α_2
postsynaptic	+ +	+
presynaptic	+	+ +
Agonists		
norepinephrine	+ +	+ +
phenylephrine	+ +	(+)
clonidine	+	+ +
Antagonists		
yohimbine	+	+ +
prazosin	+ +	(+)

Fig. 4.   Classification of adrenergic α-receptors as α_1 and α_2 receptors showing distribution of pre- and postsynaptic sites and the effects of various agonists and antagonists.

membranes, whereas corynanthine had a 36 times higher affinity for the H^3-WB 1401 than for the H^3-clonidine site. This points to a selective affinity of corynanthine for α_1 receptors and to selective action of rauwolscine and yohimbine at α_2 receptors.

The hypotensive and bradycardiac effects of clonidine in anesthetized rabbits were almost completely inhibited by pretreatment with yohimbine, but only marginally so by prazosin (Figs. 5 and 6). The blocking agents were used in equipotent doses for norepinephrine inhibition. Similar results were obtained by van Zwieten [1980] in cats that received the drugs via a vertebral artery. Low doses of yohimbine and rauwolscine (3–10 μg/kg) strongly reduced the depressor effect of clonidine, whereas higher doses were needed with corynanthine (100 μg/kg). According to these results, the hypotensive effect of clonidine may be partially due to action on α_1 receptors.

The question now arises whether clonidine reduces sympathetic tone and blood pressure by action on central pre- or postsynaptic α adrenoceptors. In keeping with the results obtained on isolated rabbit pulmonary artery strips, clonidine blocked the norepinephrine outflow of isolated cerebral cortical slices stimulated in vitro [Starke and Montel, 1973]. According to these and other findings, mentioned above, α adrenoceptors that behave like peripheral presynaptic receptors exist within the CNS and can be influenced by clonidine in the same way as at the periphery.

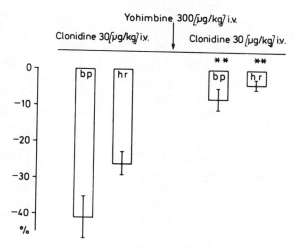

Fig. 5. Anesthetized rabbits. Influence of yohimbine on the effect of clonidine on blood pressure (bp) and heart rate (hr). Mean ± SE of four experiments. ** P <0.01.

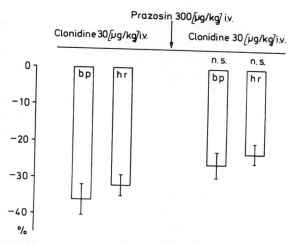

Fig. 6. Anesthetized rabbits. The influence of prazosin on the effect of clonidine on blood pressure (bp) and heart rate (hr). Mean ± SE of four experiments. n.s. = P >0.05.

Destruction of central adrenergic neurons by intraventricular injection of 6-hydroxydopamine should abolish the effects of clonidine if they are mediated by presynaptic adrenergic receptors. However, Haeusler and Finch [1972] and Warnke and Hoefke [1977] were unable to show a reduced effect of clonidine on blood pressure and heart rate after pretreatment with

6-hydroxydopamine (Fig. 7). Dollery and Reid [1973], however, reported a smaller blood pressure reduction by clonidine after 6-hydroxydopamine pretreatment. After pretreatment with reserpine and α-methyl-p-tyrosine, clonidine retained its ability to reduce synpathetic firing [Haeusler, 1974] (Fig. 8). The results of these experiments suggest that clonidine is still active after depletion of brain norepinephrine. It may be inferred that the effects of clonidine on sympathetic tone and blood pressure are not mediated by action on centrally located presynaptic receptors of adrenergic neurons but that other presynaptic sites are involved.

Experiments by Greenberg et al [1976] have shown that clonidine has a high affinity for postsynaptic α adrenoceptors of mammalian brain. Further experiments have indicated that H^3-catecholamines label the same receptor sites as clonidine [U'Prichard and Snyder, 1978]. Svensson et al [1975], however, and Cedarbaum and Aghajanian [1977] have shown that clonidine and norepinephrine inhibit the spontaneous firing of locus coeruleus (LC) neurons of the rat, which may mean that α adrenoceptors are present at this location. One should, however, be very careful not to draw definite conclusions since Crawley et al [1980], for example, after having seen that electrical stimulation of the locus coeruleus increased that activity of the peripheral sympathetic system as measured by an increase in the level of the norepinephrine metabolite 3-methoxy-4-hydroxy-phenylethyleneglycol (MHPG), were not able to reduce the increase in MPGH by electrical stimulation after neurochemical lesion with 6-hydroxydopamine, which destroyed rostral LC projections and LC cell bodies.

Another important area involved in the integration of cardiovascular regulation is the nucleus tractus solitarii, which is rich in norepinephrine terminals [Dahlström and Fuxe, 1964]. Ablation of this area leads to hypertension in rats, whereas stimulation causes hypotension and bradycardia. The same holds true for microinjection of norepinephrine. The area is involved in the carotid sinus occlusion reflex, which can be blocked by clonidine [Hoefke and Kobinger, 1966]. Infusions of clonidine into the nucleus tractus solitarii reduce blood pressure and heart rate [Sinha et al, 1975].

IV. PARASYMPATHETIC ACTION

Besides the sympathetic, the parasympathetic system is involved in cardiovascular control. Although a decrease in blood pressure and bradycardia can be produced by clonidine even after vagotomy [Hoefke and Koninger, 1966], it has been shown that clonidine enhances vagal reflexes [Hoefke, 1976; Scriabine et al, 1968, 1970]. Streller [1976, unpublished] recorded an increase of discharges in efferent vagal fibers after clonidine.

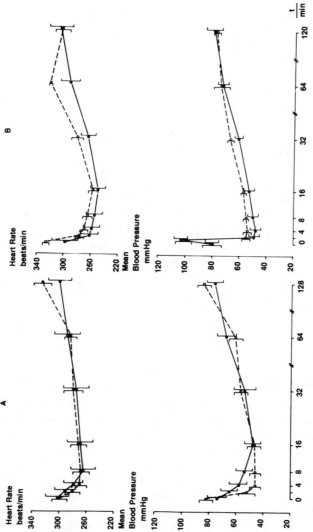

Fig. 7. Time-response curves of blood pressure and heart rate in anesthetized rabbits after administration of 1 µg/kg clonidine i.ci. (A) or 30 µg/kg IV. (B) with (●——●) or without (○----○) pretreatment with 6-OH-DA. Each point represents the mean ±SE from 4–8 experiments. (Warnke and Hoefke [1977].)

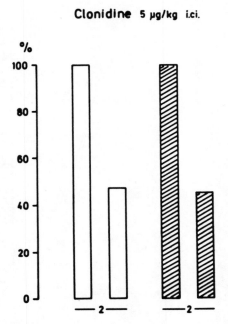

Clonidine 5 µg/kg i.ci.

Fig. 8.   Activity of the splanchnic nerve in cats, extracellular recording. Control values = 100%. Open bars = unpretreated animals; hatched bars = after pretreatment with reserpine and α-methyl-para-tyrosine, N = 2. (Hoefke and Streller [1979].)

V. SEDATIVE ACTION

One prominent effect of clonidine on the CNS is sedation, which was observed even in the initial animal experiments [Hoefke and Kobinger, 1966]. Clonidine given IV or IP decreases spontaneous activity and produces ataxia, catalepsy, and signs of increased peripheral sympathetic activity in dogs and cats, such as piloerection and exophthalmos [Hoefke and Kobinger, 1966]. At doses of 10 mg/kg and higher, clonidine induces aggressive behavior in mice [Morpurgo, 1968]. Involvement of noradrenergic mechanisms in the sedative effect of clonidine is evident—eg, in chicks 3–5 days old—in that phentolamine reduces sleep induced by clonidine to a dose-dependent degree [Fügner, 1971] (Fig. 9). According to Drew et al [1979], the sedative effect can be clocked only with α_2 antagonists and not with the α_1 antagonist prazosin.

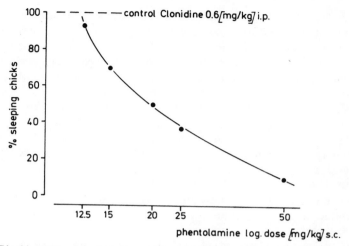

Fig. 9.   Blocking of the sleep-inducing action of clonidine by pretreatment with phentolamine injected 40–60 min before clonidine in 3–5-day-old chicks. Mean of 10–30 animals per dose. (Fügner [1971].)

Zebrowska-Lupina et al [1977] demonstrated that clonidine induced locomotor stimulation in rats instead of sedation after combined pretreatment with 6-hydroxydopamine, p-chlorophenylalanine, and α-methyl-p-tyrosine. These effects were antagonized by α-adrenoceptor antagonists. The authors concluded that clonidine normally activates presynaptic α adrenoceptors inducing sedation, but after destruction of noradrenergic neurons only postsynaptic receptors are left, and their stimulation causes hyperactivity.

One should mention that other neuronal systems can be influenced presynaptically as well. One of the effects of clonidine on central noradrenergic receptors may be that of intensifying apomorphine-induced hypermotility [Maj et al, 1972]. In EEG experiments in conscious rabbits, clonidine increased the threshold for arousal to a dose-dependent degree, whereas the spontaneous EEG was marked by slow waves of high amplitude [Gogolak and Stumph, 1966]. In rats and rabbits the clonidine-induced EEG changes were prevented by α-adrenoceptor antagonists [Florio et al, 1975].

VI. ANTINOCICEPTION AND ANTIWITHDRAWAL ACTION

Antinociceptive activity of clonidine was demonstrated in the writing and hot plate tests in mice and in the tail flick assay in rats; clonidine was more potent than morphine [Bentley et al, 1977; Schmitt et al, 1974;

Stockhaus, 1977]. The effects of morphine but not of clonidine were antagonized by naloxone in these tests, whereas the effects of clonidine were blocked by yohimbine [Fielding et al, 1978; Paalzow and Paalzow, 1976]. According to Paalzow and Paalzow [1976], reduced norepinephrine release by action on presynaptic α adrenoceptors or stimulation of epinephrine receptors are possible mechanisms of action of clonidine. Morphine and clonidine exhibited analgesic synergism in the mouse tail flick test; only the enhancement of clonidine by morphine was reversible by naloxone [Spaulding et al, 1978]. Clonidine inhibited morphine-induced running fits but not analgesia in mice [Filibeck et al, 1979]. Aghajanian [1978] noted that clonidine as well as morphine depressed the firing of neurons in the locus coeruleus. The depressant effect of morphine could be blocked by naloxone and that of clonidine by piperoxan, but not vice versa. Clonidine also inhibited the increase of neuron discharges precipitated by naloxone in morphine-dependent animals.

Golembiowska-Nikitin et al [1980] reported that neither enkephalinamide nor morphine or naloxone were able to displace clonidine from its binding site in the rat cortex. Tseng et al [1975], Vetulani and Bednarczyk [1977], and Fielding et al [1978], have shown that clonidine inhibits the signs of precipitated morphine withdrawal in rats. To obtain more insight into the mechanisms underlying the antiwithdrawal effects of clonidine, we tested four different compounds (Fig. 10).

Besides clonidine, alinidine (St 567) was chosen, which has only a weak clonidine-like effect on blood pressure and heart rate, but a marked analgesic effect [Stockhaus, 1977] and a bradycardiac effect due to peripheral action on the sinus node [Kobinger et al, 1979]. St 91 (2, 6-diethylamino-imidazolidine-HCl) does not penetrate the blood-brain barrier and shows only the peripheral effects of clonidine [Hoefke et al, 1975]. BHT 920, an azepine derivative, synthesized by Dr. Griss at Dr. K. Thomae GmbH, Biberaeh, displays clonidine-like pharmacological activity [Hammer et al, 1980; Pichler and Kobinger, in press].

The effects on blood pressure in anesthetized rabbits and the effects on pre- and postsynaptic α adrenergic receptors in pithed rats are illustrated in Figure 11, which shows that BHT 920 has a greater presynaptic effect than clonidine, whereas St 91 seems to be more active postsynaptically.

In withdrawal experiments conducted with K. Stockhaus in rats dependent on 200 mg/kg/day of morphine, morphine was withdrawn for 16–17 hours, and changes in writing attacks and wet dog shakes were recorded. Saline injection did not affect these symptoms; morphine clearly suppressed them. Clonidine blocked both symptoms to a dose-dependent degree, alinidine influenced only the writhing attacks, and St 91 was inef-

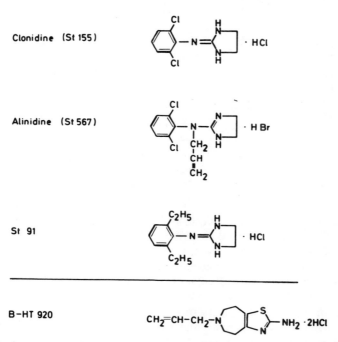

Fig. 10. Chemical structures of the imidazolidine derivatives and the thiazolo-azepine tested.

fective. Clonidine further suppressed teeth chattering, defecation, and grooming partially but had no effect on weight loss, aggressive behavior, or piloerection during withdrawal [Jennewein et al, 1980].

Other experiments were done in dogs dependent on morphine (daily morphine dosing: 2 mg/kg SC in the morning and 16 mg/kg orally in the evening for nearly 1 month). After naloxone precipitation, the symptoms of abstinence shown in Figure 12 were observed.

Blood pressure and heart rate responses were observed. After naloxone precipitation, the diastolic blood pressure as well as the heart rate increased, and the above-mentioned abstinence symptoms (AS) appeared; they were summed by a score system with 0–3 points (Fig. 13). The influence of the various compounds on these abstinence symptoms was

	anesthetized rabbit blood pressure decrease ED$_{20}$[μg/kg]	pithed rat		
		inhibition of increase in heart rate by electrical stimulation ED$_{50}$[μg/kg]	increase in diast. blood pressure	ratio bp/hr
Clonidine	10	6.0	5.5	0.9
Alinidine	3000	1400	> 3000	—
St 91	—	5.0	3.4	0.7
B-HT 920	50	8.0	40	5.0

Fig. 11.   Decrease of blood pressure in anesthetized rabbits (ED$_{20}$—20 mm Hg); inhibition of increase in heart rate after electrical stimulation and increase of diastolic blood pressure in pithed rats (ED$_{50}$ = 50% decrease or increase). Mean of four experiments.

dose-related (Fig. 14). Clonidine and BHT 920 showed a similar dose relation, alinidine decreased the symptoms at doses up to 5 mg/kg, and higher doses had smaller effects. St 91, the compound having only peripheral activity, proved ineffective.

A comparison of the effects of selected doses on the withdrawal symptoms and the heart rate is presented in Figure 15. While clonidine and BHT 920 showed equal activity in suppressing abstinence symptoms, the increase in heart rate after naloxone precipitation was blocked by clonidine only, not by BHT 920. Alinidine had smaller effects. The peripheral sup-

Abstinence Symptoms

1. autonomous nervous system

    1.1. vomiting
    1.2. salivation
    1.3. lacrimation

2. motor system

    2.1. tremor
    2.2. increased muscle tone
    2.3. increased locomotion

3. stereotypies

    3.1. yawning
    3.2. licking, grimacing
    3.3. chewing, biting-movements

Fig. 12.   Symptoms precipitated in morphine-dependent dogs by naloxone.

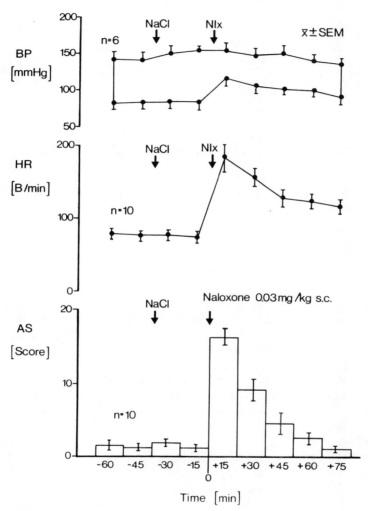

Fig. 13. Precipitation of withdrawal in morphine-dependent dogs by naloxone; abstinence syndrome (AS) and responses of blood pressure (BP) and heart rate (HR).

pression of tachycardia was noticeable even at the low dose, whereas the central inhibiting effect became evident only at the higher dose. St 91 did not influence the abstinence symptoms, but suppressed the heart rate increase after naloxone. This may be due to its vasoconstrictive activity, which induces bradycardia by a vagal reflex mechanism.

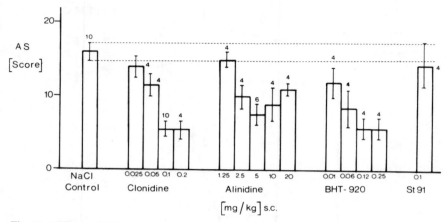

Fig. 14.   Effects of different compounds on naloxone-precipitated abstinence syndrome (AS) in morphine-dependent dogs; figures on top of the columns denote numbers of animals. $\bar{x} \pm$ SEM.

With a view to further clarification of the mechanism of action, α-adrenergic antagonists were tested regarding their ability to counteract the blockade of abstinence symptoms by clonidine and BHT 920. Yohimbine was chosen as α_2 antagonist, and prazosin was chosen as α_1 antagonist. The results obtained with clonidine are given in Figure 16. Yohimbine itself increased the withdrawal symptoms significantly; prazosin had no effect by itself. The effect of clonidine was totally blocked by yohimbine and unaffected by prazosin. This points to an α_2-agonistic action of clonidine. Preliminary experiments with BHT 920 likewise revealed an antagonistic effect of yohimbine.

That BHT 920 is as active as clonidine in suppressing the withdrawal symptoms and 5 times less active in decreasing the blood pressure may mean that it acts on different α_2 adrenoceptors located either presynaptically or postsynaptically. The blood pressure decrease may be mediated by central postsynaptic α_2 adrenoceptors. The selectivity of BHT 920 for peripheral presynaptic adrenoceptors, and the fact that the α_2 antagonist yohimbine blocks the effects of clonidine and BHT 920 on withdrawal, viewed in conjunction with evidence that BHT 920 has a greater effect on withdrawal than on blood pressure, support our hypothesis that the anti-withdrawal effects of clonidine and clonidine-like compounds are produced by an α_2-presynaptic adrenoceptor mechanism.

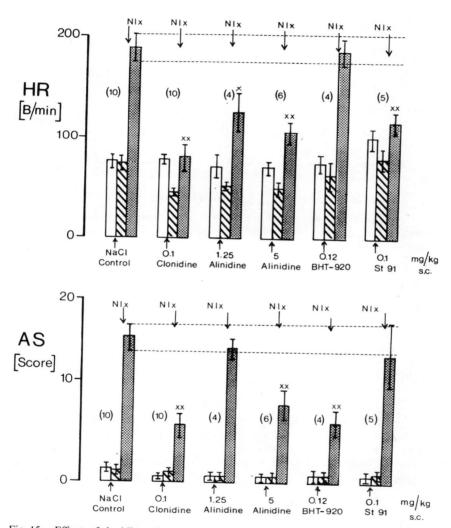

Fig. 15.   Effects of clonidine, alinidine, BHT 920, and St 91 on heart rate (HR) and abstinence syndrome (AS) in morphine-dependent dogs after naloxone precipitation; figures in parentheses denote numbers of animals. Statistics: x = P <0.05, xx = P <0.01. x̄ ±SEM.

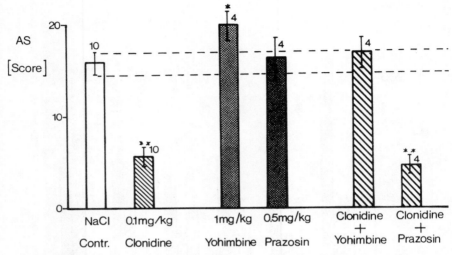

Fig. 16. Effects of the α-adrenergic blocking agents yohimbine and prazosin on naloxone-precipitated abstinence syndrome in dogs and its response to clonidine; see Figure 15 for explanations. $\bar{x} \pm$ SEM.

VII. REFERENCES

Aghajanian GK: Tolerance of locus coeruleus neurones to morphine and suppression of withdrawal response by clonidine. Nature 276:186–187, 1978.

Autret AM, Schmitt H, Fenard S, Pétillot N: Comparison of haemodynamic effects of α-sympathomimetic drugs. Eur J Pharmacol 13:208–217, 1971.

Bentley GA, Copeland IW, Starr J: The actions of some α-adrenoreceptor agonists and antagonists in an antinociceptive test in mice. Clin Exp Pharmacol Physiol 4:405–419, 1977.

Barthelsen S, Pettinger WA: A functional basis for classification of α-adrenergic receptors. Life Sci 21:595–606, 1977.

Boissier JR, Gudicelli JF, Fichelle J, Schmitt H, Schmitt H: Cardiovascular effects of 2—(2,6-dichlorphenylamino)-2-imidazoline hydrochloride (St 155). I. Peripheral sympathetic system. Eur J Pharmacol 333–339, 1968.

Cambridge D, Davey MJ, Massingham R: Further evidence for a selective post-synaptic α-adrenoceptor blockade with prazosin in vascular smooth muscle. Naunyn-Schmiedeberg's Arch Pharmacol 302:R52, 1978.

Cedarbaum JM, Aghajanian GK: Catecholamine receptors on locus coeruleus neurons: Pharmacological characterization. Eur J Pharmacol 44:375–385, 1977.

Constantine JW, McShane WK: Analysis of the cardiovascular effects of 2-(2,6,-dichlorphenylamino)-2-imidazoline hydrochloride (Catapres). Eur J Pharmacol 4:109–123, 1968.

Crawley JN, Maas JW, Roth RH: Evidence against specificity of electrical stimulation of the nucleus locus coeruleus in activating the sympathetic nervous system in the rat. Brain Res 183:301–311, 1980.

Dahlström S, Fuxe K: Evidence for the existence of monoamine-containing neurons in the central nervous system. Acta Physiol Scand 62:(Suppl) 232, 1964.

Dollery CT, Reid JL: Central noradrenergic neurones and the cardiovascular actions of clonidine in the rabbit. Br J Pharmacol 47:206–216, 1973.

Doxey JC, Everitt J: Inhibitory effects of clonidine on responses to sympathetic nerve stimulation in the pithed rat. Br J Pharmacol 61:559–566, 1977.

Drew GM: Effecats of α-adrenoceptor agonists and antagonists on pre- and postsynaptic located α-adrenoceptors. Eur J Pharmacol 36:313-320, 1976.

Drew GM: Pharmacological characterisation of the presynaptic alpha-adrenoceptor in the rat vas deferens. Eur J Pharmacol 42:123–130, 1977.

Drew GM, Gower AJ, Marriott AS: Alpha 2-adrenoceptors mediate clonidine-induced sedation in the rat. Br J Pharmacol 67:133–141, 1979.

Fielding S, Wilker J, Hynes M, Szewczak, M, Novick WJ Jr, Lal H: A comparison of clonidine with morphine for antinociceptive and antiwithdrawal actions. J Pharmacol Exp Ther 207:899–905, 1978.

Filibeck U, Castellano C, Vetulani J, Oliverio A: Inhibition by clonidine of morphine-induced running fit but not analgesia in C 57 BL/6 mice. Pol J Pharmacol 32:149–154, 1980.

Florio V, Binachi L, Longo VG: A study of the central effects of sympathomimetic drugs: EEG and behavioral investigations on clonidine and naphazoline. Neuropharmacology 14:707–714, 1975.

Fügner A: Antagonism of the drug-induced behavioral sleep in chicks. Arzneim Forsch 21:1350–1352, 1971.

Gogolak G, Stumpf Ch: Wirkung von 2-(2,6-Dichlorphenylamino)-2-imidazolinhydrochlorid auf die EEG-Weck-reaktion bei Kaninchen. Arzneim-Forsch 16:1050–1052, 1966.

Golembiowska-Nikitin R, Pilc A, Vetulani J: Opiates and specific receptor binding of ³H-clonidine. J Pharm Pharmacol 32:70–71, 1980.

Greenberg DA, U'Prichard DC, Snyder SH: Alpha-noradrenergic receptor binding in mammalian brain. Different labelling of agonist and antagonist states. Life Sci 19:69–76, 1976.

Haeusler GH: Clonidine-induced inhibition of sympathetic nerve activity: No indication for a central presynaptic or an indirect sympathomimetic mode of action. Naunyn-Schmiedeberg's Arch Pharmakol 286:97–111, 1974.

Haeusler G: Studies on the possible contribution of a peripheral presynaptic action of clonidine and dopamine to their vascular effects under in vivo conditions. Naunyn-Schmiedeberg's Arch Pharmakol 295:191–202, 1976.

Haeusler G, Finch L: On the nature of the central hypotensive effect of clonidine and α-methyldopa. J Pharmacol (Paris) 3:544–545, 1972.

Hammer R, Kobinger W, Pichler L: Binding of an imidazolidine (clonidine), an oxazolazepin (B-HT 933) and a thiazoloazepin (B-HT 920) to rat brain α-adrenoceptors and relation to cardiovascular effects. Eur J Pharmacol 62:277–285, 1980.

Hodge RL, Robinson SM: The action of clonidine on isolated arterial preparations. Aust J Exp Biol Med Sci 50:517–526, 1972.

Hoefke W: Centrally acting, antihypertensive agents. In Engelhardt EL (ed): "Antihypertensive Agents," ACS Symposium Series 27. Washington, DC: American Chemical Society, 1976, pp 27–54.

Hoefke W, Kobinger W: Pharmakologische Wirkungen des 2-(2,6-Dichlorphenylamino)-2-imidazolinhydrochlorids, einer neuen, antihypertensiven Substanz. Arzneim-Forsch 16:1038–1050, 1966.

Hoefke W, Kobinger W: Pharmakologische Wirkungen eines neuen Antihypertensivums mit Imidazolin-Struktur. Naunyn-Schmiedeberg's Arch Pharmakol 257:28–29, 1967.

Hoefke W, Kobinger W, Walland A: Relationship between activity and structure in derivatives of clonidine. Arzneim-Forsch 25:786–793, 1975.

Hoefke W, Streller I: Cardiovascular effects of α-adrenolytic agents: Indication of a central presynaptic mode of action. Naunyn-Schmiedeberg's Arch Pharmacol 308:R12, 1979.

Jennewein HM, Stockhaus K, Hoefke W: Effects of clonidine and alinidine on the morphine withdrawal syndrome in rats and dogs. Naunyn-Schmiedeberg's Arch Pharmacol 311:R66, 1980.

Kobinger W: Uber den Wirkungsmechanismus einer neuen antihypertensiven Substnaz mit Imidazolinstruktur. Naunyn-Schmiedeberg's Arch Pharmakol 258:48–58, 1967.

Kobinger W, Lillie C, Pichler W: Cardiovascular actions of N-allyl-clonidine (St 567) a substance with specific bradycardic action. Eur J Pharmacol 58:141–150, 1979.

Maj J, Sowinska H, Baran L, Kapturkiewicz Z: The effect of clonidine on locomotor activity in mice. Life Sci 11:483–491, 1972.

Medget IC, McCulloch MW, Rand MJ: Partial agonist action of clonidine on prejunctional and postjunctional alpha-adrenoceptors. Naunyn-Schmiedeberg's Arch Pharmakol 304:215–221, 1978.

Morpurgo C: Aggressive behavior induced by large doses of 2-(2,6-dichlorphenylamino)-2-imidazoline hydrochloride (St 155) in mice. Eur J Pharmacol 3:374–377, 1968.

Nayler WG, Price JM, Swann JB, McInnes I, Race D, Lowe TE: Effect of the hypotensive drug St 155 (Catapres) on the heart and peripheral circulation. J Pharmacol Exp Ther 164:45–59, 1968.

Paalzow G, Paalzow L: Clonidine antinociceptive activity: Effects of drugs influencing central monoaminergic and cholinergic mechanisms in the rat. Naunyn-Schmiedeberg's Arch Pharmakol 292:119–126, 1976.

Pichler L, Kobinger W: Centrally mediated cardiovascular effects of B-HT 920 (2-amino-6-allyl-5,6,7,8-Tetrahydro-4H-Thiazolo-[5, 4-d]-azepin-dihydrochloride), a hypotensive agent of the "clonidine type." Cardiovascular Pharmacol 3:269–277, 1981.

Robson RD, Kaplan HR: An involvement of St 155 [2-(2,6-dichlorophenylamino)-2-imidazoline hydrochloride, Catapres] in cholinergic mechanisms. Eur J Pharmacol 5:328–337, 1969.

Salt PJ: Inhibition of noradrenaline uptake in the isolated rat heart by steroids, clonidine and methoxylated phenyl-thylamines. Eur J Pharmacol 20:329–340, 1972.

Sattler RW, van Zwieten PA: Acute hypotensive action of 2-(2,6-dichlorophenylamino)-2-imidazoline hydrochloride (St 155) after infusion into the cat's vertebral artery. Eur J Pharmacol 2:9–13, 1967.

Schmitt H, Schmitt H: Localization of the hypotensive effect of 2-(2,6-dichloro-phenylamino)-2-imidazoline hydrochloride (St 155, Catapresan). Eur J Pharmacol 6:8–12, 1969.

Schmitt H, Le Douarec JC, Petillot N: Antinociceptive effects of some α-sympathomimetic agents. Neuropharmacology 13:289–294, 1974.

Scriabine A, Stavorski J, Wenger HC, Torchiana ML, Stone CA: Cardiac slowing effects of clonidine (St 155) in dogs. J Pharmacol Exp Ther 171:256–264, 1970.

Scriabine A, Stone CA, Stavorski JM: Studies on the mechanism of St 155-induced cardiac slowing in dogs. Pharmacologist 10:156, 1968.

Sherman GP, Grega GJ, Woods RJ, Buckley JP: Evidence for a central hypotensive mechanism of 2-(2,6-dichlorphenylamino)-2-imidazoline (Catapresan, St 155). Eur J Pharmacol 2:326–328, 1968.

Sinha JN, Atkinson JM, Schmitt H: Effects of clonidine and L-DOPA on spontaneous and evoked splanchnic nerve discharges. Eur J Pharmacol 24:113–119, 1973.

Sinha JN, Tangri KK, Bhargava KP, Schmitt H: Central sites of sympathoinhibitory effects of clonidine and L-DOPA. In Milliez P, Safar M (eds): "Recent Advances in Hypertension," Vol. 1 Reims: Société Aliena, 1975, pp 97–109.

Spaulding TC, Venafro JJ, Ma M, Cornfeldt M, Fielding S: Interaction of morphine and clonidine in the tail flick test: Potentiation studies. Pharmacologist 20:269, 1978.

Starke K, Montel H: Involvement of α-receptors in clonidine-induced inhibition of transmitter release from central monoamine neurons. Neuropharmacology 12:1073–1080, 1973.

Starke K, Montel H, Gayk W, Merker R: Comparison of the effects of clonidine on pre- and postsynaptic adrenoceptors in the rabbit pulmonary artery, α-sympathomimetic inhibition of neurogenic vasoconstriction. Naunyn-Schmiedeberg's Arch Pharmakol 285:133–150, 1974.

Starke K, Tanaka T, Stamm G: Evidence against agonist- and antagonist-selective α-adrenoceptor subtypes. Naunyn-Schmiedeberg's Arch Pharmacol 311:R58, 1980.

Stockhaus K: Investigations concerning the profile of action of 2-[N-allyl-N-(2,6-dichloro-phenyl)-amino]-2-imidazoline-hydrobromide (St 567-BR) a compound with analgesic activity. In "Problems of Drug Dependence." Proceedings of the 39th Annual Scientific Meeting, Committee on Problems of Drug Dependence Inc., Washington, DC: National Research Council, 1977, pp 355–366.

Svensson TH, Bunney BS, Aghajanian GK: Inhibition of both noradrenergic and serotonergic neurons in brain by the α-adrenergic agonist clonidine. Brain Res 92:291–306, 1975.

Timmermans PBMWM: A simple method for the discrimination between α_1- and α_2-adrenoceptors. Naunyn-Schmiedeberg's Arch Pharmacol 311:R59, 1980.

Tseng L, Loh HH, Wei ET: Effects of clonidine on morphine withdrawal signs in the rat. Eur J Pharmacol 30:93–99, 1975.

U'Prichard DC, Snyder SH: ^{3}H-catecholamine binding to α-receptor in rat brain: Enhancement by reserpine. Eur J Pharmacol 51:145–155, 1978.

Vetulani J, Bednarczyk B: Depression by clonidine of shaking behavior elicited by nalorphine in morphine-dependent rats. J Pharm Pharmcol 29:567–569, 1977.

Warnke E, Hoefke W: Influence of central pretreatment with 6-hydroxydopamine on the hypotensive effects of clonidine. Arzneim-Forsch 27:2311–2313, 1977.

Werner U, Starke K, Schümann HJ: Actions of clonidine and 2-(2-methyl-6-ethyl-cyclonexylamino)-2-oxazoline on postganglionic nerves. Arch Int Pharmacodyn Ther 195:282–290, 1972.

Zebrowska-Lupina J, Przegalinski E, Sloniec M, Keinrok Z: Clonidine-induced locomotor hyperactivity in rats. The role of central postsynaptic α-adrenoceptors. Naunyn-Schmiedeberg's Arch Pharmakol 297:227–231, 1977.

van Zwieten PA: Characterization of the central α-adrenoceptors involved in the hypotensive action of clonidine by yohimbine, corynanthine and rauwolscine. Naunyn-Schmiedeberg's Arch Pharmacol 311:R58, 1980.

Psychopharmacology of Clonidine, pages 99–145
© 1981 Alan R. Liss, Inc., 150 Fifth Avenue, New York, NY 10011

Psychotropic Actions of Clonidine

Harbans Lal and Gary T. Shearman

I. INTRODUCTION

Many chemical substances have proved useful in the treatment of diseases. Very few, however, become investigational tools that stimulate critical research in medicine. Clonidine is one such substance. Originally synthesized by Stähle, a medicinal chemist at Boehringer, to relieve symptoms associated with the common cold and sinusitis, clonidine was subsequently found to offer a new approach to the control of hypertension. The antihypertensive action of clonidine involves a unique mechanism. Hypertension was once thought to be caused primarily by the faulty functioning of peripheral blood vessels and had usually been treated by drugs acting at peripheral sites. However, clonidine was found to act directly on the central nervous system. The discovery that a centrally acting drug could be used to treat a peripheral malfunction aroused great interest among biomedical researchers throughout the world and led to investigation of clonidine not only as a tool of research on hypertensive diseases but also as a means of developing new treatment modalities for several other disease states.

More recently, the use of clonidine in biomedical research has led to the recognition of a new type of α-adrenergic receptor, now known as the α-2 adrenoreceptor. These receptors are pharmacologically similar to the classical α receptors except that they are visualized in presynaptic locations (autoreceptors) and are therefore considered primarily responsible for the modulation of norepinephrine (NE) release. They are present in the brain and other body organs, and stimulation or inhibition of their activity can therefore be expected to produce diverse types of effects.

Clonidine is an α-2 adrenergic receptor agonist. Consequently, most of its effects bear on various manifestations of noradrenergic activity. In the brain, the locus coeruleus (LC) is the largest nucleus of NE-containing cells. These cells show extensive dendritic arborization or axon collateralization. LC receives afferent projections from a wide variety of sensory pathways from other brain areas. In addition to NE receptors, receptors for acid (GABA) serotonin, acetylcholine, endorphins, and substance P have been found in LC. Similarly, axons from LC ascend and descend to influence wide areas in the brain and spinal cord.

Because of the central position of LC in brain functions and the extreme sensitivity of LC activity to clonidine, investigators in various countries are beginning to focus on psychopharmacological research with clonidine. It is anticipated that this research will yield important new information in many fields of psychiatry, neurology, and behavioral pharmacology. Already, dysfunctions of brain noradrenergic systems are being implicated in depression, schizophrenia, dementia, anxiety, and drug withdrawal syndromes. Because of the high specificity and potency of clonidine in modulating LC functions, there are numerous possibilities of using this drug as a tool not only to investigate the pathogenesis of many psychiatric and other illnesses, but also to explore avenues of new drug development. In order that the potential usefulness of this drug in psychopharmacological research may be fully understood, we have undertaken to review the recent literature and to present here an overview of those of its actions that influence behavior.

Effects of clonidine on cardiovascular, gastrointestinal, and endocrine systems are not considered in this chapter. Interested readers may consult many other reviews dealing with those aspects of the drug's action.

II. MOTOR BEHAVIOR

A. Spontaneous Locomotion

The study of locomotion and other types of motor behavior is an integral part of any assessment of drug effects on behavior. It is obvious that impairment or stimulation of motor functions can alter both simple and complex behavioral patterns. The dysfunctions of motor behavior due to a drug can disrupt behavior as much as the loss of discriminative functions, the drive to satisfy hunger and thirst, pleasure-seeking, or interference with memory or conditioning. In addition, exaggeration or diminution of motor tasks may interfere with other behavior through the intermediary of competing motor responses. Behaviorally toxic doses of most drugs are known to affect motor behavior as well. It is therefore imperative that any review of behavioral pharmacology take into consideration the range of doses that affect behavior. Because α-2 adrenoreceptor stimulation results from administration of low doses and α-1 adrenoreceptor stimulation is caused by high doses of clonidine, so that its behavioral effects may be biphasic, the clinically relevant effects of clonidine have to be differentiated from toxic effects produced by high doses.

The neural basis of factors affecting motor behavior is not known. In a recent review, Kelly [1977] strongly implicated the mesolimbic dopaminergic system as the major brain system regulating locomotor activity. Dopamine injected into the nucleus accumbens stimulates locomotor activity which is blocked by dopamine antagonists [Pijnenberg et al, 1973, 1975]. Serotonergic neurons that ascend from the dorsal raphe nucleus to the ventral tegmental area and to the nucleus accumbens inhibit locomotor activity [Costell et al, 1976]. GABA inhibits serotonergic neurons of the dorsal raphe nucleus [Przewlocka et al, 1979]. Norepinephrine seems to have a modulatory role in dopamine-induced activity, whereas muscarinic influences are inhibitory [Thornburg and Moore, 1973].

Locomotor activity in laboratory animals is often measured by the number of times the subject interrupts a light beam in a photocell chamber. Each time the light beam is interrupted, a count is recorded, and so the number of counts varies proportionately with the subject's locomotor activity. Systemic administration of clonidine (0.05–25.0 mg/kg) has been reported to cause a dose-dependent decrease in the locomotor activity of mice and rats measured in the above manner [Maj et al, 1972, 1975a; Strombom, 1975; Tilson et al, 1977]. The magnitude of the effect also depends on the habituation of the subject to the apparatus and on whether the animals are fed or hungry [Bednarczyk and Vetulani, 1977]. Bilateral introduction of dopamine (5–10 μg) or d-amphetamine into the nucleus accumbens stimulated locomotor activity, whereas norepinephrine (1–10 μg) or clonidine (1–10 μg) decreased locomotor activity [Pijnenburg et al, 1976a]. Clonidine (5 μg) caused only a slight reduction in the locomotor activity induced by ergotamine when both drugs were injected into the nucleus accumbens, whereas the imidazoline derivative 3,4-dihydroxyphenylamine-2-imidazoline (DPI) strongly inhibited this effect of ergotamine [Pijnenburg et al, 1976b].

The effect of clonidine on locomotor activity is antagonized by volumitine [von Voigtlander et al, 1978; Delini-Stula et al, 1979], piperoxan [Delini-Stula et al, 1979], niaserine [Delini-Stula, 1978], or atropine and scopolamine [Maj et al, 1975a]. The peripherally acting cholinolytic drugs atropine methyl nitrate and scopolamine butyl bromide were ineffective in mice but partially active in rats in antagonizing clonidine-induced motor retardation [Maj et al, 1975a]. By contrast, the action of clonidine was potentiated by imipramine and amitriptyline [Delini-Stula, 1978], and by phenoxybenzamine and phentolamine [Delini-Stula et al, 1979]. It was not affected by lithium [Berggren et al, 1978].

Although clonidine (0.5 mg/kg) was found to antagonize amphetamine stimulation in the rat in one experiment [Skolnick et al, 1978], it is usually believed to enhance locomotor stimulation caused by apomorphine [Maj et al, 1975b; Handley and Thomas, 1978] or amphetamine [Handley and Thomas, 1978]. Clonidine also stimulates activity in animals pretreated with reserpine and α-methyl-para-tyrosine, an action that is not antagonized by intraperitoneally administered GABA [Biswar and Carlsson, 1978].

The potentiating effect of clonidine on apomorphine-induced locomotor stimulation in reserpine-treated mice was almost completely blocked by phenoxybenzamine (20 mg/kg), partially antagonized by tolazoline (50 mg/kg), and not significantly affected by yohimbine (3 and 10 mg/kg) [Anden et al, 1976] or FLA-63 [Dolphin et al, 1976]. Similarly, Zebrowska-Lupina et al [1977] reported that the α-receptor blockers phenoxybenzamine, phentolamine, aceperone, as well as yohimbine (10 mg/kg) antagonized the clonidine-induced locomotor stimulation of rats pretreated with 6-hydroxydopamine plus reserpine. The dopamine receptor antagonists spiroperidol and pimoside had no antagonistic effect [Zebrowska-Lupina et al, 1977].

While clonidine (1–25 mg/kg) potentiated the decrease in locomotor activity caused by pretreatment with the neuroleptic spiroperidol [Maj et al,

1972], it did not influence the depression of locomotor activity due to pre-treatment with reserpine [Anden et al, 1970a, 1973, 1976; Maj et al, 1972; Menon et al, 1977], α-methyl-para-tyrosine [Anden et al, 1972; Maj et al, 1972], FLA-63, or phenoxybenzamine [Maj et al, 1972], despite marked sympathomimetic signs. However, clonidine (1–25 mg/kg) did potentiate the partial reversal of locomotor activity produced by apomorphine or piribedil in mice pretreated with reserpine [Anden et al, 1970b, 1973, 1976; Jenner and Marsden, 1975; Jenner and Pycock, 1976; Maj et al, 1972; Dolphin et al, 1976; Menon et al, 1977], α-methyl-para-tyrosine [Anden et al, 1970b; Maj et al, 1972], and FLA-63 [Maj et al, 1972] at doses not interfering with the metabolism of apomorphine [Anden et al, 1973]. Furthermore, increased locomotor activity induced by the dopamine receptor stimulant meta-tyrosine [Anden et al, 1973] or LSD [Menon et al, 1977] in reserpine-treated mice was enhanced by pretreatment with clonidine (1.0 mg/kg IP). Caffeine (25 mg/kg) caused a fourfold increase in the locomotor activity-reversing effect of ET-495 plus clonidine in reserpinized mice [Waldeck, 1973]. Subcutaneous administration of clonidine (0.0125–0.5 mg/kg) promoted intense locomotor activity in rats pretreated with 6-hydroxydopamine plus reserpine [Zebrowska-Lupina et al, 1977]. Similar but less intensive hyperactivity was observed when rats were given clonidine after combined pretreatment with 6-hydroxydopamine plus p-chlorophenylalanine plus α-methyl-p-tyrosine or with reserpine plus yohimbine (3 mg/kg) [Zebrowska-Lupina et al, 1977]. Clonidine (5 and 25 mg/kg) did not potentiate the apomorphine antagonism of a phenoxybenzamine-induced decrease in locomotor activity but, on the contrary, decreased the effect of apomorphine [Maj et al, 1972].

Repeated application of electroconvulsive shocks (ECS) to mice increased the locomotor stimulatory effect of clonidine (1.5 mg/kg) in reserpinized mice treated with apomorphine [Modigh, 1975]. Furthermore, administration of clonidine (1.5 mg/kg) to mice receiving only ECS pretreatment resulted in increased locomotor activity [Modigh, 1975], suggesting that repeated ECS increases the sensitivity of noradrenergic receptors.

Administration of clonidine (100 or 500 μg/kg but not 25 μg/kg) to mice during withdrawal from long-term haloperidol treatment resulted in marked locomotor stimulation as compared with vehicle-treated mice, suggesting that the long-term haloperidol treatment led to development of supersensitive noradrenergic receptors [Dunstan and Jackson, 1976, 1977].

Chronic treatment with clonidine has been shown to produce changes in sensitivity to other drugs. After treatment with clonidine (0.1 mg/kg) given twice daily for 12 days, Svensson and Strombom [1977] showed that locomotor stimulation produced by apomorphine plus clonidine in reserpinized mice was enhanced. The motor effects of apomorphine alone were not affected, indicating that noradrenergic responsiveness was enhanced. Overstreet et al [1979] treated rats with clonidine (0.1 or 0.5 mg/kg) twice daily for 21 days. This treatment reduced the depressive effect of oxotremorine on locomotor activity. They also observed reduced binding of cholinergic agonists in certain brain areas. These findings make it appear that chronic treatment with clonidine may reduce sensitivity to cholinergic stimulation.

In conclusion, these studies have demonstrated that clonidine causes a dose-dependent decrease in the locomotor activity of both mice and rats. However, clonidine may potentiate the increase in locomotor activity produced by other drugs under certain pharmacological conditions such as destruction of presynaptic nerve endings or depletion of brain neurotransmitters. Results of studies on the mechanism by which clonidine affects locomotor activity suggest involvement of the noradrenergic and cholinergic systems. These studies also appear to demonstrate that stimulation of both the dopaminergic and the noradrenergic system is required for optimal locomotor activity and that any imbalance in these systems will cause changes in this activity.

B. Exploratory Activity

The exploratory motor activity of laboratory animals is often measured in the open field and in hole tests. In the open field situation, rats are placed individually in a circular arena and the frequency of diameter crossing ("ambulation score") and of rearings ("rearing score") is recorded. Similarly, the number of fecal pellets excreted over the observation period is recorded ("defecation score") [Janssen et al, 1960]. In the hole test, laboratory animals are placed in a box containing several round holes. The number of times the animals put their heads in the holes ("peeping") is recorded as a measure of exploratory activity [File and Pope, 1974].

Dandiya and Patni [1973] reported that intraventricular administration of clonidine decreased the ambulation and rearing of rats in an open field situation. Similarly, Herman et al [1976] found that clonidine (0.1 mg/kg but not 0.05 mg/kg) decreased ambulation, rearing, and defecation in the open field and reduced the peeping of rats in the hole test. Intracerebroventricular administration of 6-hydroxydopamine potentiated the depressant action of clonidine [Herman et al, 1976].

Strombom [1975] reported that clonidine (0.025–0.8 mg/kg) depressed the exploratory behavior of mice in a Y-shaped runway maze and appeared to break the pattern of adaptation.

These data suggest that clonidine depresses exploratory activity in small laboratory animals. Norepinephrine may be important in exploratory behavior, and clonidine may inhibit the release of NE to the receptor site.

C. Rotorod Test

The Rotorod test measures the ability of an animal to stay on a revolving drum or cylinder for a certain time. This test has often been used to evaluate general sedation or muscle relaxation by drugs. Clonidine (1.0 mg/kg IP) reduced Rotorod performance in rats [Laverty and Taylor, 1969] and mice (ED$_{50}$: 0.24 mg/kg SC) [Cornfeldt et al, 1978]. These findings indicate that clonidine in doses far beyond the pharmacological range will produce general sedation and confound the interpretation of other behavioral data obtained with the use of such doses.

III. EXPERIMENTAL ABNORMAL BEHAVIOR

A. Compulsive Circling

Compulsive circling or rotating activity in rats is produced by unilateral lesions of the nigrostriatal pathway in studies of dopamine-dependent behavior. Drugs that increase dopaminergic activity in the central nervous system after lesioning provoke rotational behavior [Ungerstedt et al, 1969].

By using a rotometer to measure the number of full turns a subject makes in unit time, Satoh et al [1976] found that in rats with unilateral 6-hydroxy-dopamine-induced lesions of the substantia nigra, intraventricular injection of apomorphine, dopamine, and norepinephrine in doses of 64 μg caused the rats to turn toward the intact side, whereas intraventricular injection of methamphetamine (250 μg) caused them to turn toward the damaged side. However, intraventricular injection of clonidine (64 μg) did not induce any turning. It was suggested by Satoh et al that dopamine, norepinephrine, and apomorphine directly stimulate the supersensitive dopamine receptors on the side of the lesion, whereas methamphetamine indirectly stimulates dopamine receptors on the intact side. Since clonidine is considered to be an α-noradrenergic agonist but did not cause the rats to turn, the turning induced by NE was attributed to a nonspecific stimulation of dopamine receptors.

Direct injection of clonidine (100 μg) into one striatum of rats with intact nigrostriatal systems did not cause circling, nor did this pretreatment result in circling after the subcutaneous administration of the dopamine agonist apomorphine (0.5 mg/kg) [Jenner and Pycock, 1976]. However, circling behavior induced by either apomorphine (0.25 mg/kg SC) or d-amphetamine (3 mg/kg IP) in mice with unilateral lesions of the nigrostriatal pathway was potentiated by pretreatment with clonidine (0.06–2.0 mg/kg IP) [Jenner and Pycock, 1976; Pycock et al, 1977]. In contrast to this latter finding, Cornfeldt et al [1978] reported that clonidine (ED$_{50}$: 0.08 mg/kg IP) blocked amphetamine-induced circling but did not block apomorphine-induced circling in rats with striatal lesions.

Unilateral electrolytic destruction of the locus coeruleus in rats results in spontaneous ipsilateral turning, which is soon replaced by contralateral turning [Pycock et al, 1975]. One week after locus coeruleus lesioning, when spontaneous turning had stopped, intraperitoneal administration of the dopamine agonists apomorphine, d-amphetamine, and piribedil, but not of the noradrenergic agonist clonidine (0.05–0.5 mg/kg), led to contralateral circling [Donaldson et al, 1976]. Donaldson et al suggested that circling behavior seen after unilateral locus coeruleus lesions is caused by supersensitive striatal dopamine receptors in the nigrostriatal pathway on the side of the lesion. Recently, Arnt and Scheel-Kruger [1979] observed contralateral turning after unilateral injection of clonidine (10 μg) into the pars reticulata of the substantia nigra.

The results of the above studies of the effects of clonidine on rotational behavior indicate that clonidine does not stimulate dopamine receptors, and they provide further evidence that rotational behavior depends on dopaminergic rather than noradrenergic mechanisms. However, it appears that rotational behavior induced by dopaminergic agonists may be modified by clonidine through its adrenergic stimulating mechanisms.

B. Stereotypy

Stereotypic behavior consists of repeated spontaneous motor responses within the animal's normal behavior pattern. Usually they include licking, sniffing, biting, gnawing, and head bobbing, which are apparently aimless and repeated at the expense of normal adaptive functions. Stereotypic behavior is believed to be the result of heightened dopaminergic activity in the corpus striatum, although many other brain areas have been implicated in apomorphine-induced stereotypy [Lal and Gianutsos, 1980]. Both direct and indirect dopaminergic agonists, such as apomorphine and d-amphetamine, elicit stereotypic behavior. Some signs of stereotypy can also be produced by anticholinergic drugs. The stereotypy thus elicited is blocked by typical neuroleptics.

Intraperitoneal administration of clonidine (0.5 mg/kg) to rats did not produce stereotyped behavior and did not affect the stereotyped behavior induced by apomorphine (0.1–5.0 mg/kg SC) in rats [Jenner and Pycock, 1976; Pycock et al, 1977]. At doses as high as 1.25 mg/kg, clonidine failed to inhibit stereotypy induced by either amphetamine (10 mg/kg IV) or apomorphine (1.25 mg/kg SC) [Cornfeldt et al, 1978]. It therefore appears that clonidine does not stimulate striatal dopamine receptors. The action of drugs on the striatum is generally considered to underlie their extrapyramidal side effects in man.

C. Catalepsy

In the state of catalepsy the experimental animal ceases all motor activity and allows itself to be placed in abnormal positions for long periods [Fielding and Lal, 1978]. Usually, neuroleptic drugs cause this condition, which is considered related to the neurological deficits underlying Parkinson like extrapyramidal reactions in patients. Potent neuroleptics with high antidopaminergic activity in the striatum and no anticholinergic actions are more effective in causing catalepsy than the low-potency neuroleptics with anticholinergic activity. Centrally acting antimuscarinic drugs reverse neuroleptic catalepsy.

Clonidine causes no catalepsy, even at high doses (0.5 mg/kg). However, it has been reported to potentiate the cataleptic action of haloperidol [Jenner and Pycock, 1976; Pycock et al, 1977]. This action is probably nonspecific and due to sedation, particularly in view of a recent report by Al-Shabibi and Dogget [1978] who found that in doses up to 0.5 mg/kg clonidine antagonized haloperidol-induced catalepsy in the rat. Since yohimbine (1–10 mg/kg) also antagonized haloperidol catalepsy, this effect of clonidine is attributed to postsynaptic α-1 stimulation.

D. Abnormal Body Shakes

"Wet-dog-like body shakes" observed in rats have been ascribed to narcotic withdrawal [Gianutsos et al, 1976], exposure to intense cold [Wei et al, 1974], and treatment with certain drugs. They are considered to be exaggerated reflexes in response to certain stresses. Clonidine has been reported to inhibit the "wet-dog shakes" produced in rats by immersion in ice-cold water [Wei, 1975], by administration of the drug AG-3-5 [1-hydroxyphenyl]-4(3-nitrophenyl)-1,2,3,6-tetrahydropyrimidin-2-one] [Wei, 1976], or by withholding narcotics from an addicted animal [Fielding et al, 1977, 1978]. Jahn and Mixich [1976] reported that clonidine (0.01–0.1 mg/kg SC) caused a dose-dependent reduction of "wet-dog shakes" induced by the benzylidene-aminooxycarbonic acid derivative Sqd 8473. The ability of clonidine to reduce "wet-dog shakes" was considered nonspecific since several other drugs, including narcotics, narcotic antagonists, psychosedatives, cocaine, dl-amphetamine, and apomorphine, were also found effective in this regard [Jahn and Mixich, 1976].

Cowan and Watson [1979] reported that clonidine (0.1 mg/kg), haloperidol, and LSD, but not morphine, reduced body shakes induced by RX 336-M (7,8-dihydro-5′,6-dimethyl-cyclohex-5′-eno-1′,2′,8′,14-codein one). The clonidine action was not blocked by naloxone. Recently, Kruse et al [1980] showed that drug-induced body shakes were related to the analgesic or possible antiheadache effects of drugs. The activity of clonidine in this test may show a potential for the treatment of migraine. It is interesting to note that clonidine inhibits hard twitches produced by intraventricular injections of 5-hydroxytryptophan or IP injections of 5-methoxytryptamine. The ED_{50} values were less than 0.1 mg/kg. Clonidine was still effective after chemical destruction of catecholaminergic or serotonergic neurons [Bednarczyk and Vetulani, 1978].

IV. OPERANT BEHAVIOR

Responses that are controlled through their consequences have been termed operants. Since the environmental and organismal control can be objectively defined, operants are often employed to analyze subtle behavioral influences of drugs. With the aid of operant behavior paradigms, different components of behavior can be discretely examined as targets for drug action. In this section effects of clonidine on operant behavior will be reviewed. Operants used as tools to study a particular aspect of drug action are discussed separately in other sections of this chapter.

Administration of clonidine (0.006–0.3 mg/kg) causes a dose-dependent suppression of operant behavior maintained by fixed-ratio [Colelli et al, 1976; Sparber and Meyer, 1978; Harris et al, 1978], fixed-interval [Harris et al, 1976, 1977, 1978], and differential reinforcement of low-rate [Tilson et al, 1977] schedules of food reinforcement. In one study, tolerance was found to develop to the depressant effect of clonidine on food-reinforced responding after 5 days of administration. No sedative effect of clonidine was seen after 2 weeks [Meyer et al, 1977]. Termination of clonidine treatment of the tolerant rats resulted in a suppression of normal operant behavior for as long as 1 week [Meyer et al, 1977]. Clonidine antagonized the disruption of fixed-ratio operant behavior produced by naloxone injection in morphine-dependent rats [Colelli et al, 1976; Sparber and Meyer, 1978].

Whereas the rate-decreasing effect of apomorphine in a fixed-interval schedule of food reinforcement was potentiated by naloxone, the effect of clonidine was unaltered [Harris et al, 1976, 1977]. At doses capable of suppressing operant behavior in morphine-dependent rats [Gellert and Sparber, 1977], naloxone failed to disrupt operant behavior in clonidine-tolerant rats [Meyer et al, 1977].

Suppression of fixed-ratio food-reinforced operant behavior in rats caused by depletion of brain catecholamines with α-methyl-para-tyrosine or tetrabenazine was not antagonized by apomorphine or clonidine; L-dopa reversed the suppression caused by α-methyl-para-tyrosine but not that caused by tetrabenazine [Ahlenius et al, 1971b].

A dose-dependent suppression of water-reinforced responding in rats trained on a fixed-interval schedule occurs after both apomorphine (0.25–10.0 mg/kg) and clonidine (0.002–0.1 mg/kg). Frontal cortical lesions increased the sensitivity to apomorphine but not to clonidine [Glick and Cox, 1976].

Intraventricular administration of 1-norepinephrine (10 μg), but not of clonidine (0.5 μg), restored the dose-related decrease in the rate of substantia nigra self-stimulation caused by diethyl dithiocarbamate inhibition of nor-epinephrine synthesis [Belluzi et al, 1975].

These findings indicate that clonidine suppresses operant behavior maintained by different schedules of food reinforcement and by a fixed-interval schedule of water reinforcement. Since clonidine also reduces food intake [Le Douarec et al, 1972], water intake [Le Douarec et al, 1971], and loco-motor activity [Tilson et al, 1977] in rats, it is not certain whether clonidine suppresses operant behavior based on food and water reinforcement by virtue of its anorexic and adipsic effect or its sedative effect. Inasmuch as a reduction in operant behavior is observed after a reduction in noradrenergic transmission [Belluzi et al, 1975], the suppressant effect of clonidine on operant behavior may be related to its stimulation of presynaptic α-adrenergic receptors, which reduces noradrenergic transmission. This assumption is supported by the finding that norepinephrine, but not clonidine [Belluzi et al, 1975], will restore operant behavior suppressed by inhibition of norepinephrine synthesis. Finally, the suppressant action of clonidine on operant responding is not related to any action on endorphin mechanisms, since naloxone fails to alter the effect of clonidine [Harris et al, 1976, 1977; Gellert and Sparber, 1977].

V. CONDITIONED AVOIDANCE RESPONSE

In the paradigm of conditional avoidance responding (CAR), animals are trained to avoid an aversive consequence by responding to a stimulus preceding the onset of the aversive event. If the subject responds to the warning stimulus, the oncoming aversive events can be avoided. Failing that, a response designed to terminate the aversive stimulus is known as an escape response. Both dopamine and norepinephrine are considered to be involved in the mediation of avoidance responses [for review, see Seiden and Dykstra, 1977]. Neuroleptic drugs selectively disrupt avoidance responding at doses which do not disrupt escape behavior [for review, see Fielding and Lal, 1978].

Laverty and Taylor [1969] reported that intraperitoneal administration of clonidine (0.1–1.0 mg/kg) to rats trained to climb a pole to avoid a shock caused a dose-dependent inhibition of the conditioned avoidance behavior. Similarly, Cornfeldt et al [1978] reported inhibition of conditioned avoidance by clonidine in rats (ED_{50} = 0.4 mg/kg IP) and monkeys (ED_{50} = 0.5 mg/kg orally). These may be nonspecific effects resulting from sedation, since these doses have been reported to decrease locomotor activity and operant responding [Maj et al, 1972; Tilson et al, 1977]. Delbarre and Schmitt [1974] found that subcutaneous administration of clonidine (0.15 mg/kg) depressed an avoidance-conditioned reflex in the rat but did not influence the escape response. However, Izquierdo and Cavalhiero [1976] reported that clonidine (0.2 mg/kg IP) depressed both avoidance and escape responding of rats in a two-way shuttle avoidance paradigm. Clonidine (0.2–0.4 mg/kg) further decreases conditioned avoidance responses already depressed by haloperidol [Taboada et al, 1979].

Pretreatment with atropine (10 mg/kg), yohimbine (1–2 mg/kg), and piperoxan (10 mg/kg) antagonized the depression of the conditioned avoidance reflex produced by clonidine [Delbarre and Schmitt, 1974].Phenoxybenzamine (10 mg/kg) blocked a clonidine-induced depression of avoidance and escape responding in the shuttle-avoidance paradigm [Izquierdo and Cavalhiero, 1976]; however, Delbarre and Schmitt [1974] reported that phenoxybenzamine alone also depressed the conditioned avoidance reflex. Yohimbine antagonized avoidance suppression caused by clonidine (0.1–0.3 mg/kg) in another experiment in which methysergide was found inactive [Robson et al, 1978].

In contrast to the above studies demonstrating a suppression of CAR by clonidine, Ruiz and Monti [1975] and Lenard and Beer [1975] reported that suppression of a previously learned conditioned avoidance response in rats produced by intraventricular administration of 6-hydroxydopamine was reversed by intraventricular administration of norepinephrine, dopamine, L-dopa, or by intraperitoneal administration of amphetamine, phenelzine, desipramine, apomorphine, and clonidine. Pretreatment with the neuroleptic spiroperidol prevented the recovery induced by the above drugs; however, clonidine-induced recovery was affected the least [Lenard and Beer, 1975]. Hawkins and Monti [1979], using a shuttle box avoidance device, noted that clonidine (0.1–0.4 mg/kg) produced a dose-dependent decrease in conditional avoidance responding. This effect was considerably reduced by 6-hydroxydopamine treatment. Yohimbine and phentolamine antagonized clonidine; propranolo enhanced its effect.

In conclusion, these studies have demonstrated that clonidine may depress or restore conditioned avoidance responses, depending upon the physiological state of the subject and the doses of clonidine used. The depressant effects are caused by high doses. Furthermore, the action of clonidine on CAR appears to be mediated by catecholaminergic and cholinergic mechanisms. Usually, the selective suppression of conditional avoidance responding is considered predictive of neuroleptic activity [Fielding and Lal, 1978]. However, with clonidine the neuroleptic effect requires behaviorally toxic doses.

VI. SELF-STIMULATION OF BRAIN REWARD SYSTEMS

It is a well-established fact that experimental animals will perform a task such as lever pressing to obtain electrical stimulation of brain sites along the medial forebrain bundle that extend from the "limbic midbrain" through the lateral hypothalamus to the limbic forebrain structures and neocortex. The most intense self-stimulation is derived from implants in the paramedian region of the midbrain and the lateral hypothalamic areas. In view of the specific anatomical sites that are sensitive to brain self-stimulation and the types of drugs that attenuate this behavior, both noradrenergic and dopaminergic systems seem to provide a substrate for such self-stimulation [Fibiger, 1978; Wauquier, 1979].

It is believed that the stimulation of sensitive brain sites provides reinforcements variously termed pleasure sensation, reward, arousal, or activation of memory. Many efforts have been made to identify drugs which enhance or suppress brain self-stimulation. Clonidine is one of the drugs investigated in this regard.

Wauquier et al [1980] compared the effect of clonidine on intracranial self-stimulation (ICSS) with that of spiperone, haloperidol, and apomorphine. They compared lever pressing during sessions in which the stimulus parameters were varied from low to high intensity. They also trained their rats to walk to opposite sides of a shuttle box in order to turn the brain stimulation on or off. Clonidine inhibited ICSS, as did haloperidol and spiperone. Apomorphine had a biphasic action, based upon the doses used. Dopamine antagonists reduced ICSS at all brain sites tested and under all experimental conditions. The authors concluded that dopamine antagonists interfere with the reinforcing effect of the stimulation. Most of the inhibition of ICSS by clonidine was attributed to the mild sedation it produces. However, some interference with the reinforcement was at play. According to Wauquier et al [1980], dopaminergic systems are indispensable for reinforcement mechanisms, and noradrenergic systems cause general arousal. Franklin [1978] reported that clonidine (0.03 and 0.15 mg/kg) reduced the reinforcing component of lateral hypothalamic or ventral tegmental self-stimulation by the doses used and also depressed motor performance. By contrast, pimozide (0.2–0.9 mg/kg) reduced the reward without reducing motor performance. Piperoxan antagonized the effect of clonidine in suppressing reward but potentiated the motor deficit. These data suggest dopamine is involved in producing the reward.

Utilizing a shuttle box technique providing a rate-independent index of the rewarding and aversive components of ICSS, Hunt et al [1976] found that intraperitoneal administration of clonidine (0.004–0.063 mg/kg) led to a dose-dependent increase in the latency of initiation of lateral hypothalamic ICSS, whereas the latency of escape from ICSS was largely unaffected except at doses that depressed performance. The peripheral α-adrenergic agonist 1-phenylephrine (0.05–1.0 mg/kg) was ineffective in this regard, indicating that inhibition of reward by clonidine is a central effect [Hunt et al, 1976]. Clonidine acted synergistically with the catecholamine synthesis inhibitor α-methyl-para-tyrosine (250 mg/kg), greatly increasing (>500%) the magnitude of the latency of initiation and prolonging the duration of inhibition of reward while leaving the magnitude of the escape latency largely unaffected [Hunt et al, 1976]. Whereas administration of clonidine (0.016–0.064 mg/kg) or α-methyl-para-tyrosine alone 24 hours before testing had no effect, their concomitant administration resulted in complete elimination of the initiating behavior, while escape behavior remained unaffected [Hunt et al, 1976]. More recently, Hunt et al [1978] reported that clonidine (0.0125–0.05 mg/kg) caused a dose-dependent increase in the latency of lateral hypothalamic self-stimulation without affecting escape behavior. Yohimbine (0.5–2 mg/kg) increased both latencies. Phenoxybenzamine potentiated the effect of clonidine. Amphetamine (0.25–0.5 mg/kg) reversed it to a dose-dependent degree, and this reversal was blocked by inhibition of catecholamine synthesis by α-methyl-tyrosine. These findings represent additional evidence that activation of α-adrenergic receptors mediates the reward component of lateral hypothalamic self-stimulation.

High-rate lateral hypothalamic ICSS in squirrel monkeys was blocked by clonidine (0.1 mg/kg), whereas in the same animal caudate ICSS was much less affected at this dose [Spencer and Revzin, 1976]. A higher dose of clonidine (0.25 mg/kg), which produced sedation, depressed ICSS to equal degrees at both sites [Spencer and Revzin, 1976]. By contrast, amphetamine (10 mg/kg) and chlorpromazine (0.5 or 1.0 mg/kg) had significantly greater effects on caudate ICSS than on lateral hypothalamic ICSS [Spencer and Revzin, 1976].

Depression of lateral hypothalamic ICSS by clonidine (0.15 mg/kg) was antagonized by doses of piperoxan (1.7–15.0 mg/kg), which selectively block presynaptic α-adrenergic or epinephrine receptors, whereas higher doses of piperoxan (45 mg/kg), phentolamine (0.55–15.0 mg/kg), and phenoxybenzamine (0.1–10.0 mg/kg), which block both pre- and postsynaptic receptors, were ineffective [Franklin and Herberg, 1977].

Vetulani et al [1977] reported that intraperitoneal administration of clonidine to rats in doses producing no motor deficit (0.05–0.20 mg/kg) resulted in a dose-dependent depression of medial forebrain bundle ICSS. Furthermore, clonidine (0.10 mg/kg) blocked the facilitation of medial forebrain bundle ICSS by d-amphetamine (0.5 mg/kg) [Vetulani et al, 1977]. Since d-amphetamine has been reported to release norepinephrine, it was suggested that the blockade of medial forebrain bundle ICSS by clonidine is due to its stimulatory action at presynaptic α-noradrenergic receptors or its blockade of postsynaptic noradrenergic receptors [Vetulani et al, 1977].

In view of the demonstrated suppression of ICSS by clonidine in the above experiments, it is not surprising that inhibition of substantia nigra ICSS in rats by the norepinephrine synthesis inhibitor diethyl dithiocarbamate [Belluzi et al, 1975] or inhibition of lateral hypothalamic ICSS by the norepinephrine synthesis inhibitor disulfiram [Shaw and Rolls, 1976] was not reversed by clonidine (0.5–3.0 μg intraventricularly or 0.037–3.0 mg/kg IP).

In conclusion, the findings suggest that clonidine weakly attenuates the rewarding component of ICSS. This action appears to be mediated by its stimulatory action at central presynaptic α-noradrenergic receptors, which decreases noradrenergic transmission [Hunt et al, 1976; Franklin and Herberg, 1974; Vetulani et al, 1977]. This assumption has been given credence by other investigators [Wise et al, 1973; Hastings and Stutz, 1973; Franklin and Herberg, 1974; German and Bowden, 1974; Belluzi et al, 1975; Shaw and Rolls, 1976; Wauquier et al, 1980], who showed that reduced noradrenergic transmission inhibits self-stimulation. It must be noted, however, that inhibition of ICSS has been reported at doses that do produce some motor deficits [Tilson et al, 1977]. Lower doses affect ICSS very minimally. The suppression of brain reward mechanisms is an integral property of all antipsychotic drugs [Fielding and Lal, 1978]. It is interesting to note, therefore, that Freedman et al [1980] recently reported preliminary evidence that clonidine may possess antipsychotic activity.

VII. DRUG-INDUCED DISCRIMINATIVE STIMULI

It is now well recognized that the discriminative stimuli induced by drugs [Lal and Shearman, 1980; Lal, 1977] are a good measure of their CNS-mediated subjective effects. By evaluation of such discriminative stimuli, both the quality and the quantity of the subjective effects of drugs can be readily predicted. Unlike classical procedures of behavioral pharmacology, the drug discrimination approach does not focus on the behavioral effects of drugs; rather, a behavioral measure is used to assay the animal's perceptual realization that the drug is acting in the body. The drug actions permitting this perception are known as interoceptive discriminative stimuli (IDS). The IDS [Lal, 1979] produced by a number of psychotropic drugs have been established [Lal and Shearman, 1980].

For evaluation of drug-induced IDS, experimental animals are trained to give one response when treated with a drug and an alternative response when treated with the drug vehicle, another dose of the same drug, or a different drug. When such a response differentiation has been reliably learned, the training drug is said to produce an IDS that determines the type of responding shown by the trained subject.

Interest in the CNS manifestations of clonidine action sparked a number of experiments designed to define the discriminatively stimulating properties of this drug. Bennett and Lal [1981] found that rats can readily learn to discriminate between clonidine and saline at an approximate ED_{50} of 0.02 mg/kg. This finding suggests that clonidine exercises reliably detectable preceptual effects that can be measured in laboratory animals. In order to establish the nature of the interoceptive stimuli produced by clonidine, Miksic et al [1978] trained rats to discriminate between morphine and saline and tested their rats for generalization of the morphine stimulus to clonidine. They observed that intraperitoneal administration of clonidine (0.08–0.64 mg/kg) failed to generalize with morphine (10 mg/kg). The rats given clonidine selected the lever appropriate for saline. Since the discriminative stimulus produced by morphine is considered to be related to its subjective effect in man [Lal and Gianutsos, 1976; Lal et al, 1977], lack of generalization to morphine IDS suggests that clonidine produces no morphine-like subjective effect. These observations assume special significance, in view of the fact that clonidine produces analgesia (see Analgesia section) and reduces narcotic withdrawal symptoms in animals and humans (see Analgesia section), for they imply that clonidine may provide a nonnarcotic treatment for pain and opiate addiction without the psychotomimetic effects of morphine or any potential for morphine-like abuse. This suggestion was recently seconded by Washton et al [1980], who found that clonidine displayed no euphorigenic activity in individuals maintained on methadone.

Shearman and Lal (unpublished data) trained rats to discriminate between pentylenetetrazol and saline and tested clonidine for generalization to the pentylenetetrazol stimulus. Clonidine failed to generalize with pentylenetetrazol. The interoceptive stimuli produced by pentylenetetrazol are considered to represent anxiety [Shearman and Lal, unpublished data; Lal and Shearman, 1980]. It may therefore be inferred that clonidine does not evoke anxiety-related experiences. In the same rats clonidine showed no antipentylenetetrazol-type anxiety. In view of the positive effect of clonidine on conflict behavior (see section on Punished Behavior), which also reflects anxiety, one may conclude that the anxiolytic potential of clonidine-type drugs is limited to certain types of anxiety.

Bennett and Lal [1982] trained rats to discriminate between hydralazine and saline. Hydralazine is a potent vasodilator used clinically as an antihypertensive agent. Clonidine failed to generalize the hydralazine response, suggesting that "affective" manifestations of vasodilation are not mimicked by clonidine.

In sum, clonidine can be shown to produce an IDS that is readily perceived. However, the nature of this IDS is not known. It is not euphorigenic like that of morphine, anxiety-producing like that of pentylenetetrazol, or hydralazine-like. Further data are needed to characterize the central subjective effects of clonidine.

VIII. DRUG-REINFORCED BEHAVIOR

Drugs of several pharmacological classes are self-administered because of their positive reinforcing properties. It is now believed that in most cases the reinforcing action of drugs is related to the euphoria they produce. The nature of this euphoria is not known, but it seems to be characteristic of a drug class. Investigations into the neurochemical basis of reinforcement produced by narcotics and psychomotor stimulants have implicated the stimulation of central catecholaminergic and peptidergic systems. Studies to differentiate between noradrenergic and dopaminergic mechanisms have led to the conclusion that noradrenergic mechanisms are involved in opiate reinforcement, and that both dopaminergic and noradrenergic mechanisms are apparently involved in psychomotor stimulant reinforcement.

Davis and Smith [1977] noted that clonidine (15 μg/kg but not 1 μg/kg/injection) was self-administered by rats when its availability was made contingent on lever pressing. They believe that the reinforcing effect of clonidine results from its stimulatory action at postsynaptic α-noradrenergic receptors since intraperitoneal pretreatment with phenoxybenzamine (15 mg/kg) prevented the reinforcement associated with clonidine administration. They also found that intraperitoneal pretreatment with phenoxybenzamine (15 mg/kg), but not haloperidol (5 mg/kg), prevented the establishment of stimulus paired with injections of clonidine as a conditioned reinforcer. The authors suggest that stimulation of α-noradrenergic receptors by clonidine results in positive reinforcement. However, the high dose of haloperidol used by Davis and Smith is known to produce not only dopaminergic but also α-adrenergic blockade [Davis et al, 1975; Davis and Smith, 1975]. Moreover, this dose is known to cause catalepsy, which interferes with operant responding. Since haloperidol failed to block clonidine self-administration in their study, the mechanisms of self-administration in the rat could not be clarified.

Shearman et al [1977] further investigated clonidine self-administration in the rat. They found that a particular dose (15 μg/kg/injection) of clonidine was readily self-administered and, furthermore, that clonidine self-administration was not attenuated by naloxone, showing that opiate mechanisms were not involved. Moreover, in their experiment, clonidine self-administration was completely abolished by the dopaminergic antagonist haloperidol and the adrenergic antagonist azaperone, which points to catecholamine involvement in self-administration.

These studies have demonstrated that clonidine can be used as a tool for the study of brain reinforcement mechanisms that are dependent on catecholamine medication.

IX. AROUSAL AND SLEEP MECHANISM

Because of the involvement of arousal mechanisms in learning, sleep, wakefulness, and many other body functions, a great deal of effort has been devoted to their investigation. Both serotonin and catecholamines appear to play a role in the neurochemical processes leading to arousal.

Open-field behavior is considered to be a measure of exploratory activity indicative of high or low arousal levels. In this test individual rats are placed in a circular open space, and the number of times the animal crosses the diameter (ambulation) and the number of rearings are recorded. In addition, defecations are counted [Janssen et al, 1960]. Another measure of exploratory activity is the hole test. The apparatus is a box containing many round holes. Animals are placed in the box individually, and the frequency with which they place their heads in the holes is counted [File and Pope, 1974].

Dandiya and Patni [1973] observed that intraventricular administration of clonidine decreased the ambulation and rearing of rats in an open-field situation. Similarly, Herman et al [1976] found that clonidine (0.1 but not 0.05 mg/kg) decreased ambulation, rearing, and defecation in the open field and reduced the peeping of rats in the hole test. Intracerebroventricular administration of 6-hydroxy-dopamine potentiated the depressant effect of clonidine [Herman et al, 1976]. Strombom [1975] reported that clonidine (0.025–0.8 mg/kg) depressed the exploratory behavior of mice in a Y-shaped runway maze and appeared to break the pattern of adaption. These findings suggest that norepinephrine may be of importance for exploratory behavior, and that clonidine may be used as a tool to study this symptom.

Clonidine has been found to have somnifacient and sedative effects when administered by several routes to young chicks, mice, rats, cats, rabbits, and man [Zaimis, 1970; Delbarre and Schmitt, 1971; Holman et al, 1971a, b; Florio et al, 1975; Marley and Nistico, 1974, 1975; Walland, 1977; Autret et al, 1976, 1977; Ashton and Rawlins, 1978]. Sleep induced by clonidine given intravenously was considered similar to normal sleep or sleep induced by intravenous epinephrine or norepinephrine [Holman et al, 1971a, b].

The somnifacient effect of clonidine has been reported to be antagonized by the following α-noradrenergic receptor-blocking agents: Phentolamine [Delbarre and Schmitt, 1971; Holman et al, 1971a, b; Fugner, 1971; Marley and Nistico, 1974; Drew et al, 1977]; tolazoline [Delbarre and Schmitt, 1973; Drew et al, 1977]; piperoxan [Delbarre and Schmitt, 1971; Drew et al, 1977]; and dibenamine [Delbarre and Schmitt, 1971]. However, several α-adrenergic blockers including dibozane, ethoxane, azapetine, mosixylite [Delbarre and Schmitt, 1973], thymoxamine, and labetalol [Drew et al, 1977] did not antagonize the sleep-inducing effect of clonidine. Since postsynaptic α adrenoreceptors are more sensitive to the antagonistic effects of thymoxamine and labetalol [Drew, 1977; Drew et al, 1977], the α adrenoreceptors that moderate the clonidine-induced sedation may more closely resemble the peripheral presynaptic α receptors than the postsynaptic α receptors. Whereas Marley and Nistico [1974] reported that phenoxybenzamine antagonized the sedative effect of clonidine, Delbarre and Schmitt [1971] and Fugner [1971] found that phenoxybenzamine did not antagonize this effect of clonidine. These discrepant findings may be related to procedural differences.

Sleep induced by clonidine was not antagonized by several β blockers [Delbarre and Schmitt, 1973; Marley and Nistico, 1974], atropine [Marley and Nistico, 1974], methysergide [Holman et al, 1971a, b], or p-chlorophenylalanine [Holman et al, 1971a, b; Marley and Nistico, 1974]. However, pretreatment with lysergic acid diethylamide (LSD) effectively prevented the induction of sleep by clonidine [Holman et al, 1971a, b].

Clonidine (0.1–2.5 mg/kg) prolonged the chloral hydrate sleeping time in rats [Laverty and Taylor, 1969], chicken, and mice [Delbarre and Schmitt, 1971, 1972, 1973]. Tolazoline, phentolamine, piperoxan, dibenamine [Delbarre and Schmitt, 1971], and yohimbine, but not phenoxybenzamine, antagonized this effect [Delbarre and Schmitt, 1973].

Clonidine induced electroencephalographic (EEG) synchronization and increased spindle activity [Hukuhara et al, 1978; Tran Quang Loc et al, 1974]. Kleinlogel et al [1975] reported that clonidine abolished paradoxical sleep (PS) in rats and reduced slow-wave sleep (SWS). This report was corroborated by Putkonen et al [1977] who found that clonidine (5–20 μg/kg IP) caused a dose-dependent inhibition of PS in cats, a depression of SWS, and produced a synchronized rhythmic EEG. Ashton and Rawlins [1978] also reported a dissociation of the EEG and behavioral effects of clonidine. Yohimbine (3 mg/kg) pretreatment antagonized the PS-suppressing action of clonidine (10 μg/kg) [Putkonen et al, 1977]. In man, clonidine (0.04 μg/kg) does not affect paradoxical sleep and antagonizes the enhancement of paradoxical sleep by chlorpromazine (0.5 mg/kg). However, high doses of clonidine (1.6 μg/kg) decrease paradoxical sleep [Gaillard and Kafi, 1979].

Behavioral depression and EEG synchronization induced by clonidine (0.1 mg/kg) in rats, cats, and rabbits were attenuated by pretreatment with the α-noradrenergic receptor-blocking agents phentolamine (10 mg/kg), tolazoline, (10 mg/kg), and yohimbine (0.5 mg/kg), but not by phenoxybenzamine (10 mg/kg). Pretreatment with α-methyl-para-tyrosine ester (100 mg/kg, 3 days) or reserpine (2 mg/kg) potentiated clonidine (0.1 mg/kg)-induced sedation and EEG synchronization [Florio et al, 1975]. Amphetamine (1 or 2 mg/kg) reversed the behavioral depression and EEG synchronization produced by clonidine (0.2 mg/kg) [Florio et al, 1975]. Furthermore, clonidine abolished the behavioral activation and EEG desynchronization induced by amphetamine [Florio et al, 1975; Marley and Nistico, 1974, 1975] and methamphetamine [Gogolak and Stumpf, 1969]; however, the EEG arousal produced by physostigmine was unaffected by clonidine [Gogolak and Stumpf, 1969].

Ponto-geniculo-occipital (PGO) waves induced by the benzoquinolizine derivative RO4-1248 or the tryptophan hydroxylase inhibitor p-chlorophenylalamine (PCPA) were suppressed by clonidine [Ruth-Monachon et al, 1976]. Bilateral lesions of the locus coeruleus increased the density of the PGO waves induced by PCPA so that their suppression by clonidine may be due to stimulation of locus coeruleus neurons, which depress neurons in the pontine reticular formation that is involved in the generation of PGO waves [Ruth-Monachon et al, 1976].

Clonidine increased the threshold of the EEG arousal reaction evoked by reticular stimulation [Gogolak and Stumpf, 1969]. Behavioral and electrocortical sleep induced by intraventricular administration of clonidine (5–15 μg) was easily interrupted by an arousing stimulus [Holman et al, 1971a], and presentation of sensory stimuli during clonidine-induced sleep caused behavioral and phasic electrocortical arousal [Marley and Nistico, 1975]. Fletcher [1974] observed that clonidine (0.125 or 0.25 mg/kg) depressed the amplitude of the acoustic startle response when administered to reserpinized rats. This observation was confirmed by Davis et al [1977], who found that intraperitoneal administration of clonidine (0.01–2.0 mg/kg) led to a dose-dependent depression of startle amplitude when rats were exposed to startle-eliciting tones. Pretreatment with piperoxan (10 mg/kg) antagonized this effect; phentolamine (10 mg/kg) did not [Davis et al, 1977]. Clonidine also depressed startle in acutely decerebrated rats and in rats with bilateral lesions of the locus coeruleus; this effect may therefore be produced by stimulating central epinephrine rather than norepinephrine receptors [Davis et al, 1977]. The depression of startle by clonidine was related to its ability to improve habituation rather than to a reduction of sensitization, or impairment, of motor function [Davis et al, 1977]. Handley and Thomas [1979] observed that clonidine (0.5 mg/kg) reduced the startle amplitude to a puff of air but potentiated the increased startle amplitude produced by d-amphetamine. Norepinephrine and α-methylnorepinephrine, but not apomorphine, had the same effects as clonidine. Serotonin, p-chlorophenylalanine, and atropine also potentiate the effect of amphetamine on startle amplitude.

In conclusion, several studies have demonstrated a sedative or sleep-inducing effect of clonidine. Indications are that this effect of clonidine results from a stimulatory action of this drug at central α-noradrenergic receptors. It does not seem to depend on serotonergic [Holman et al, 1971a, b] or cholinergic [Marley and Nistico, 1974] transmission.

X. LEARNING AND MEMORY

The debilitating effects of poor learning or dementia have spawned a great deal of interest in drugs that improve learning and memory. While an important role for each of the central neurotransmitters has been postulated in learning and memory processes, the exact function of each remains unclear. Studies measuring the effect of pharmacological agents on learning and memory processes must be interpreted with caution, since factors such as sedation and impairment of motor function can seriously affect the results.

Gazzani and Izquierdo [1976] reported a study in which posttrial intraperitoneal administration of clonidine (0.1 mg/kg) or haloperidol (0.5 mg/kg) to rats trained in a shuttle avoidance paradigm resulted in lower retention of this task in a retest session carried out 7 days later, as compared with animals that received a posttrial saline injection. This effect of clonidine was prevented by pretreatment with either phenoxybenzamine (10 mg/kg) or phentolamine (10 mg/kg), whereas the effect of haloperidol was prevented by pretreatment with apomorphine (4 mg/kg, but not 0.5 mg/kg). These workers suggested that clonidine impaired memory consolidation. However, the deficit in performance may have been due to state-dependent learning rather than to an action of clonidine on memory or learning processes per se. Animals trained to perform a task under the influence of a number of drugs are known to show performance deficits when tested without the training drugs, and this has been thought to be unrelated to any drug effect on learning. More recently, Freedman et al [1979] reported that IP injection of clonidine (0.001–0.5 mg/kg), but not d-amphetamine, produced a dose-dependent reversal of amnesia caused by the dopamine-β-hydroxylase inhibitor diethyl dithiocarbamate in a multiple food-motivated discrimination trial. This effect was blocked by phentolamine. These observations show that brain noradrenergic mechanisms are important in memory processes and that clonidine can be used to reactivate memory processes made deficient by noradrenergic depletion. Similar findings have been made in human subjects.

McEntee and Mair [1980] reported that administration of clonidine to patients with Korsakoff's syndrome (who had low CSF levels of methoxyhydroxyphenylglycol correlating with memory impairment) resulted in a consistent improvement of memory. Since clonidine is presumed to be an α-noradrenergic agonist in the central nervous system, its action in improving memory is additional evidence of an important role of norepinephrine in learning and memory processes. In the same study other CNS stimulants such as amphetamine and methylphenidate were inactive.

In light of these studies, drugs such as clonidine may prove useful in the treatment of memory deficits encountered in conditions such as senile dementia and mental retardation as well as Korsakoff's syndrome.

XI. ANXIETY-RELATED BEHAVIOR

Two approaches have been used to investigate antianxiety effects of drugs preclinically. In one, the reinforced operant behavior is suppressed by response-contingent punishment and in the other, anxiogenic chemicals are injected to elicit behavior reflecting anxiety.

The Geller conflict procedure uses a behavioral response sequence consisting of a punished component and a nonpunished component. During the punished component of this procedure, punishment (usually an electric grid shock) is made contingent upon previously reinforced behavior (usually lever pressing for food reward), whereas during the nonpunished component the reinforcement is available without punishment. Behavior is suppressed during the punished component. Anxiolytic drugs disinhibit behavior that has been suppressed by punishment [for review, see Fielding and Lal, 1978], and the Geller conflict procedure is therefore widely used as a preclinical predictive test for anxiolytic activity.

Bullock et al [1978] tested clonidine by the Geller conflict procedure to determine a possible anxiolytic component in the pharmacological profile of clonidine. They found that intraperitoneal administration of clonidine (0.025–0.10 mg/kg) to rats caused a significant increase in responding during the punishment component, whereas responding during the nonpunished component was unaffected at the lower doses and markedly suppressed at the higher doses, at which sedation was observed. These results suggest a possible anxiolytic effect of clonidine.

In the same laboratory, in a new group of rats, Kruse et al [1980] replicated the clonidine-induced (0.025–0.10 mg/kg) release of suppressed bar pressing due to foot shock. Furthermore, to elucidate the mechanism of this anxiolytic action, various noradrenergic, cholinergic, and serotonergic antagonists were given concomitantly with clonidine, administered in IP doses of 0.10 mg/kg. The anticonflict effect of clonidine was prevented by yohimbine (a presynaptic α antagonist), 5 mg/kg SC, and partially antagonized by phenoxybenzamine (a postsynaptic α blocker) at a higher dose (2.5 mg/kg) but not at the usual dose (1 mg/kg). Atropine (5 mg/kg), methysergide (5 mg/kg), or naloxone (10 mg/kg) also failed to block the action of clonidine. However, since neither phenoxybenzamine at 2.5 mg/kg nor yohimbine at 5 mg/kg had any significant influence on the anxiolytic effect of diazepam in this paradigm, the effect of clonidine was obviously different from that of diazepam. Therefore, the anxiolytic effect of clonidine may come about through presynaptic and/or postsynaptic stimulation of α-noradrenergic neurons.

Redmond and Huang [1979] injected yohimbine to cause anxiety-related behavior in primates and found that the symptoms thus produced were attenuated by clonidine. Lal and Shearman [1980], who administered pentylenetetrazol as an anxiogenic agent, did not observe an antianxiety effect of clonidine. This may mean that clonidine is potentially anxiolytic in certain situations and not in others.

Svensson and co-workers [1978] recently reported that clonidine proved effective in relieving anxiety in six out of 14 patients. Six of the eight nonresponders to clonidine were depressed patients. The authors concluded that clonidine is an effective anxiolytic drug in patients not suffering from depression.

Fear and anxiety reactions are important symptoms of narcotic withdrawal. Clonidine has been found to be very effective in eliminating those symptoms [Gold et al, 1978a,b]. Similarly, an antianxiety effect of clonidine in patients undergoing alcohol withdrawal has been reported [Bjorkvist, 1975].

XII. PAIN AND ANALGESIA

In recent years, increasing interest has been shown in the development of nonnarcotic analgesics. Clonidine has given evidence of antinociceptive effects in several animal species in different tests designed to cause pain in laboratory animals. These tests, in many of which clonidine proved an effective analgesic, will be described below. The analgesic effectiveness of clonidine has also been studied in terms of its interaction with noradrenergic and peptidergic mechanisms. Clonidine has shown no resemblance whatever to narcotic agents.

A. Abdominal Constriction Assay

Abdominal constriction tests measure the ability of drugs to alter abdominal constriction in response to abdominal pain caused by injection of noxious chemical agents. A drug is considered to produce analgesia in this test if the number of abdominal constrictions induced by the chemical agent is significantly decreased.

Subcutaneous administration of clonidine (0.0125–0.05 mg/kg) to mice resulted in dose-dependent inhibition of writhing induced by phenyl-p-benzoquinone, which was not antagonized by naloxone or phenoxybenzamine [Fielding et al, 1977, 1978]. Similarly, clonidine (ED_{50} = 0.025 mg/kg) prevented abdominal constrictions caused by hydrochloric acid, which were antagonized by yohimbine and by imipramine [von Voigtlander et al, 1978]. Clonidine, oxymetazoline, and 1-norepinephrine bitartrate were equally effective in antagonizing the nociceptive action of acetic acid or acetylcholine when administered subcutaneously to mice, whereas phenylephrine was ineffective [Bentley et al, 1977]. Piperoxan (8 and 16 mg/kg) antagonized the antinociceptive action of oxymetazoline and norepinephrine, and partially antagonized the antinociceptive effect of clonidine, whereas phentolamine (16 mg/kg) had no antagonistic effect on any of the three drugs [Bentley et al, 1977]. Clonidine and oxymetazoline were more potent when administered intracisternally; however, their antinociceptive effects by this route were not antagonized by piperoxan (16 mg/kg) administered subcutaneously (50 μg/kg) or intracisternally [Bentley et al, 1977].

B. Hot Plate Test

The hot plate test measures the ability of drugs to inhibit reflex responses of mice placed on a plate that is maintained at a constant temperature of 55°C. A drug is said to produce analgesia if the time of reaction to the heat is significantly increased. Schmitt et al [1974] observed that intraperitoneal (0.1 and 1.0 mg/kg) and intraventricular (0.3–1.0 μg) administration of clonidine increased the reaction time to heat. The antinociceptive activity of clonidine in the hot plate test appears to be mediated centrally since other α-sympathomimetics of the imidazoline series (naphazoline, tetryzolin, and oxymetazoline) which do not cross the blood brain barrier show antinociceptive activity only when administered intracerebroventricularly [Schmitt et al, 1974].

C. Tail Withdrawal Test

The tail withdrawal test measures the ability of drugs to alter the time within which mice or rats withdraw their tails from hot water, usually maintained at 55°C. A drug is said to produce analgesia in this test if the delay in tail withdrawal is significantly increased [for details, see Miksic and Lal, 1977]. Using the tail withdrawal test in mice, Sewell and Spencer [1975] found that subcutaneous administration of clonidine (0.3 mg/kg) produced analgesia. However, when clonidine (0.5 mg) was injected intracerebroventricularly, it not only showed merely marginal antinociceptive activity, but it substantially reduced the analgesic effect of morphine (3 mg/kg SC) when given concurrently [Sewell and Spencer, 1975]. The antinociceptive activity of subcutaneously administered clonidine (0.3 mg/kg) was significantly antagonized by concurrent intraventricular administration of phentolamine (10 μg) [Sewell and Spencer, 1975]. Intraventricular administration of propranolol (10 μg) did not potentiate the antinociceptive effect of concurrent SC administration of morphine (2.5 mg/kg), pentazocine (15 mg/kg), or clonidine (0.3 mg/kg) [Sewell and Spencer, 1975].

Intraperitoneal administration of clonidine (2.5 and 10.0 mg/kg) to rats was effective in inhibiting tail withdrawal from hot water, which was not antagonized by naloxone [Fielding et al, 1977, 1978].

D. Tail Flick Test

The tail flick test measures the ability of drugs to alter the time in which mice or rats remove their tails from a radiant heat source. A drug is considered to produce analgesia in this test if the delay in removal of the tail from the heat is significantly increased.

Subcutaneous administration of clonidine was reported to result in a dose-dependent (ED_{50}: 0.7 mg/kg) inhibition of the tail flick response in mice [Fielding et al, 1977, 1978]. The antinociceptive action of clonidine in this test was not antagonized by naloxone (1.0 mg/kg) or phenoxybenzamine (10.0 mg/kg) [Fielding et al, 1978]. Whereas the analgesic ED_{50} of morphine for mice in the tail flick test was increased 4–7 times following spinal transection, the ED_{50} of clonidine was not significantly altered [Spaulding et al, 1978b]. These findings indicate that clonidine and morphine have different action sites in this test.

Subcutaneous administration of clonidine (0.016 mg/kg) increased the analgesic effect of morphine in the tail flick test approximately fivefold, and morphine (0.16 mg/kg) increased the antinociceptive effect of clonidine four times [Spaulding et al, 1978a]. Naloxone reversed the morphine-induced increase in the effect of clonidine [Spaulding et al, 1978a]. No tolerance to the antinociceptive action of clonidine has been observed in the tail withdrawal and tail flick procedures [Fielding et al, 1977]. Cross-tolerance to the antinociceptive action of clonidine in morphine-pelleted mice also has not been observed [Spaulding et al, 1978a].

E. Randall-Selitto Inflammatory Pain Assay

The Randall-Selitto test measures the ability of drugs to alter the reaction to gradually increasing pressure applied to an inflamed paw by an "analgesia meter." A drug is considered to produce analgesia in this procedure if the pressure required to induce a reaction is significantly increased.

In a modified version of the Randall-Selitto test, Fielding et al [1977, 1978] observed that subcutaneous administration of clonidine (0.125–1.0 mg/kg) produced a dose-dependent increase in the pain threshold.

F. Electrical Stimulation of Tail

Paalzow [1974] measured the changes in the threshold for vocalization in mice and the threshold for motor response (spinal reflex), vocalization, and vocalization after discharge induced in mice and rats by electrical stimulation of the tail. Subcutaneous administration of clonidine (0.08–1.25 mg/kg) led to a dose-dependent increase (100–500%) of the threshold for vocalization and vocalization after discharge in rats, whereas the threshold for motor response was unaffected [Paalzow, 1974]. The threshold for a motor response was raised by 100% at a dose of 10 mg/kg; however, this dose caused sedation and marked sympathomimetic signs [Paalzow, 1974]. Clonidine also increased the threshold for vocalization in mice; however, the dose was higher (2.5–10.0 mg/kg) than that required to cause a similar increase in rats [Paalzow, 1974]. Tolerance to the antinociceptive action of clonidine in raising the threshold for vocalization in rats was observed after chronic treatment [Paalzow, 1979]. Acute administration of clonidine (0.5 mg/kg SC) simultaneously with morphine (5.0 mg/kg) greatly augmented the morphine-induced increase of the threshold for vocalization in rats [Paalzow, 1979].

Pretreatment with chlorpromazine (5 mg/kg SC), atropine (1 mg/kg SC), and p-chlorophenylalanine (400 mg/kg IP) increased the antinociceptive effect of clonidine (0.625 mg/kg SC) on both the threshold for vocalization and the threshold for vocalization after discharge, whereas pretreatment with phenoxybenzamine (10 mg/kg IP) and reserpine (10 mg/kg IP) increased the effect on the threshold for vocalization, only the threshold for vocalization after discharge remaining unaffected [Paalzow and Paalzow, 1976]. Yohimbine (2 mg/kg IP) pretreatment decreased the antinociceptive effect of clonidine on both thresholds, whereas pretreatment with 5-hydroxy-tryptophan (50 mg/kg IP) and α-methyl-p-tyrosine (250 mg/kg IP) decreased the effects on the threshold for vocalization after discharge only [Paalzow and Paalzow, 1976]. Naloxone (8 mg/kg SC) pretreatment or concomitant LSD (50 μg/kg SC) did not alter the antinociceptive effect of clonidine on either of the pain responses studied [Paalzow and Paalzow, 1976]. Schmitt et al [1974] reported the effect of clonidine on four types of behavioral reaction to electrical stimulation of the rat tail: Startle, flight, vocalization, and biting of electrodes. Intraperitoneal administration of clonidine (0.5–3.0 mg/kg) resulted in a dose-dependent reduction of the startle, cry, and biting of electrodes; clonidine was only weakly effective against flight [Schmitt et al, 1974]. Intraventricular administration of clonidine (30 μg) reduced the vocalization and the biting of electrodes but was less effective in terms of startle and flight [Schmitt et al, 1974]. Intraventricular clonidine was 5–7 times as potent as clonidine administered intraperitoneally [Schmitt et al, 1974].

G. Sites and Mechanism of Action

Clonidine-induced analgesia does not seem to be the result of an impairment of motor function, since the threshold for a motor response [Paalzow, 1974] or flight reaction [Schmitt et al, 1974] is unaffected at doses that produce analgesia. The antinociceptive action of clonidine appears to be mediated centrally, since other imidazolines such as xylazine, tetryzolin and oxymetazoline, which do not cross the blood brain barrier, exercise antinociceptive effects only when administered intracerebroventricularly. The analgesic activity of these compounds after systemic administration depends on their lipid solubility, hence their capacity to pass the blood brain barrier. Apparently, clonidine is the best in this class.

It is possible that the antinociceptive action of clonidine in writhing tests may be due to its stimulatory action on α-adrenoceptors located at sensory nerve endings in the peritoneum, since other peripherally acting α-agonists are also antinociceptive in these tests. Depending on the dose, route of administration, and species, it appears that clonidine may increase or decrease the analgesic action of morphine. It follows that the analgesic activities of clonidine and morphine may have a common neuronal pathway. However, in contradistinction to narcotics, neither tolerance to the antinociceptive action of clonidine nor cross-tolerance in morphine-dependent mice has been observed. It is apparent that α-adrenergically mediated analgesia is not due to an opiate receptor interaction, since naloxone consistently failed to antagonize the action of clonidine. The results of studies of the effects of other drugs on clonidine-induced analgesia indicate that several neurochemical systems may mediate the antinociceptive action of clonidine.

The processing of noxious inputs and the associated responses have been studied at the spinal and supraspinal levels. The anatomical locations of morphine-sensitive areas associated with a decrease in pain responding have been reviewed. The postulation that clonidine is active in reducing nociceptive responding through an α-adrenergic mechanism associated with morphine-sensitive sites is based on experiments with ascending and descending projections in pain-related pathways. The noradrenergic-sensitive sites related to nociception have been localized in the locus coeruleus [Price and Fibiger, 1975; Redmond, 1977], nucleus raphe magnus [Lobatz, 1976], and the bulbospinal n. reticularis gigantocellularis [Takagi et al, 1976, 1979].

It is common practice to compare the antinociceptive effectiveness of a compound that is active in the tail flick test with that of opiates. The anatomical and pharmacological distinctions between clonidine and morphine have been investigated with pithed mice and adrenergic antagonists. In terms of the agonistic activity of clonidine, no differences in ED_{50} could be found in the tail flick test between pithed (T6 transection) and intact mice, whereas morphine activity was significantly reduced. Therefore, in contrast to morphine, clonidine acts entirely at the spinal level. In other words, interaction with descending neuronal pathways is not necessary to account for the effect of clonidine on the spinal reflex as measured in the tail flick test.

Moreover, just as naloxone is selective in reducing morphine-induced analgesia, yohimbine effectively blocks clonidine-induced analgesia. The antagonism is present at doses that cause little or no blockade of morphine activity. These findings in conjunction with the observation that phenoxybenzamine was not effective in antagonizing clonidine activity support the concept of a presynaptic adrenergic site for clonidine-induced antiociception in the tail flick test.

XIII. REGULATION OF HUNGER, THIRST, AND SEX DRIVES

Gustatory and sex drives are the basic drives for survival in mammals. It is not clear how clonidine affects eating, drinking, and sexual functions. In dogs, low doses of clonidine increased food intake, whereas high doses reduced it [Le Douarec et al, 1972]. In rats, parenteral administration of clonidine (0.15–0.3 mg/kg) reduced food intake [Le Douarec et al, 1972; Atkinson et al, 1978]. However, chronic subcutaneous administration of clonidine (0.3 mg/kg/day) to rats had an appetite-stimulating effect, suggesting that tolerance develops to the anorectic effect of clonidine. Yim et al [1978] found that clonidine (5–50 μg/kg) increased food intake in satiated rats 3–6 times without increasing intake in nonsatiated rats. Piperoxan antagonized the inhibitory effect of clonidine on food intake in rats, whereas yohimbine and phentolamine proved partially antagonistic [Le Douarec et al, 1972]. However, many α-adrenergic receptor blockers such as tolazoline, dibenamine, and phenoxybenzamine were ineffective, as were β-adrenergic receptor blockers [Le Douarec et al, 1972].

Holman et al [1971a] reported that after intraventricular administration of clonidine (25–75 μg/kg) to rats, approximately one-third of the rats began eating continuously, and occasionally periods of eating alternated with periods of sleep. Ritter et al [1975] also found that rats ate voraciously after intraventricular injection of clonidine (0.05–5 μg) and that clonidine facilitated feeding with a potency 100 times greater than that of norepinephrine. Intraventricular administration of clonidine reversed the anorectic effect of intraperitoneally administered d-amphetamine. Intrahypothalamic administration of clonidine (1 μg) strongly increased food consumption in satiated rats [Le Douarec et al, 1972; Broekkamp and van Rossum, 1972]. The clonidine-induced eating response was completely blocked by the α-antagonist phentolamine [Broekkamp and van Rossum, 1972].

In an investigation of the effect of clonidine on behavior associated with food intake, Poignant and Rismondo [1975] observed that clonidine (0.05–0.2 mg/kg) increased the time for intake of standard alimentary material in hamsters without affecting the associated hoarding behavior. By contrast, amphetamine (1 and 2 mg/kg) modified both intake time and hoarding behavior [Poignant and Rismondo, 1975].

Clonidine (0.0375–0.3 mg/kg) reduced water intake and induced diuresis in water-deprived and water-satiated rats [Le Douarec et al, 1971; Atkinson et al, 1978]. The antidipsogenic effect of clonidine was followed by a delayed increase in water consumption, apparently due to the diuretic effect of the drug since this was suppressed by nephrectomy [Atkinson et al, 1978]. Lower doses of clonidine that are not themselves effective potentiate effects of isoproterenol on drinking and diuresis [Kelleherj and Fregly, 1978]. The reduction in water intake was antagonized by piperoxan, tolazoline, and phentolamine; however, other α-adrenergic receptor blockers such as dibenamine and phenoxybenzamine were ineffective [Le Douarec et al, 1971]. Beta-adrenergic blockers as well as the anticholinergic drugs atropine and mecamylamine were devoid of any antagonistic activity [Le Douarec et al, 1971].

Schlemmer et al [1979] recently reported the observation that clonidine increased food intake in primates. The hyperphagia induced by clonidine resulted in weight gain.

Since clonidine does not increase water intake and in some cases decreases it, the increase in food intake is clearly not associated with fluid intake. Usually, drugs that increase food intake also increase fluid intake. Clonidine must therefore affect hunger or satiation directly. Central noradrenergic systems are known to play important roles in the mediation of feeding behavior. Therefore, a drug with central noradrenergic action is expected to mimic the natural role of the neurotransmitter. Since blockers of α-2 but not of α-1 adrenoreceptors inhibit the effect of clonidine on feeding, the effect is plainly due to α-2 stimulation. It is known that bilateral lesions of the locus coeruleus cause hyperphagia and weight gain [Redmond et al, 1977]. This effect is correlated with a reduction in the cerebral metabolism of norepinephrine. The effect of clonidine is thus evidently due to inhibition of the locus coeruleus noradrenergic system.

Not much is known about the effect of clonidine on the sexual drive. Ahlenius et al [1971a] have suggested that sexual behavior is under the control of both catecholaminergic and serotonergic systems. Malmnas [1973] examined the effects of LSD, clonidine, and apomorphine on testosterone-activated heterosexual copulation of castrated male rats. The percentage of subjects that displayed copulatory behavior was decreased by LSD (30 and 100 μg/kg) and increased by apomorphine (30–300 μg/kg). Clonidine (3–30 μg/kg) did not change the percentage of subjects engaging in copulation.

Michanek [1979] noted that clonidine (20 μg/kg) inhibited the lordotic response of ovariectomized rats to exogenous estrogen. Crowley et al [1978] found that clonidine facilitated lordotic behavior in female guinea pigs. In a number of clinical studies on the use of clonidine in the treatment of hypertension, the incidence of male impotence has ranged from 0.1% to 5.0% [McMahon, 1978].

The few available data do not allow any inferences to be drawn about a possible effect of clonidine on sexual behavior.

XIV. AGGRESSIVE BEHAVIOR

In experimental pharmacology, aggression has been used to determine neurotransmitter involvement in drug action. Aggression is induced in the laboratory animal through a variety of stimuli, and drugs are tested regarding their effect on the aggression. It has been suggested that central catecholamines and serotonin are involved in the mediation of aggressive behavior [for review, see Gianutsos and Lal, 1976]. Morpurgo [1968] was the first to report that intraperitoneal administration of extremely high doses (10 and 50 mg/kg) of clonidine induced aggression (biting attacks) in mice but not in rats or rabbits. This behavior was also produced when clonidine was administered orally, intravenously, or subcutaneously. Intracerebral injection of an 0.5%-solution of clonidine immediately provoked biting attacks [Morpurgo, 1968]. More recently, Razzak et al [1975] also reported that clonidine (50 mg/kg IP) induced automutilation in mice; however, this behavior was seen only when the mice were housed individually in the absence of objects to bite. Ozawa et al [1975] reported that clonidine (40 mg/kg) induced aggressive behavior in mice without altering the brain levels of serotonin, norepinephrine, or dopamine. By contrast, Razzak et al [1977] observed that a large dose of clonidine that induced automutilation in mice markedly increased brain norepinephrine, slightly increased brain dopamine levels, and did not change cerebral serotonin levels.

Other imidazoline derivatives (maphazoline, oxymetazoline) with peripheral sympathomimetic effects similar to those of clonidine did not induce biting even when administered intracerebrally [Morpurgo, 1968]. This is particularly interesting in view of the finding that the imidazoline derivatives, including naphazoline and oxymetazoline, which do not cross the blood brain barrier, cause analgesia when administered intracerebroventricularly [Schmitt et al, 1974].

Pretreatment with neuroleptic drugs (eg, haloperidol: ED$_{50}$, 1.6 mg/kg) inhibited clonidine-induced biting attacks. However, pretreatment with the α-adrenergic blocking agent phentolamine or the anticholinergic atropine was ineffective in preventing aggressive behavior [Morpurgo, 1968]. Since the sympathomimetic effects of clonidine were still evident following neuroleptic pretreatment, the findings of Morpurgo [1968] suggest that clonidine-induced aggression in mice is independent of its α-adrenergic action. Ozawa et al [1975], however, have reported that aggressive behavior in mice induced by intraperitoneal administration of clonidine (40 mg/kg) was markedly inhibited by intraperitoneal pretreatment with the α-blocking agent phenoxybenzamine (20 mg/kg). Similarly, Razzak et al [1977] reported that auto-mutilation induced by a large dose of clonidine was inhibited by prior treatment with reserpine, α-methyl-para-tyrosine, phenoxybenzamine, phentolamine, or chlorpromazine. Pretreatment with amitriptyline, parachlorophenylalanine, L-dopa, 5-hydroxytryptophan, or glycine had no effect on the clonidine-induced aggression and self-mutilation [Ozawa et al, 1975; Stern and Catovic, 1975; Razzak et al, 1977]. Aggression and automutilation induced by clonidine were reported to be potentiated by disulfiram, lithium chloride [Ozawa et al, 1975], nalorphine, mephensin [Stern and Catovic, 1975], methamphetamine, caffeine, and theophylline [Razzak et al, 1977]. These results imply that central noradrenergic mechanisms are involved in the mediation of aggression and automutilation by clonidine. However, the megadoses used in the above experiments make the real meaning of these data questionable.

In rats, aggression can be induced by sufficiently high doses of the dopaminergic agonist apomorphine [McKenzie, 1971] or by termination of chronic narcotic administration [Lal, 1975]. It has been suggested that both these forms of aggression are due to hyperstimulation of dopaminergic neurons in the central nervous system [Lal, 1975; Lal et al, 1975]. Clonidine by itself, administered subcutaneously in doses of 0.25 and 0.5 mg/kg, did not cause aggression in drug-naive rats; however, it enhanced aggression caused by a subthreshold (for aggression) dose (2.5 mg/kg) of apomorphine to a dose-dependent degree (0.0625–0.25 mg/kg), and it enhanced aggression when administered to rats from which morphine had been withdrawn 72 hours previously [Gianutsos et al, 1976]. It has also been reported that irritability and violent aggressive behavior occur in rats after chronic treatment with clonidine [Laverty and Taylor, 1969; Paalzow, 1979] and that rats become irritable and aggressive on receiving clonidine (5 μg/ml) in their drinking water [Dix and Johnson, 1977].

While all of the above studies suggest that clonidine may promote aggressive behavior in mice and rats, Laverty and Taylor [1969] observed that subcutaneous administration of clonidine (0.2–1.0 mg/kg) resulted in a dose-dependent inhibition of aggressive behavior induced by application of painful electric shocks to the grid floor of a cage in which a pair of rats were placed. Cornfeldt et al [1978] reported that clonidine (ED_{50}: 3.8 mg/kg orally) inhibited foot shock-induced aggression in mice. However, clonidine is known to produce analgesia (see Analgesia section) as measured by an increase in the threshold for vocalization [Paalzow, 1974; Schmitt et al, 1974] and vocalization after discharge [Paalzow, 1974; Paalzow and Paalzow, 1976] after electrical stimulation of the rat's tail and several other procedures [Fielding et al, 1978]. Therefore, clonidine-induced inhibition of fighting induced by application of an electrical shock to the grid floor may be due to its analgesic action rather than to an ability to modulate aggressive behavior. However, Buss-Lassen [1978] found that clonidine (0.05–0.16 mg/kg) inhibited aggressive behavior in mice provoked by isolation.

Simultaneous administration of the α-antagonist piperoxan in a dose (5 mg/kg) that selectively blocks presynaptic α-adrenergic receptors prevented the antiaggressive effect of clonidine, suggesting that this effect of clonidine is mediated by its stimulatory action at presynaptic α-adrenergic receptors [Buss-Lassen, 1978].

In conclusion, it has been demonstrated that clonidine may promote, inhibit, or have no effect on aggressive behavior. Its effect on aggressive behavior appears to depend on several factors, including species, dose, treatment regimen (acute vs chronic), and the method of inducing aggression. Induction of aggressive behavior by clonidine appears to depend on postsynaptic stimulation of both dopaminergic and noradrenergic receptors [Morpurgo, 1968; Ozawa et al, 1975; Razzak et al, 1977], whereas inhibition of aggressive behavior by clonidine appears to depend on presynaptic noradrenergic stimulation [Buss-Lassen, 1978].

XV. NARCOTIC AND ALCOHOL WITHDRAWAL SYNDROMES

The aversive nature of syndromes provoked by the withdrawal of abused drugs from dependent subjects has been the main factor discouraging patients from ending drug abuse. The blocking of withdrawal symptoms by drugs that are themselves addictive is counterproductive. Efforts have therefore been concentrated on finding nonaddicting drugs for the treatment of withdrawal syndromes. Earlier research with haloperidol and its analogs revealed that certain α-receptor blockers such as azaperone are effective in blocking heroin withdrawal symptoms [Hynes and Lal, 1981]. More recently, it was noted [for review, see Redmond, 1979] that the effects of electrical or pharmacological activation of the locus coeruleus in monkeys were in certain respects similar to those experienced during opiate withdrawal.

On the basis of observations with azaperone and locus coeruleus research, Fielding et al [1977, 1978] investigated the effect of clonidine on narcotic withdrawal.

Wet-dog-like shakes are reliable signs of narcotic withdrawal in the rat, which are widely used to evaluate the effectiveness of new drugs against symptoms of narcotic withdrawal generally [Gianutsos et al, 1976]. Using this sign and other observations, Fielding et al [1977, 1978] noted that clonidine (0.01–0.16 mg/kg) given IP suppressed narcotic withdrawal signs to a dose-dependent degree. This effect of clonidine was not reversed by naloxone. Other investigators [Tseng et al, 1975; Vetulani and Bednarczyk, 1977] employed higher and more sedative doses (0.1–0.8 mg/kg) to block narcotic withdrawal signs precipitated by the administration of narcotic antagonists to rats. Lipman and Spencer [1978], who recently confirmed the above studies, also observed, similarly to earlier observations of Gianutsos et al [1976], that high doses (0.8 mg/kg) of clonidine caused stereotypy in rats subjected to narcotic withdrawal. These authors reported increased aggression in morphine-addicted but detoxified rats. Lipman and Spencer [1978] observed augmented morphine withdrawal signs after injecting clonidine directly into the ventricles.

Redmond et al [1976] and Redmond [1977], stimulating the locus coeruleus in the monkey, observed that some signs such as autonomic hyperactivity and aural reactions were similar to those observed in animals undergoing narcotic withdrawal, but that many other typical withdrawal signs were absent. The effects of locus coeruleus stimulation as simulated by piperoxan injection were antagonized by either clonidine or morphine, suggesting that certain of the withdrawal signs may be related to locus coeruleus activity.

Opiates administered systemically or applied microiontophoretically turn off the firing of locus coeruleus neurons [Korf et al, 1974]. Tolerance can be developed to this effect of morphine, and in withdrawal, hyperactivity of the cells is demonstrable. Clonidine reverses this morphine withdrawal sign [Aghajanian, 1978] at the neuronal level.

The effectiveness of clonidine in relieving the withdrawal syndrome was recently confirmed in opioid-dependent patients by two independent research teams [Gold et al, 1978a, b, 1979; Washton et al, 1978, 1980]. They reported that clonidine effectively blocks as well as reverses the heroin or methadone withdrawal symptoms of confirmed addicts. Withdrawal symptoms and signs were measured with the use of a variety of rating scales and by physical examination of the patients. The syndrome induced by abrupt withdrawal of the narcotic is both prevented [Washton et al, 1980] and reversed [Gold et al, 1979] by a single dose of clonidine (about 0.005 mg/kg). This dose causes some hypotension in some patients, but this effect is minimal and easily tolerated. Both physical signs and the "affect" associated with narcotic withdrawal are relieved. Clonidine acts to relieve the high anxiety usually present during drug-free detoxification procedures. Washton et al [1980] have summarized several studies in which patients were maintained on clonidine alone for several days in order to achieve opioid-free detoxification as tested by the absence of naloxone-precipitated withdrawal signs at the end of this treatment. They found that clonidine proved effective in achieving complete detoxification from heroin or methadone. Similar results have recently been reported by Gold et al [1979].

The ability of clonidine to relieve symptoms of narcotic withdrawal does not seem to be directly related to action on opiate receptors. Naloxone, an effective opiate antagonist, did not inhibit the ability of clonidine to decrease withdrawal signs in animals [Fielding et al, 1978] or human patients [Washton et al, 1978]. Similarly, the Narcon test does not promote the withdrawal syndrome in addicts who are maintained on clonidine [Washton et al, 1980]. Clonidine does not show any affinity for opioid or endorphin receptors. The mechanism by which it relieves the narcotic withdrawal syndrome is not known at present.

In addition to relieving the symptoms of narcotic withdrawal, clonidine has been found to lessen sweating, tremor, and anxiety associated with alcohol withdrawal in humans [Bjorkqvist, 1975]. The mechanism of its action in alcoholism remains to be investigated.

It seems therefore that clonidine may be an effective treatment of the narcotic withdrawal syndrome, after which the patients may be treated with a long-acting narcotic antagonist concomitantly with rehabilitation therapy. These observations open a new approach toward the development of nonnarcotic drugs for the treatment of addiction.

XVI. THERMOREGULATION

Thermoregulation normally involves the integration of both behavioral and physiological mechanisms. Studies on the role of central neurotransmitters in thermoregulation point to involvement of both catecholamines and serotonin [Stricker and Zigmond, 1976; Cooper et al, 1978]. The role of norepinephrine has been studied in many experiments by use of clonidine.

Wendt and Caspers [1968] reported a suppression of sweating in man during exposure to heat and exercise after oral administration of 75 and 150 μg (about 1 and 2 μg/kg) of clonidine, whereas Laverty and Taylor [1969] observed a fall in body temperature when clonidine (0.1–2.5 mg/kg) was subcutaneously administered to rats. Similarly, Tsoucaris-Kupfer and Schmitt [1972] found that subcutaneous or intraperitoneal administration of clonidine (0.5–1.5 mg/kg) induced hypothermia in rats, the intensity and duration of which were dose-dependent.

Maskrey et al [1970] reported that intraventricular administration of clonidine (0.067–0.107 μg/kg) lowered or raised body temperature in sheep and goats, depending on whether the ambient temperature was above or below thermoneutrality. Intraventricular injection of clonidine in a dose of 15 μg [Tseng et al, 1975], but not in doses of 2–3 μg [Tsoucaris-Kupfer and Schmitt, 1972], lowered the body temperature of rats and produced a dose-dependent (0.02–0.4 μM) degree of hypothermia in young chicks and adult fowl [Marley and Nistico, 1974, 1975] at thermoneutrality. Intrahypothalamic administration of clonidine (3 μg or 0.04 μM) was also found to cause hypothermia [Tsoucaris-Kupfer and Schmitt, 1972; Marley and Nistico, 1975].

The hypothermia produced by clonidine administration was found to be antagonized by the α-blocking agents phentolamine, phenoxybenzamine, piperoxan, tolazoline, and dibenamine [Tsoucaris-Kupfer and Schmitt, 1972; Reid et al, 1975; Marley and Nistico, 1974, 1975]. Piperoxan was the most effective antagonist [Tsoucaris-Kupfer and Schmitt, 1972]. The β-adrenergic receptor antagonists propranolol, pindolol, and bunitrolol were also reported to be effective in decreasing the hypothermic effect of clonidine [Tsoucaris-Kupfer and Schmitt, 1972]. However, Reid et al [1975] and Marley and Nistico [1974, 1975] observed that propranolol did not alter the hypothermic effect of clonidine. Similarly, Tsoucaris-Kupfer and Schmitt [1972] noted that atropine and haloperidol were effective in decreasing the hypothermic effect of clonidine, whereas mecamyline and imipramine were ineffective. Maj et al [1975] and Marley and Nistico [1974, 1975], on the other hand, reported that atropine did not affect clonidine-induced hypothermia, and Reid et al [1975] found that the relatively selective dopamine receptor antagonist pimozide did not modify the hypothermic effect of clonidine. Marley and Nistico [1975] reported that haloperidol did not attenuate the hypothermic effect of clonidine. Other α-sympathomimetic imidazolines such as naphazoline, tetryzoline, and oxymetazoline, which do not cross the blood brain barrier [Walland, 1977], were also effective in producing hypothermia after peripheral administration [Tsoucaris-Kupfer and Schmitt, 1972]. Depletion of brain catecholamines by intracisternal administration of 6-OHDA failed to alter the hypothermic response to clonidine [Reid et al, 1975]. Therefore, the hypothermic effect of clonidine may be due to action at both central and peripheral sites.

Scheel-Kruger and Hasselager [1974] found that the hypothermia induced by clonidine (0.5 mg/kg) in rats could be antagonized by apomorphine (2 × 2.5 mg/kg). These authors suggested that the hypothermic effect of clonidine might be due to its action on serotonin turnover since apomorphine also significantly antagonized the clonidine-induced decrease of 5-hydroxyindoleacetic acid levels, and the time course of this action of apomorphine correlated with its antagonism of clonidine-induced hypothermia. However, Marley and Nistico [1974, 1975] found that intraventricular pretreatment with the serotonin receptor blocker methysergide (0.1 μM) or the serotonin depletor PCPA methyl ester did not attenuate the hypothermic effect produced by intraventricular injection of clonidine (0.05–0.2 μm).

Finally, Tseng et al [1975] noted that intraperitoneal (0.1–0.4 mg/kg) or intraventricular (5 and 15 μg) administration of clonidine inhibited precipitated shakes and potentiated escape attempts induced by naloxone in morphine-dependent rats. These symptoms of morphine withdrawal were previously thought [Wei et al, 1974] to be related to heat gain and heat loss mechanisms, respectively.

In conclusion, these findings demonstrate that clonidine produces hypothermia via several routes of administration. In view of the antagonism of clonidine-induced hypothermia by α-adrenergic blocking agents, it appears that the hypothermic action of clonidine is mediated by its stimulatory action at α-adrenergic receptors. This assumption is supported by the finding that hypothermia induced by intraventricular administration of norepinephrine is antagonized by phentolamine [Burks, 1972]. However, as suggested by Scheel-Kruger and Hasselager [1974], the hypothermic effect of clonidine may be secondary to its action on noradrenergic receptors and may be the result of the clonidine-induced decrease in serotonin turnover [Anden et al, 1970; Scheel-Kruger and Hasselager, 1974; Rochette and Bralet, 1975]. According to Feldberg and Myers [1964], intraventricular administration of serotonin causes hyperthermia. It would follow, therefore, that a reduction in serotonin turnover by clonidine results in hypothermia. Finally, we cannot be certain whether or not the hypothermic effect of clonidine is produced at central or peripheral α-adrenergic receptors or both since other imidazoline sympathomimetics that do not cross the blood brain barrier also cause hypothermia when administered peripherally.

XVII. CONCLUSIONS

Clonidine exhibits a spectrum of psychotropic activity that extends to many areas of research on brain physiology and therapeutics. Accordingly, many new topics for preclinical and clinical research are suggested by a review of the drug's psychotropic effects.

The area of research attracting the most attention is the physiology of the nucleus locus coeruleus (LC) and the role this nucleus plays in mental illness. The LC is a relatively homogeneous group of catecholamine-containing nerve cell bodies with projections throughout the central nervous system [Moore and Bloom, 1979]. Besides, this pontine nucleus is innervated by nerve terminals that contain many of the known neurotransmitters such as serotonin, GABA, acetylcholine, and the more recently identified opioid peptides. Drugs that act specifically on the locus coeruleus may therefore be of unique significance in medicine, since they provide opportunities to influence selected brain functions. Clonidine is a specific agonist for σ_2-adrenoreceptors in the locus coeruleus. The availability of this drug for research greatly assists the discovery of LC functions and their control. Clonidine is thus helping us to establish the role of the LC in health and disease, just as research with haloperidol helped to elucidate the functions of the striatum and the limbic system. The effects of clonidine on anxiety, learning, and memory, and on symptoms of heroin and alcohol withdrawal may well be related to its action on the LC.

Other brain areas that have a high concentration of clonidine-binding sites are the nucleus tractus solitarii of the hypothalamus, rapha nucleus, periventricular nucleus of the thalamus, the arcuate nucleus of the median eminence, and the substantia gelatinosa in the spinal cord. These areas of the central nervous system are associated with many important brain functions, and many pharmacological effects of clonidine may be attributed to actions at these sites. Among them may be antihypertensive, antinociceptive, and endocrinological effects as well as effects on thermoregulation and hunger drives.

Areas of research of immediate therapeutic significance in neuropsychiatry include the treatment of drug addiction, anxiety, pain, dementia, and perhaps psychoses. The effects of clonidine on pain and the narcotic withdrawal syndrome have been investigated more extensively. All indications are that clonidine treatment will be found useful as a nonnarcotic chemotherapeutic method of narcotic detoxification. Its usefulness for the treatment of acute or chronic pain, which gave very encouraging results in preclinical studies, still remains to be established in clinical settings. On an experimental basis, clonidine is being used to treat dementia related to alcoholism and to control anxiety in certain situations.

Clonidine is being used predominantly to control hypertension. This effect can be a liability for use of the drug in psychiatry and neurology. While the doses used in these fields cause only minimal hypotension and sedation, efforts should be made to evaluate analogs of clonidine that possess psychotropic activity without exerting any hypotensive or sedative effects.

Clonidine has opened the door to an understanding of the neuropathology of many disease states. In a general way, this is reminiscent of the opportunities afforded by the advent of reserpine in the early 1950s and of haloperidol in the early 1960s. Both these drugs represented immensely important research tools without which neuropsychopharmacology would not have progressed this far. We now entertain similar hopes for research with clonidine, which is still in its infancy. This review has been presented to provide a broader perspective on the frontiers to be explored.

XVIII. REFERENCES

Aghajanian GK: Tolerance of locus coeruleus neurons to morphine and suppression of withdrawal response by clonidine. Nature 276:186–188, 1978.

Ahlenius S, Eriksson H, Larsson K, Modigh K, Sodersten P: Mating behavior in the male rat treated with p-chlorophenylalanine methyl ester alone and in combination with pargyline. Psychopharmacologia 20:383–388, 1971a.

Ahlenius S, Anden NE, Engel J: Importance of catecholamine release by nerve impulses for free operant behavior. Physiol Behav 7:931–934, 1971b.

Al-Shabibi UMH, Doggett NS: On the central noradrenergic mechanism involved in haloperidol-induced catalepsy in the rat. J Pharm Pharmacol 30:529–531, 1978.

Anden NE, Corrodi H, Fuxe K, Hokfelt B, Rydin C, Svensson T: Evidence for a central noradrenaline receptor stimulation by clonidine. Life Sci 9:513–523, 1970a.

Anden NE, Butcher SG, Engel J: Central dopamine and noradrenaline receptor activity of the amines formed from m tyrosine, alpha-methyl-m-tyrosine and alpha-methyldopa. J Pharm Pharmacol 22:548–550, 1970b.

Anden NE, Strombom U, Svensson TH: Dopamine and noradrenaline receptor stimulation: Reversal of reserpine-induced suppression of motor activity. Psychopharmacologia 29:289–798, 1973

Anden NE, Gabrowska M, Strombom U: Different alpha adrenoceptors in the central nervous system mediating the biochemical and functional effects of clonidine and receptor blocking agents. Naunyn Schiedebergs Arch Pharmacol 292:43–52, 1976.

Arnt J, Scheel-Kruger J: GABAergic and glycinergic mechanisms within the substania nigra: Pharmacological specificity of dopamine-independent contralateral turning behavior neuro-transmitters.Psychopharmacologia 62:267–277, 1979.

Ashton H, Rawlins M: Central nervous system depressent actions of clonidine and UK-14, 304: Partial dissociation of EEG and behavioral effects. Br J Clin Pharmacol 5:135–140, 1978.

Atkinson J, Kirchertz E, Peters-Haefeli L: Effects of peripheral clonidine on ingestive behavior. Physiol Behav 21:73–77, 1978.

Autret A, Minz M, Beillevaire T, Cathala HP, Castaigne P: Suppression of paradoxal sleep by clonidine in man. CR Acad Sci D 283:955–957, 1976.

Autret A, Minz M, Beillevaire T, Cathala HP, Schmitt H: Effect of clonidine on sleep patterns in man. Eur J Clin Pharmacol 12:319–322, 1977.

Bednarczyk B, Vetulani J: Stimulatory and inhibitory action of clonidine on locomotor activity in the rat. Pol J Pharmacol Pharm 29:219–229, 1977.

Bednarczyk B, Vetulani J: Antagonism of clonidine to shaking behavior in morphine abstinence syndrome and to head twitches produced by serotonergic agents in the rat. Pol J Pharmacol Pharm 30:307–322, 1978

Belluzi JD, Ritter S, Wise CD, Stein L: Substantia nigra self-stimulation: Dependence on noradrenergic pathways. Behav Biol 13:103–111, 1975.

Bennett D, Lal H: Yohimbine blockade of discriminative stimuli produced by clonidine in the rat. Fed Proc 40:292, 1981.

Bennett D, Lal H: Discriminative stimulus properties of the vasodilator, hydralazine: Differential generalization with alpha$_1$ and alpha$_2$ adrenoreceptor drugs. Prog Neuropsychopharmacol (1982, in press).

Bentley GA, Bennett D, Lal H, Copeland IW, Starr J: The actions of some alpha-adrenoceptor agonists and antagonists in an antinociceptive test in mice. J Clin Exp Pharmacol Physiol 4: 405–419, 1977.

Berggren U, Tallstedt L, Ahlenius S, Engel J: The effect of lithium on amphetamine-induced locomotor stimulation. Psycho Pharmacol 59:41–45, 1978.

Biswas B, Carlsson A: Effect of intraperitoneally administered GABA on the locomotor activity of mice. Psychopharmacol 59:91–94, 1978.

Bjorkqvist SE: Clonidine in alcohol withdrawal. Acta Psych Scand 52:256–263, 1975.

Broekkamp C, van Rossum J: Clonidine-induced intrahypothalamic stimulation by eating in rats. Psychopharmacol 25:162–168, 1972.

Bullock SA, Kruse H, Fielding S: The effect of clonidine on conflict behavior in rats: Is clonidine an anxiolytic agent? Pharmacologist 20:223, 1978.

Burks TF: Central alpha-adrenergic receptors in thermoregulation. Neuropharmacol 11:615–624, 1972.

Buss-Lassen J: Piperoxane reduces the effects of clonidine on aggression in mice and on noradrenaline-dependent hypermotility in rats. Eur J Pharmacol 47:45–49, 1978.

Colelli B, Meyer DR, Sparber SB: Clonidine antagonizes disruption of fixed ratio operant behavior in morphine-pelleted rats given naloxone. Pharmacologist 18:236, 1976.

Cooper JR, Bloom FF, Roth RH: "The Biochemical Basis of Neuropharmacology." New York: Oxford University Press, 1978.

Cornfeldt ML, Fielding S, Kruse H, Billey-Nichuck J, Dobson C, Wilker J: Clonidine: Inhibition of amphetamine-induced circling and other psychopharmacological effects. Pharmacologist 20:162, 1978.

Costell B, Naylor RJ, Marsden CD, Pycock CJ: Serotonergic modulation of the dopamine response from the nucleus accumbens. J Pharm Pharmacol 28:523–526, 1976.

Cowan A, Watson T: The effect of naloxone on compounds that attenuate chemically-induced shaking in rats. Fed Proc 38:682, 1979.

Crowley W, Nock B, Feder H: Facilitation of lordosis behavior by clonidine in female guinea pigs. Pharmacol Biochem Behav 8:207–209, 1978.

Dandiya P, Patni S: Influence of substances acting on the central adrenergic receptor on open-field behavior in rats. Ind J Med Res 61:891–895, 1973.

Davis WM, Smith SG: Effect of haloperidol on (+)amphetamine self-administration. J Pharm Pharmacol 27:540–542, 1975.

Davis WM, Smith SG: Catecholaminergic mechanisms of reinforcement: Direct assessment by drug self-administration. Life Sci 20:483–492, 1977.

Davis M, Cedarbaum J, Aghajanian G, Gendelman D: Effects of clonidine on habituation and sensitization of acoustic startle in normal, decerebrate and locus coeruleus-lesioned rats. Psychopharmacol 51:243–253, 1977.

Davis WM, Smith SG, Khalsa JH: Noradrenergic role in the self-administration of morphine and amphetamine. Pharmacol Behav 3:477–484, 1975.

Delbarre B, Schmitt H: Sedative effects of alpha-sympathomimetic drugs and their antagonism by adrenergic and cholinergic blocking drugs. Eur J Pharmacol 13:356–363, 1971.

Delbarre B, Schmitt H: A further attempt to characterize sedative receptors activated by clonidine in chickens and mice. Eur J Pharmacol 22:355–359, 1973.

Delbarre B, Schmitt H: Effects of clonidine and some alpha-adrenoreceptor blocking agents on avoidance-conditioning reflexes in rats: Their interactions and antagonism by atropine. Psychopharmacol 35:195–202, 1974.

Delini-Stula A: Effect of single and repeated treatment with antidepressants on clonidine-induced hypoactivity in the rat. Navryn-Schmied Arch Pharmacol Suppl 302:53, 1978.

Delini-Stula A, Baumann P, Buch O: Depression of exploratory activity by clonidine in rats as a model for the detection of relative pre- and postsynaptic central noradrenergic receptor selectivity of x-adrenolytic drugs. Navryn Schmied Arch Pharmacol 307:115–122, 1979.

Dix R, Johnson E Jr: Withdrawal syndrome upon cessation of chronic clonidine treatment in rats. Eur J Pharmacol 44:153–159, 1977.

Dolphin A, Jenner P, Marsden C: The relative importance of dopamine and noradrenaline receptor stimulation for the restoration of motor activity in reserpine or alpha-methyl-p-tyrosine pre-treated mice. Pharmacol Biochem Behav 4:661–670, 1976.

Donaldson I, Dolphin A, Jenner P, Marsden C, Pycock C: The roles of noradrenaline and dopamine in contraversive circling behavior seen after unilateral electrolytic lesions of the locus coeruleus. Eur J Pharmacol 39:179–191, 1976.

Drew GM: Pharmacological characterization of pre-synaptic alpha adrenoceptors which regulate cholinergic activity in the guinea pig ileum. Br J Pharmacol 61:468, 1977.

Drew G, Gower A, Marriott A: Pharmacological characterization of alpha-adrenoceptors which mediate clonidine-induced sedation. Br J Pharmacol 61:468, 1977.

Dunstan R, Jackson DM: The demonstration of a change in adrenergic receptor sensitivity in the central nervous system of mice after withdrawal from long-term treatment with haloperidol. Psychopharmacol 48:105–114, 1976.

Dunstan R, Jackson D: The effect of apomorphine and clonidine on locomotor activity in mice after long-term treatment with haloperidol. Clin Exp Pharmacol Physiol 4:131–141, 1977.

Feldberg W, Myers RD: Effects on temperature of amines injected into the cerebral ventricles. A new concept of temperature regulation. J Physiol 173:226–237, 1964.

Fibiger HC: Drugs and reinforcement mechanisms. A critical review of the catecholamine theory. Ann Rev Pharmacol Toxicol 18:37–56, 1978.

Fielding S, Lal H: Behavioral pharmacology of neuroleptics. In Iversen L, Snyder S (eds): "Handbook of Psychopharmacology." New York: Plenum Press, 1978, pp 91–148.

Fielding S, Wilker J, Hynes M, Szewzak M, Novick W, Lal H: Antinociceptive and withdrawal actions of clonidine: A comparison with morphine. Fed Proc 36:1024, 1977.

Fielding S, Wilker J, Hynes M, Szewczak M, Novick W, Lal H: A comparison of clonidine with morphine for antinociceptive and antiwithdrawal actions. J Pharmacol Exp Ther 207:899–905, 1978.

File SE, Pope JH: The action of chlorpromazine on exploration in pairs of rats. Psychopharmacol 37:249–254, 1974.

Flechter L: The effects of lodopa, clonidine, and apomorphine on the acoustic startle reaction in rats. Psychopharmacol 39:331–344, 1974.

Florio V, Bianchi L, Lonogo VG: A study of the central effects of sympathomimetic drugs: EEG and behavioral investigations of clonidine and naphazoline. Neuropharmacol 14:707–714, 1975.

Franklin KBJ, Herberg LJ: Presynaptic alpha-adrenoceptors: The depression of self-stimulation by clonidine and its restoration by piperoxane but not by phentolamine or phenoxybenzamine. Eur J Pharmacol 43:33–38, 1977.

Franklin KBJ: Catecholamines and self-stimulation's reward and performance effects dissociated. Pharmacol Biochem Behav 9:813–820, 1978.

Franklin KBJ, Herberg LJ: Self-stimulation and catecholamines: Drug-induced mobilization of the "reserve" pool re-established responding in catecholamine-depleted rats. Brain Res 67: 429–437, 1974.

Freedman LS, Backman MZ, Quatermahn D: Clonidine reverses the amnesia induced by dopamine beta hydroxylase inhibition. Pharmacol Biochem Behav 11:259–263, 1979.

Freedman R, Bell J, Kirch D: Clonidine therapy for coexisting psychosis and tardive dyskinesia. Am J Psychiatr 137:629–630, 1980.

Fugner A: Antagonism of the drug-induced behavioral sleep in chicks. Arzneim Forsch 71: 1350–1356, 1971.

Gaillard JM, Kafi S: Involvement of pre- and postsynaptic receptors in catecholaminergic control of paradoxical sleep in man. Eur J Clin Pharmacol 15:83–89, 1979.

Gazzani JL, Izquierdo I: Possible peripheral adrenergic and central dopaminergic influences on memory consolidation. Psychopharmacol 49:109–112, 1976.

Gellert VF, Sparber SB: A comparison of the effects of naloxone upon body weight loss and suppression of fixed-ratio operant behavior in morphine-dependent rats. J Pharmacol Exp Ther 201:44–54, 1977.

German DC, Bowden DM: Catecholamine systems as the neural substrate for intracranial self-stimulation: A hypothesis. Brain Res 73:381–419, 1974.

Gianutsos G, Hynes MD, Lal H: Enhancement of morphine-withdrawal and apomorphine-induced aggression by clonidine. Psychopharm Commun 2:165–171, 1976.

Gianutsos G, Lal H: Drug-induced aggression. In Valzelli L, Essman W (eds): "Current Developments in Psychopharmacology." Jamaica, NY: Spectrum, 1976, pp 199–220.

Glick SD, Zimmerberg B, Charap AD: Effects of alpha-methyl-para-tyrosine on morphine dependence. Psychopharmacol 32:365–371, 1973.

Glick SD, Cox R: Differential sensitivity to apomorphine and clonidine following frontal cortical damage in rats. Eur J Pharmacol 36:241–245, 1976.

Gogolak VG, Stumpf C: The effects of 2-(2,6-dichlorophenylamino)-2-imidazoline hydrochloride on the EEG-arousal reaction in rabbits. Arzneim Forsch 16:1050–1052, 1969.

Gold MS, Redmond DE Jr, Kleber HD: Clonidine in opiate withdrawal. Lancet 1:929–930, 1978a.

Gold MS, Redmond DE Jr, Kleber HD: Clonidine in opiate-withdrawal symptoms. Lancet 2:599–602, 1978b.

Gold M, Redmond D, Kleber H: Noradrenergic hyperactivity in opiate withdrawal supported by clonidine reversal of opiate withdrawal. Am J Psychiatry 136:100–102, 1979.

Handley SL, Thomas KV: Influence of catecholamines on dexamphetamine-induced changes in locomotor activity. Psychopharmacol 58:283–288, 1978.

Handley SL, Thomas KV: Potentiation of startle response by d- and l-amphetamine: The possible involvement of pre- and postsynaptic alpha-adrenoceptors of a tactile startle response. Psychopharmacol 64:105–111, 1979.

Harris RA, Snell D, Loh HH: Effects of stimulants, anorectics, and related drugs on schedule-controlled behavior. Psychopharmacol 56:49–55, 1978.

Harris R, Snell D, Loh HH, Way EL: Behavioral interactions of apomorphine, clonidine and naloxone: Possible presynaptic involvement. Proc West Pharmacol Soc 19:448–451, 1976.

Harris RA, Snell D, Loh HH, Way EL: Behavioral interactions between naloxone and dopamine agonists. E J Pharmacol 43:243–246, 1977.

Hastings L, Stutz RM: The effect of alpha- and beta-adrenergic antagonists on the self-stimulation phenomenon. Life Sci 13:1253–1259, 1973.

Hawkins M, Monti JM: Effects of pretreatment with 6-hydroxydopamine or noradrenergic receptor blockers or the clonidine-induced disruption of conditioned avoidance responding. Eur J Pharmacol 58:53–58, 1979.

Herman ZS, Brus R, Drybanski A, Szkilnik R, Slominska-Zurek J: Influence of 6-hydroxydopamine on the behavioral effects induced by apomorphine or clonidine in rats. Psychopharmacol 50:73–80, 1976.

Hill RT, Tedeschi DH: Animal testing and screening procedures in evaluating psychotropic drugs. In Rech R, Moore K (eds): "An Introduction to Psychopharmacology." New York: Raven Press, 1971, pp 237–279.

Holman RB, Shillito EE, Vogt M: Sleep-produced clonidine (2-(2,6-dichlorophenylamino)-2-imidazoline hydrochloride). Br J Pharmacol 43:685–695, 1971a.

Holman R, Shillito E, Vogt M: Sleep elicited by clonidine and its relation to neurons containing 5-hydroxy tryptamine. J Physiol (Lond) 217:51P–52P, 1971b.

Hukuhara T Jr, Otsuka Y, Takeda R, Sakai F: Synchronization of EEG and increased spindle activity following clonidine in cats. Arzneim Forsch 18:1147, 1968.

Hunt GE, Atrens DM, Becker FT, Paxiros G: 2-Adrenergic modulation of hypothalamic self-stimulation: Effects of phenoxybenzamine, yohimbine, dexamphetamine and their interactions with clonidine. Eur J Pharmacol 53:1–8, 1978.

Hunt GE, Atrens DM, Chechet GB, Becker FT: A noradrenergic modulation of hypothalamic self-stimulation: Studies employing clonidine, 1-phenulephrine and alpha-methyl-p-tyrosine. Eur J Pharmacol 37:105–111, 1976.

Hynes M, Lal H: A comparison of butyrophenone and tricyclic neuroleptics with narcotics in blocking withdrawal signs in rats continuously infused with morphine. Drug Dev Res 1: 1981.

Izquierdo I, Cavalhiero EA: Three main factors in rat shuttle behavior: Their pharmacology and sequential entry in operation during a two-way avoidance session. Psychopharmacol 49: 145-157, 1976.

Jahn U, Mixich G: Wet dog shake behavior in normal rats elicited by benzylidenamino-oxycarbonic acid derivatives. Psychopharmacol 46:191-196, 1976.

Janssen PAJ, Jageneau AHM, Schellekens KHL: Chemistry and pharmacology of compounds related to 4/4-hydroxy-phenyl-piperidinobutyrophenone. Part IV. Influence of haloperidol (R 16251) and chlorpromazine on the behavior of rats in an unfamiliar "open field" situation. Psychopharmacol 1:389-392, 1960.

Jenner P, Marsden DC: The influence of piribedil (ET 495) on components of locomotor activity. Eur J Pharmacol 33:211-216, 1975.

Jenner PG, Pycock CJ: Interaction of clonidine with dopamine dependent behaviors in rodents. Br J Pharmacol 58:469, 1976.

Kelleherj DL, Fregly MJ: The acute effect of clonidine on various dipsegernic stimuli in rats. Fed Proc 37:815, 1978.

Kelly PH: Drug-induced motor behavior. In Iversen LL, Iversen SD, Snyder SH (eds): "Handbook of Psychophecology," vol 8. "Drug, Neurotransmitters, and Behavior." New York: Plenum Press, pp 295-331, 1977.

Kleinlogel H, Scholtysik G, Sayer A: Effects of clonidine and BS 100-141 on the EEG sleep pattern in rats. Eur J Pharmacol 33:159-163, 1975.

Korf J, Bunney BS, Aghajanian GK: Noradrenergic neurons: Morphine inhibition of spontaneous activity. Eur J Pharmacol 25:165-169, 1974.

Kruse H, Thevrer KL, Dunn RW, Novick WJ, Shearman GT: Attenuation of conflict-induced suppression by clonidine: Indication of anxiolytic activity. Drug Dev Res 1980 (in press).

Kruse H, Moller J: Thyroliberin (TRH)-induced shaking behavior in rats: Inhibition by antinociceptive compounds. Drug Dev Res 1980 (in press).

Lal H: Interoceptive stimuli as tools of drug development. Drug Dev Ind Pharmacol S:133-149, 1979.

Lal H: Morphine-withdrawal aggression. In Ehrenpreis S, Neidle EA (eds): "Methods in Narcotic Research." New York: Marcel Dekker, 1975, pp 149-169.

Lal H (ed): "Discriminative Stimulus Properties of Drugs." New York: Plenum Press, 1977.

Lal H, Gianutsos G: Alterations in neuropharmacology of apomorphine by chronic treatment with haloperidol. In Fann WE, Smith RS, Davis JM, Domino EF (eds): Tardive Dysiness. New York: SP Medical and Scientific Brshs., 1958, pp 14, 51-64.

Lal H, Gianutsos G: Discriminable stimuli produced by narcotic analgesics. Psychopharmacol Commun 2:311-314, 1976.

Lal H, Gianutsos G, Puri SK: Comparison of narcotic analgesics with neuroleptics on behavioral measures of dopaminergic activity. Life Sci 17:29-34, 1975.

Lal H, Gianutsos G, Miksic S: Discriminable stimuli produced by analgesics. In Lal H (ed): "Discriminative Stimulus Properties of Drugs." New York: Plenum Press, 1977, pp 23-45.

Lal H, Shearman GT: Interoceptive discriminative stimuli in the development of CNS drugs. A case of an animal model of anxiety. Ann Rep Med Chem 15:51-58, 1980.

Laverty R, Taylor KM: Behavioral and biochemical effects of 2-(2,6-dichlorophenylamino)-2-imidazoline hydrochloride (ST 155) on the central nervous system. Br Pharmacol 35:253-264, 1969.

Le Douarec JC, Schmitt H, Lucet B: Effect of clonidine and alpha-sympathomimetics on water intake in rats deprived of water. J Pharmacol (Paris) 2:435-444, 1971.

Le Douarec JC, Schmitt H, Lucet B: Effects of clonidine and other alpha-sympathomimetic agents on food intake: Antagonism by adrenolytics. J Pharmacol (Paris) 3:187–198, 1972.

Lenard LG, Beer B: Modification of avoidance behavior in 6-hydroxydopamine-treated rats by stimulation of central noradrenergic and dopaminergic receptors. Pharmacol Biochem Behav 3:887–893, 1975.

Lipman J, Spencer P: Clonidine and opiate withdrawal. Lancet 2:521, 1978.

Lobatz MK, Proudfit HK, Anderson EG: Effects of noxious stimulation, iontophoretic morphine and norepinephrine on neurons in nucleus raphe magnus. Pharmacol 18(2):213, 1976.

Maj J, Sowinska H, Baran L, Kapturkiewicz Z: The effect of clonidine on locomotor activity in mice. Life Sci 11:483–491, 1972.

Maj J, Baran L, Sowinska H, Zielinski M: The influence of cholinolytics on clonidine action. Pol J Pharmacol 27:17–26, 1975a.

Maj J, Moglinicka E, Palider W: Serotoninergic mechanism of clonidine and apomorphine interaction. Pol J Pharmacol Pharm 27:27–35, 1975b.

Malmnas C: Effects of LSD-25, clonidine and apomorphine on copulatory behavior in the male rat. Acta Physiol Scand 395:96–116, 1973.

Marley E, Nistico G: Sleep and hypothermic effects of clonidine in fowls. Br J Pharmacol 52:434–435, 1974.

Marley E, Nistico G: Central effects of clonidine, 2-(2,6-dichlorophenylamino)-2-imidazoline hydrochloride in fowls. Br J Pharmacol 55:459–473, 1975.

Maskrey M, Vogt M, Bligh J: Central effects of clonidine (2-(2,6-dichlorophenylamino)-2-imidazoline hydrochloride, ST 155) upon thermoregulation in the sheep and goat. Eur J Pharmacol 12:297–302, 1970.

McEntee WJ, Mair RG: Memory enhancement in Korsakoff's psychosis by clonidine: Further evidence for a noradrenergic deficit. Am Neurol 7:466–470, 1980.

McKenzie GM: Apomorphine-induced aggression in the rat. Brain Res 34:323–330, 1971.

McMahon FW: Clondine (Catapres). In McMahon FW (ed): "Management of Essential Hypertension." New York: Futura, 1978, pp 151–174.

Menon MK, Clark WG, Masvoka DT: Possible involvement of the central dopaminergic system in the antireserpine effect of LSD. Psychopharmacol 52:291–297, 1977.

Meyer DR, El-Azhary R, Bierer D, Hanson SK, Robbins MS, Sparber SB: Tolerance and dependence after chronic administration of clonidine to the rat. Pharmacol Biochem Behav 7:227–231, 1977.

Michanek A: Potentiation of d- and l-amphetamine effects on copulatory behavior in female rats by treatment with alpha-adrenoreceptor blocking drugs. Arch Int Pharmacodyn 239:241–256, 1979.

Miksic S, Lal H: Tolerance to morphine-produced discriminative stimuli and analgesia. Psychopharmacol 54:217–221, 1977.

Miksic S, Shearman G, Lal H: Generalization study with some narcotic and non-narcotic drugs in rats trained for morphine–saline discrimination. Psychopharmacol 60:103–104, 1978.

Modigh K: Electroconvulsive shock and postsynaptic catecholamine effects: Increased psychomotor stimulant action of apomorphine and clonidine in reserpine pretreated mice by repeated ECS. J Neural Transm 36:19–32, 1975.

Moore RY, Bloom FE: Central catecholamine neuron systems: Anatomy and physiology of the dopamine systems. Ann Rev Neurosci 1:129–169, 1978.

Morpurgo C: Aggressive behavior induced by large doses of 2-(2,6-dichlorophenylamino)-2-imidazoline hydrochloride (ST 155) in mice. Eur J Pharmacol 3:374–377, 1968.

Overstreet D, Reisire T, U'Prichard D, Yamamura H: Changes in cholinergic activity following chronic treatment with the alpha-noradrenergic receptor agonist clonidine. Pharmacol 21:150, 1979.

Ozawa H, Miyanchi T, Sugawara K: Potentiating effect of lithium chloride on aggressive behavior induced in mice by nialamide plus L-dopa and by clonidine. Eur J Pharmacol 34:169–179, 1975.

Paalzow L: Analgesia produced by clonidine in mice and rats. J Pharm Pharmacol 26:361–363, 1974.

Paalzow G: Development of tolerance to the analgesic effect of clonidine in rats: Cross-tolerance to morphine. Naunyn Schmiederberg Arch Pharmacol 304:1–4, 1979.

Paalzow G, Paalzow L: Clonidine antinociceptive activity: Effects of drugs influencing central monoaminergic and cholinergic mechanisms in the rat. Naunyn Schmiederberg Arch Pharmacol 292:119–126, 1976.

Pijnenburg AJJ, Honig WMM, van Rossum JM: Effects of antagonists upon locomotor stimulation induced by injection of dopamine and noradrenaline into the nucleus accumbens of nialamide-pretreated rats. Psychopharmacologia 41:175–180, 1975.

Pijnenburg A, Honig W, van der Hoyden J, van Rossom J: Effects of chemical stimulation of the mesolimbic dopamine system upon locomotor activity. Eur J Pharmacol 35:45–58, 1976a.

Pijnenburg A, Honig W, Boudier H, Cools A, van der Heyden J, van Rossum J: Further investigations on the effects of ergometrine and other ergot derivatives following injection into the nucleus accumbens of the rat. Arch Int Pharmacodyn Ther 222:103–115, 1976b.

Pijnenburg AJJ, Woodruff GN, van Rossum JM: Ergometrine induced locomotor activity following intracerebral injection into the nucleus accumbens. Brain Res 59:289–302, 1973.

Poignant JC, Rismondo N: Influence of the administration of psychopharmacological compounds on the take-up time of an alimentary material in the hamster and a study of the associated behavior. Psychopharmacol 43:47–52, 1975.

Price TC, Fibiger HC: Ascending catecholamine systems and morphine analgesia. Brain Res 99:189–193, 1975.

Przewlocka B, Stala B, Scheel-Kruger J: Evidence that GABA in the nucleus dorsalis raphe induces stimulation of locomotor activity and eating behavior. Life Sci 25:937–946, 1979.

Putkonen P, Leppavour A, Stenberg D: Paradoxical sleep inhibition by central alpha-adrenoceptor stimulant clonidine antagonized by alpha-receptor blocker yohimbine. Life Sci 21:1059–1065, 1977.

Pycock C, Donaldson IM, Marsden CD: Circling behavior produced by unilateral lesions of the locus coeruleus in rats. Brain Res 97:317–323, 1975.

Pycock CJ, Jenner PG, Marsden CD: The interaction of clonidine with dopamine-dependent behavior in rodents. Naunyn Schmiederberg Arch Pharmacol 297:133–141, 1977.

Razzak A, Fujiwara M, Veki S: Automutilation induced by clonidine in mice. Eur J Pharmacol 30:356–360, 1975.

Razzak A, Fujiwara W, Oishi R, Veki S: Possible involvement of a central noradrenergic system in automutilation induced by clonidine mice. Jpn J Pharmacol 27:145–152, 1977.

Redmond DE Jr: New and old evidence for the involvement of a brain norepinephrine system in anxiety. In Fann WE, Karacan I, Pokorny AD, Williams RL (eds): "Phenomenology and Treatment Anxiety." Jamaica, New York: Spectrum, 1979, pp 153–203.

Redmond DE Jr, Huang YH, Snyder DR, Maas JW: Behavioral effects of stimulation of the nucleus locus coeruleus in the stump-tailed monkey Macaca arctoides. Brain Res 116:502–510, 1976.

Redmond DE, Huang YH, Snyder DR, Maas JW: Hyperphagia and hyperdipsia after locus coeruleus lesions in the stump-tailed monkey. Life Sci 20:1619–1628, 1977.

Redmond DE, Huang YH: New evidence for a locus coeruleus-norepinephrine connection with anxiety. Life Sci 25:2144–2162, 1979.

Redmond DE Jr: Alterations in the function of the nucleus locus coeruleus: A possible model for studies of anxiety. In Hanin I, Usdir E (eds): "Animal Models in Psychiatry and Neurology." Oxford: Pergamon Press, 1977, pp 293–305.

Reid JL, Lewis PJ, Meyers MG: Role of central dopaminergic mechanisms in piribedil and clonidine induced hypothermia in the rat. Neuropharmacol 14:215–220, 1975.

Ritter S, Wise D, Stein L: Neurochemical regulation of feeding in the rat: Facilitation by alpha-noradrenergic but not dopaminergic, receptor stimulants. J Comp Physiol Psychol 88:778–784, 1975.

Robson RD, Antoraccio MJ, Saelers JK, Liebman J: Antagonism by Miarserin and classical 2-adrenoceptor blocking drugs of some cardiovascular and behavioral effects of clonidine. Eur J Pharmacol 47:431–442, 1978.

Rochette L, Bralet J: Effect of the norepinephrine receptor stimulating agent "clonidine" on the turnover of 5-hydroxytryptamine in some areas of rat brain. J Neural Trans 37:259–267, 1975.

Ruiz M, Monti JM: Reversal of the 6-hydroxydopamine-induced suppression of CAR by drugs facilitating central catecholaminergic mechanisms. Pharmacol 13:281–286, 1975.

Ruth-Monachon M, Jaffre M, Haefely W: Drugs and PGO waves in the lateral gericulate body of the curarized cat. III. PGO wave activity and brain catecholamines. Arch Int Pharmacodyn Ther 219:287–307, 1976.

Satoh H, Satoh Y, Notsu Y, Honda F: Adenosine 3',5'-cyclic monophosphate as a possible mediator of rotational behavior induced by dopaminergic receptor stimulation in rats lesioned unilaterally in the substantia nigra. Eur J Pharmacol 39:365–377, 1976.

Scheel-Kruger J, Hasselager E: Studies of various amphetamines, apomorphine and clonidine on body temperature and brain. Psychopharmacologia 36:189–202, 1974.

Schlemmer RF, Casper RC, Narasinhachri N: Clonidine induced hyperphagia and weight gain in monkeys. Psychopharmacol 61:233–234, 1979.

Schmitt H, Le Douarec JC, Petillot N: Antinociceptive effects of some alpha-sympathometic agents. Neuropharmacol 13:289–294, 1974.

Seiden LS, Dykstra LA: Dopamine, norepinephrine and behavior. In Seiden LS, Dykstra LA (eds): "Psychopharmacology: A Biochemical and Behavioral Approach." New York: Van Nostrand Reinhold, 1977, pp 117–171.

Sewell RDE, Spencer PSJ: Antinociceptive activity in mice after central injections of alpha- and beta-adrenoceptor antagonists. Br J Pharmacol 54:256–257, 1975.

Shaw SG, Rolls ET: Is the release of noradrenaline necessary for self-stimulation of the brain? Pharmacol Biochem Behav 4:375–379, 1976.

Shearman G, Hynes M, Fielding S, Lal H: Clonidine self-administration in the rat: A comparison with fentanyl self-administration. Pharmacologist 19:171, 1977.

Skolnick P, Daly J, Segal D: Neurochemical and behavioral effects of clonidine and related imidazolines: Interaction with alpha-adrenoceptors. Eur J Pharmacol 47:451–455, 1978.

Sparber S, Meyer D: Clonidine antagonizes naloxone induced suppression of conditioned behavior and body weight loss in morphine-dependent rats. Pharmacol Biochem Behav 9:319–325, 1978.

Spaulding TC, Fielding S, Venafro JJ, Lal H: Antinociceptive activity of clonidine and its potentiation of morphine analgesia. Eur J Pharmacol 58:19–25, 1979.

Spaulding TC, Venafro J, Ma MG, Cornfeldt M, Fielding S: Interaction of morphine and clonidine in the tail flick test: Potentiation studies. Pharmacologist 20:269, 1978a.

Spaulding TC, Venafro JJ, Ma MG, Fielding S: The dissociation of the antinociceptive effort of clonidine from supraspinal structures. Neuropharmacol 103–105, 1978b.

Spencer J, Revzin A: Amphetamine, chlorpromazine and clonidine effects on self-stimulation in caudate or hypothalamus of the squirrel monkey. Pharmacol Biochem Behav 5:149–156, 1976.

Stern P, Catovic S: Brain glycine and aggressive behavior. Pharmacol Biochem Behav 3:723–726, 1975.

Stricker EM, Zigmond MJ: Recovery of function following damage to central catecholamine-containing neurons: A neurochemical model of the lateral hypothalamic syndrome. In Sprague JM, Epstein AN (eds): "Progress in Psychobiology and Physiological Psychology." New York: Academic Press, 1976.

Strombom U: Effects of low doses of catecholamine receptor agonists on exploration in mice. J Neural Transm 37:229-235, 1975.

Strombom U, Svensson T, Carlsson A: Antagonism of ethanol's central stimulation in mice by small doses of catecholamine–receptor agonists. Psychopharmacol 51:293-299, 1977.

Svensson TH, Persson R, Wallin L, Walinder J: Anxiolytic action of clonidine. Nordisk Psychiatr Tidskr 32:439-441, 1978.

Svensson TH, Strombom U: Discontinuation of chronic clonidine treatment: Evidence for facilitated brain noradrenergic neurotransmission. Naunyn Schmied Arch Pharmacol 299: 83-87, 1977.

Svensson TH, Bunney BS, Aghajanian GK: Inhibition of both noradrenergic and serotonergic neurons in brain by the alpha-adrenergic antagonist clonidine. Brain Res 92:291-306, 1975.

Taboada ME, Souto M, Hawkins H, Monti JM: The actions of dopaminergic and noradrenergic antagonists on conditioned avoidance responses in intact and 6-hydroxydopamine-treated rats. Psychopharmacol 62:83-88, 1979.

Takagi H, Shiomi H, Kursishi Y, Fubui K, Udea H: Pain and the bulbospinal noradrenergic system: Pain-induced increase in normetanephrine content in the spinal cord and its modification by morphine. J Pharmacol 54:99-107, 1979.

Takagi H, Doi T, Akaike A: Microinjection of morphine into the medial part of the bulban reticular formation in rabbit and rat: Inhibition effects on lamina V cells of spinal dorsal horn and behavioral analgesia. In Kosterlitz HW (ed): "Opiates and Endogenous Opioid Peptides." Amsterdam: Elsevier, pp 191-198, 1976.

Thornburg JE, Moore KE: Inhibition of anticholinergic drug-induced locomotor stimulation in mice by d-methyltyrosine. Neuropharmacol 12:1179-1185, 1973.

Tran Quang Loc D, Tsoucaris-Kupfer Y, Bogaievsky D, Delbarre B, Schmitt H: Antagonisme de l'action sedative de la clonidine par quelques α-adrenolytiques: Etude electrocorticographique et comportement ale chez le lapin et le chat. J Pharmacol (Paris) 5:51-55, 1974.

Tilson HA, Chamberlain JH, Gylys JA, Boyniski JP: Behavioral suppressant effects of clonidine in strains of normotensive and hypertensive rats. Eur Pharmacol 43:99-105, 1977.

Tseng LF, Loh HH, Wei ET: Effect of clonidine on morphine withdrawal signs in the rat. Eur Pharmacol 30:93-99, 1975.

Tsoucaris-Kupfer D, Schmitt H: Hypothermic effect of alpha-sympathomimetic agents and their antagonism by adrenergic and cholinergic blocking drugs. Neuropharmacol 11:625-635, 1972.

Ungerstedt U, Butcher LL, Butcher SG, Anden NE, Fuxe K: Direct chemical stimulation of dopaminergic mechanism in the neostriatum of the rat. Brain Res 14:461-468, 1969.

Vetulani J, Bednarczyk B: Depression by clonidine of shaking behavior elicited by nalorphine in morphine-dependent rats. J Pharm Pharmacol 29:567-568, 1977.

Vetulani J, Leith NJ, Stawarz RJ, Sulser F: Effect of clonidine on the noradrenergic cyclic AMP generating system in the limbic forebrain and on medial forebrain self-stimulation behavior. Experientia 33:1490-1491, 1977.

von Voigtlander PF, Triezenberg HJ, Losey EG: Interactions between clonidine and antidepressant drugs. Neuropharmacol 17:375-381, 1978.

Waldeck B: Sensitization by caffeine of central catecholamine receptors. J Neural Transm 34: 61-72, 1973.

Walland A: Clonidine. In Goldberg ME (ed): "Pharmacological and Biochemical Properties of Drug Substances." Washington, DC: Assoc Amer Pharm, 1977, pp 67-107.

Washton AM, Resnick RB, LaPlaca RA: Clonidine hydrochloride: A nonopiate treatment for opiate withdrawal. Abstract ACNP, 1978.

Washton AM, Resnick RB, Rawson RA: Clonidine for outpatient opiate detoxification. Lancet, 1980.

Washton AM, Resnick RB, Rawson RA: Clonidine hydrochloride: A nonopiate treatment for opiate withdrawal. Proceedings of the 41st Annual Scientific Meeting of the Committee on Problems of Drug Dependence, Philadelphia, 1979. NIDA Research Monograph, US Government Printing Office.

Wauquier A: Neuroleptics and brain self-stimulation behavior. Int Rev Neurobiol 21:335–403, 1979.

Wauquier A, Clincke G, Fransen J: Brain reinforcement mechanisms: Alpha-adrenergic and dopaminergic agonists–antagonists. In Lal H, Fielding S (eds): "Psychopharmacology of Clonidine." New York: Alan R. Liss, 1981.

Wei ET: Resemblance of morphine antinociception to the central depressant actions of norepinephrine. Life Sci 17:17–18, 1975.

Wei ET: Chemical stimulants of shaking behavior. J Pharm Pharmacol 28:722–723, 1976.

Wendt F, Caspers I: Koppertemperateur und schweiss-sekretin vei koperlicker belastung unter dem einflurs von 2-(2,6-dichlorophenylamino)-2-imidazolin hydrochlorid. In Heilmeyer L, Holtmeier HJ, Pfeiffer EP (eds): "Hochdruck-Therapie, Symposium uben 2(2,6-dichloro-phenylamino)-2-imidazolin hydrochlorid." Stuttgart: George Thieme, 1968.

Wise CD, Bergen BP, Stein L: Evidence of alpha-noradrenergic reward receptors and serotonergic punishment receptors in the rat brain. Biol Psychiatr 6:3–11, 1973.

Yim GKW, Pfister WR, Yau ET, Mennear JH: Comparison of appetite stimulation by chlordiazepoxide, chlordimeform, clonidine and cyproheptadine in rats. Fed Proc 37:860, 1978.

Zaimis E: The pharmacology of Catapres (ST 155). In Conolly ME (ed): "Catapress in Hypertension." London: Butterworth, 1970, pp 9–22.

Zebrowska-Lupina I, Pregdinski E, Sloniec M, Kleinrok Z: Clonidine-induced locomotor hyperactivity in rats. The role of central postsynaptic alpha-adrenoceptors. Naunyn Schmiedebergs Arch Pharmacol 297:227–231, 1977.

Psychopharmacology of Clonidine, pages 147–163
© 1981 Alan R. Liss, Inc., 150 Fifth Avenue, New York, NY 10011

Clonidine and the Primate Locus Coeruleus: Evidence Suggesting Anxiolytic and Anti-Withdrawal Effects

D. Eugene Redmond, Jr.

I. INTRODUCTION

Studies of the contribution of noradrenergic brain systems to primate behavior were begun at Yale University in 1973 in an attempt to understand the extensive inferential pharmacological and biochemical evidence implicating catecholamine involvement in affective and emotional processes [Schildkraut and Kety, 1967; Friedhoff, 1975]. Previous studies with non-human primates had suggested that quantitative analysis of primate behavior might provide unique data relevant to the understanding of human emotional processes [Redmond et al, 1971, 1973], and histochemical fluorescence studies of the anatomy of noradrenergic brain systems revealed the importance of the nucleus locus coeruleus as a means of studying noradrenergic brain function (see Chapter 1 for a review).

II. EFFECTS OF LOCUS COERULEUS STIMULATION

A reliable method of implanting electrodes or making lesions in this nucleus was developed [Huang et al, 1975], and its effectiveness in decreasing levels of norepinephrine (NE) or its metabolite 3-methoxy-4-hydroxy-phene-thylene glycol (MHPG) in known projection areas of the locus coeruleus (LC) was tested. Histologically confirmed lesions of the LC decreased MHPG concentrations in lesioned monkeys as compared with normal control animals, whereas low-intensity electrical stimulation increased concentrations of MHPG ipsilateral to the stimulating electrodes as compared either with the contralateral side or with normal control monkeys.

The behavioral effects of stimulation were most extensively evaluated because activation of short duration could be studied over periods of several months and compared with the animal's own baseline and control periods between stimulations. Behavioral effects on chair-conditioned and restrained animals were quantitated by videotape recording and computer-generated timing and marking signals, which allowed subsequent categorization of the behavioral effects for computer analysis by raters blinded to the specific experimental conditions. Carefully defined patterns of movement were used as behavioral categories, which were then analyzed by their temporal sequences following stimulation (for specific definitions and more details on the methods used see Redmond and Huang [1979]). Preliminary experiments revealed consistent increases after low-intensity electrical stimulation (bipolar, biphasic square waves of 0.3–0.6 mA intensity, 0.5 msec pulse widths, at 50 Hz) in a particular behavioral pattern that included yawning, chewing, scratching, startling, wringing of hands, pulling of hair or skin, tongue movement, grasping of chair, struggling, self-mouthing, and self-clasping [Redmond et al, 1976b]. There were also a number of physiological effects, such as pupillary dilatation, piloerection, alerting, and increases in blood pressure and heart rate. These original findings have now been replicated in 15 monkeys, and the interactions between LC stimulation and various noradrenergic agonists and antagonists have been characterized [Redmond and Huang, 1979].

III. CLONIDINE BLOCKS EFFECTS OF LOCUS COERULEUS STIMULATION

We were interested, first of all, in determining whether stimulation effects are produced by activation of the LC or its projections rather than of adjacent non-noradrenergic pathways. It was in this context that the effects of clonidine on locus coeruleus-associated behavior in the primate were first studied. Clonidine had been shown to reduce NE turnover [Starke and Altman, 1973; Starke and Montel, 1973] in rats and, specifically, to reduce the firing rate of LC neurons when applied iontophoretically or systemically in low doses [Svensson et al, 1975; Cedarbaum and Aghajanian, 1976, 1977]. In the same studies, low doses of piperoxan, an α-adrenergic antagonist, had effects opposed to those of clonidine. Piperoxan, therefore, increased LC activity and MHPG outflow from the brain, presumably by antagonizing the action of endogenous NE or epinephrine (E) at regulatory α-2-adrenergic autoreceptors [Cedarbaum and Aghajanian, 1977; Aghajanian et al, 1977] (for more details, see Chapter 1). We postulated that behavioral effects of stimulation that were related to LC function should be increased or decreased in keeping with the demonstrated effects on LC neurons in the rat and on MHPG outflow from cerebral circulation in M. arctoides [Maas et al, 1976].

Clonidine, 10 μg/kg, administered intravenously to chair-restrained monkeys from outside a sealed experimental chamber, reduced the behavioral effects of LC stimulation (Fig. 1), whereas piperoxan produced effects identical to those provoked by electrical stimulation. Clonidine also blocked the effects of piperoxan, as predicted. We further postulated that the effects of stimulation, or of other stimuli that increase LC activity, should be blocked by postsynaptic α- or β-adrenergic receptor antagonists since neuronal blockade had been demonstrated in the characterization of LC projections to several areas (for a review, see Chapter 1). This hypothesis was confirmed by reduction of the behavioral effects of stimulation by the beta-adrenergic antagonist propranolol [Huang et al, 1977; Redmond, 1977]. However, the specific effects of the α blocker phenoxybenzamine, in doses reported to produce α-1-adrenergic blockade, could not be evaluated because of hypotension, extreme sedation, or loss of consciousness following its administration.

IV. OPIOIDS BLOCK EFFECTS OF LOCUS COERULEUS STIMULATION

Morphine has also been found to reduce LC neuronal activity in rats [Korf et al, 1974]. The demonstration of specific opiate receptor binding on the cell bodies of the LC [Pert et al, 1975] and the existence of endogenous opioid neurotransmitters [Hughes, 1975; Pasternak et al, 1975] made it clear that endorphinergic and α-2-adrenergic receptors may interact in a variety of conditions. In the studies that followed, morphine was found to block the effects of LC stimulation or piperoxan administration and vice versa [Redmond, 1977]. In addition, the synthetic pentapeptide FK 33-824 produced naloxone-reversible effects similar to those of morphine [Redmond et al, 1978], consistent with effects predictable from single-neuron studies of the LC [Bird and Kuhar, 1977]. These biochemical studies, along with the experimental elucidation of other stimuli producing effects similar to those of LC stimulation,

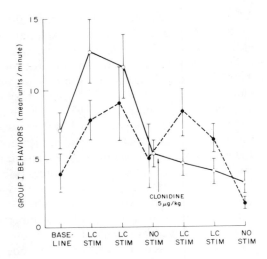

Fig. 1. The effect of clonidine on behavior associated with increased LC activity (Group I behavior, as detailed in Redmond and Huang [1979]) is compared in one male and two female adult stump-tailed macaque monkeys. Data were recorded on two experimental days under the following conditions: "Baseline" was recorded for 5 minutes prior to "LC stim," a very low-intensity electrical stimulation of a unilateral LC electrode (0.6–1.5 mA intensity, 0.5 msec pulse duration, 50 Hz) for 10 seconds each minute under computer program control. A second 5-minute period of identical "LC stim" was followed by a 5-minute "no stim" poststimulation period. The entire stimulation was then repeated, with clonidine (5 mcg/kg IV) administered on the "clonidine day." Significant differences were determined by a correlated t-test. Clonidine appeared to prevent the increases induced by LC stimulation alone.

pointed to the importance of NE-endorphin receptor interactions in regulating whatever processes underlie the behavioral and physiological effects seen in monkeys. Some data that may serve as a basis for speculation about the nature of these processes are on hand.

V. A BRAIN "ALARM SYSTEM" ACTIVATED BY FEAR-PROVOKING STIMULI AND BY OPIATE WITHDRAWAL

Initially, it was noted that the exact sequence of behavioral effects of LC stimulation was reproduced by threats of attack from humans [Redmond et al, 1976b], and that several of the principal types of behavior also occurred in natural situations of impending conflict, aggression, or uncertainty [Bertrand, 1969], and during withdrawal from morphine in the monkey [Seevers,

1936] and man [Himmelsbach, 1939]. These associations were specifically tested by comparison of the effects of fear, anxiety, and the naloxone-precipitated opiate abstinence syndrome. Four raters blinded to the experimental conditions could not distinguish the fear or anxiety induced by reintroduction into a situation in which noxious stimuli had been experienced previously from the effects of LC stimulation or piperoxan administration [Redmond et al, 1979]. These effects were also similar to those produced by a stimulus previously paired with a noxious electrical shock [Redmond and Huang, 1979]. (See Table I.) LC lesions appeared to have the effect of counteracting activities intensified by LC stimulation and associated with fear-provoking stimuli in the previous studies [Huang et al, 1976; Redmond et al, 1976a; Redmond, 1979b]. There were also some similarities in old-world monkeys between the effects of LC lesions and effects of treatment with opioids, specifically methadone, although there were significant differences as well [Crowley et al, 1975].

Evidence of the effects of several drugs tested in monkeys supported the interpretation that the LC is related to human fear. Piperoxan and yohimbine cause anxiety or fear in humans [Goldenberg et al, 1947; Soffer, 1954; Holmberg and Gershon, 1961], whereas morphine [Mirin et al, 1976] and propranolol [Kielholz, 1977] reduce anxiety or fear in humans. In addition, the most widely used anxiolytic drug, diazepam, was found to reduce the behavioral effects of LC stimulation in monkeys [Redmond, 1977]. (See Redmond [1979a] for a review of the human data indicating involvement of NE in alarm or fear).

Natural anxiety or fear and the morphine withdrawal syndrome were studied to test further the hypothesis of common neuronal mechanisms underlying these conditions in monkeys. Striking similarities were seen between the behavioral effects of stimuli of varying intensity that are expected to induce fear and those caused by increasing doses of naloxone in morphine-tolerant monkeys (Fig. 2). Both types of effect were similar to the effects of central NE activation (Redmond, unpublished data). A review of these and other physiological and pharmacological findings provided strong support for the hypothesis that there are similarities between opiate withdrawal, anxiety, or fear, and the results of central NE activation (see Table II).

Two predictions from these studies appear to have clinical implications and have provided the impetus for further work regarding the neuronal substrates for anxiety and opiate withdrawal syndromes. Clonidine should have both anxiolytic and antiwithdrawal effects in humans, in view of the primate and human data described above. Reports by Tseng et al [1975], Gianutsos et al [1976], and Paalzow [1974] suggested that α-1 agonist doses of clonidine worsened some measured withdrawal symptoms in the rat, whereas other groups of investigators found NE hyperactivity to be involved both in cloni-

TABLE I. Effects of Activation of NE Systems by LC Stimulation, by Blockade of Autoregulatory α Receptors With Piperoxan, or With Stimuli Previously Paired With Mildly Painful Electrical Shock or With LC Stimulation

Minutes	Baseline N3		Piperoxan N4		LC stim N3		Constant LC stim N3		Signal of LC stim N3		Signal of shock N3	
	Mean	SEM	Mean	SEM	Mean	SEM	Mean	SEM	Mean	SEM	Mean	SEM
0–5	0.7	0.3	9.4	1.7	31.8	7.1	91.8	11.6	22.2	4.0	42.5	7.4
5–10	5.1	1.4	17.2	2.2	30.9	9.7	60.9	8.7	22.6	3.7		
10–15	3.7	1.2	10.1	2.1	32.7	7.1	38.4	6.3	20.2	3.5		

Baseline: After 1 month of chair training without any experimentation or drug administration. Piperoxan: 1 mg/kg IV administered from outside a closed experimental chamber. LC stim: Four 1-second trains/minute of low-intensity biphasic, bipolar stimulation at 0.2–0.6 mA, 1 msec, and 50 Hz frequency, to unilateral LC electrode. Constant LC stim: Continuous stimulation of unilateral LC electrode at above parameters, but frequency from 30 to 50 Hz. Signal of LC stim: A signal previously paired with the LC stim condition, but with no current flow. Signal of shock: A signal that a mild electrical shock program was operating, but never actually presented with the shock during the session observed.

dine withdrawal and in "antiwithdrawal" effects of clonidine [Montel et al, 1975; Meyer and Sparber, 1976; Vetulani and Bednarczyk, 1977; Llorens et al, 1978; Lipman and Spencer, 1978; Fielding et al, 1978]. These findings might eventually have led to clinical studies of clonidine treatment for opiate withdrawal. However, we proceeded directly from the monkey locus coeruleus experiments to human clinical studies, testing the opiate withdrawal hypothesis. These studies have progressed much faster than those testing the anxiety hypothesis, and many additional study reports have now been published. Inasmuch as the antiwithdrawal actions of clonidine in animals will be reviewed by Lal et al [1981], and our original clinical studies of the effects of clonidine on methadone withdrawal [Gold et al, 1978a, b] and other clinical studies conducted thereafter are being reviewed by Gold et al [1981] and Washton and Resnick [1981], the remainder of this chapter will focus on the possible anxiolytic effects of clonidine.

VI. DOES CLONIDINE HAVE ANXIOLYTIC EFFECTS?

Following the primate studies reviewed above, which suggested anxiolytic properties of clonidine [Redmond, 1977], there have been two other animal studies which point in the same direction. Davis et al [1977, 1979] and Davis and Astrachan [1978] have shown that increased acoustic startle amplitudes in the presence of a cue that had been previously paired with an electrical shock ("potentiated startle") are a sensitive measure of classically conditioned fear that is selectively decreased by sodium amytal, diazepam, and

TABLE II. Common Symptoms, Signs, or Physiological Correlates of Opiate Abstinence and Fear or Anxiety. References Indicate Sources for the Inclusion of the Item, and its Alteration by Locus Coeruleus Stimulation or Lesions or by Pharmacologic Agents that Act on 2-Noradrenergic Receptors.

Symptom, sign or physiological change	Fear or anxiety reference	Opiate abstinence reference	LC stim or *lesion	Piperoxan or yohimbine	Clonidine
Subjective fear or anxiety	5, 18, 45	3, 9, 11, 17, 44	23	12, 42	8, 10, 25, 43
Restlessness	5, 22	3, 11, 17, 40	30, 33	12	8
Irritability	22	11, 17, 40, 44		12	8
Yawning	2, 5, 34	3, 11, 17, 34, 40	29, 30, 32	29, 32	14, 33
Chewing, grinding of teeth	5	34	30, 32	29, 32	29, 32
Effects on sleep increased waking	22	3, 11, 17	21, 30	7, 29, 32	8, 13, 16
Increased temperature	5	3, 11, 17	33	12	37
Mydriasis	5, 15	3, 11, 17	30	12, 19	8
Tachycardia	4, 5, 45	3, 11, 17	28, 33, 41, 46	12, 19, 29, 39, 42	8, 10, 13, 25
Hypertension	4, 5	3, 11, 17	28, 33, 46	12, 39, 42	8, 10, 13, 25
Tachypnea	5, 45	3, 11, 17	33	12, 29, 42	8
Piloerection (goose flesh)	5	3, 11, 17		19, 29	8
Cold sweats (perspiration)	5, 45	3, 11, 17		12, 29	8
Desynchronization of EEG	18, 48	48	21*	7	16
Increased ACTH or 17-OHCS	4	6	47		
Tremor	5, 18, 22, 45	1, 3, 11, 17, 40		12, 33	8
Gastrointestinal motility	5, 18, 22	3, 11, 17, 40	33	12, 19	10, 13, 25
Nausea, vomiting	5, 22	1, 3, 11, 17, 40		12, 19	10, 25
Spontaneous ejaculation	49	3, 11, 17			26
Priapism				12, 26	26
Lacrimation		3, 11, 17, 40		12	26
Rhinorrhea		3, 11, 17, 40			26
Restless sleep (?REM rebound)	22	3, 11, 17	33		16
Anorexia (decreased eating)	5, 22	3, 11, 17, 40	20, 31		26, 38
Pain threshold — aches and pains	22, 36	3, 11, 17	35*		24
Wavelike paroxysm of symptoms reported or observed	5	11, 27	33	33	

[1]Aceto et al, 1977; [2]Bertrand, 1969; [3]Blackly, 1966; [4]Bridges et al, 1968; [5]Darwin, 1872; [6]Eisenman et al, 1969; [7]Fuxe et al, 1974; [8]Gold et al, 1978; [9]Goldstein 1972; [10]Hansson et al, 1973; [11]Himmelsbach, 1941; [12]Holmberg and Gershon, 1961; [13]Hoobler and Sagstume, 1971; [14]Huang et al, 1977; [15]Janisse, 1976; [16]Kleinlogel et al, 1975; [17]Kolb and Himmelsbach, 1938; [18]Lader, 1973; [19]Lang and Gershon, 1963; [20]Leverenz et al, 1978; [21]Lidbrink, 1974; [22]Lief, 1967; [23]Nashold et al, 1974; [24]Paalzow, 1974; [25]Pettinger, 1975; [26]Physicians Desk Reference, 1975; [27]Pradbam and Dutta, 1977; [28]Przuntek and Philipu, 1973; [29]Redmond 1977; [30]Redmond et al, 1976; [31]Redmond et al, 1977; [32]Redmond et al, 1978; [33]Redmond et al, unpublished data; [34]Redmond, this paper; [35]Samanin et al, 1975; [36]Schalling, 1976; [37]Scheel-Kruger and Hasselager, 1974; [38]Schlemmer et al, 1979; [39]Schmitt et al, 1973; [40]Seevers, 1936; [41]Snyder et al, 1977; [42]Soffer, 1954; [43]Svensson, personal communication; [44]Tatum et al, 1929; [45]Tyrer and Lader, 1974; [46]Ward and Gunn, 1976; [47]Ward et al, 1976; [48]Wikler, 1954; [49]Feldman, 1951.

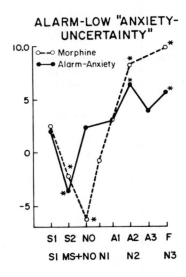

Fig. 2. Two groups of 3 C. aethiops monkeys are compared during morphine and naloxone treatment in one group, with alarm or fear stimuli in the other group, using a behavioral factor derived from 1,587 observation sessions of 23 monkeys. The specific conditions in the morphine group were 72 5-minute sessions of saline injections (S1) or 72 sessions of morphine sulfate (MS) 2 hours before observation, 9 sessions of saline injection 5 minutes before observation to control for the effects of naloxone injection with MS 2 hours beforehand (MS + N0), and 9 sessions each of three doses of naloxone, 0.00057 mg/kg (N1), 0.0057 mg/kg (N2), and 0.13 mg/kg (N3) 5 minutes before observation. In the alarm-anxiety group there were two groups of 72 5-minute sessions of saline injection 2 hours before observation (S1 and S2) and 9 sessions of saline injection matching the naloxone administration (N0). Nine sessions each of four conditions predicted to produce increasing alarm (A1-A3) or fear (F) were recorded using unfamiliar human observers (A1-A3) or a feral dog (F) as alarm or fear stimuli. These were plotted at arbitrary points against comparable intensities of abstinence based on pilot data. The asterisks represent significant deviations from the expected value under the Ho hypothesis using the Wilcoxon procedure.

morphine [Chi, 1965; Davis et al, 1977, 1979; Davis and Astrachan, 1978]. In this model, piperoxan and yohimbine, which are associated with increased anxiety in humans, enhanced the magnitude of the potentiated startle effect. Clonidine had the opposite effect of decreasing potentiated startle, consistent with the action of other known human anxiolytic agents. Neither of these effects was explained by general decreases in baseline startle amplitudes or in the rates of extinction during testing [Davis et al, 1979], but the clonidine effect was blocked by piperoxan [Davis et al, 1977], suggesting the involvement of α-2 receptors in these effects on startle. The significant decrease in potentiated startle due to the β antagonist propranolol is consistent with the involvement of postsynaptic β receptors also because β antagonists have no effect on α-2 receptors at these doses [Cedarbaum and Aghajanian, 1976].

Another widely used animal screening test for anxiolytic activity is the "conflict-induced suppression" paradigm [Geller and Seifter, 1960], which accurately identifies many anxiolytic compounds [Cook and Davidson, 1973, 1978; Cook and Sepinwall, 1975]. In this procedure, clonidine increased lever pressing for a sweetened condensed milk reward during a period when each lever pressing was punished by an electrical floor shock [Bullock et al, 1978]. This effect occurred at IP doses of 12.5, 25, and 50 μg/kg without significant reductions in the responses during no-punishment periods, which usually indicate sedation, motor impairment, and other effects irrelevant to anxiety [Kruse et al, 1980]. Doses of 100 and 200 μg/kg had the non-anxiety-specific effect of reducing the response rate during the no-punishment period. The effect of clonidine in this procedure was blocked by 5 mg/kg yohimbine and reduced by 2.5 mg/kg phenoxybenzamine, suggesting an adrenergic receptor-mediated mode of action; no effects mediated by the cholinergic, serotonergic, or endorphinergic systems were demonstrable. These dose effects of yohimbine and phenoxybenzamine also suggest the involvement of α-2 receptors, but further studies are required to delineate the involvement of α-1 and β receptors in the effect of clonidine on the conflict suppression test. The effects of clonidine revealed by this study are similar to those of diazepam and other human anxiolytic agents [Cook and Davidson, 1973, 1978; Geller and Seifter, 1960].

In the light of human studies, Svensson suggested that the psychological symptoms that occur upon discontinuation of chronic clonidine treatment, including anxiety [Hansson et al, 1973; Hunyor et al, 1973; Stokes, 1976], may be due to facilitated NE neurotransmission [Svensson and Strombom, 1977]. This observation is noteworthy especially in the absence of any convincing report of anxiolytic clonidine effects in hypertensive patients, who report "sedation" instead [Kellett and Hamilton, 1970; Onesti et al, 1971; Seedat et al, 1971; Amery et al, 1972; Hoobler and Sagastume, 1971; Putzeys and Hoobler, 1972; Simpson, 1973; Pettinger, 1975; Kellaway, 1976]. This is consistent with the finding in normal human subjects studied experimentally [Leckman et al, 1980] that the effect of clonidine (1, 2, 5, μg/kg) is experienced as sedative rather than "anxiolytic," similarly to the effects of other drugs, both anxiolytic and nonanxiolytic, in normal subjects in whom anxiety is not a target symptom. However, Svensson et al reported that in six out of fourteen patients with severe anxiety, daily clonidine doses of 150-225 mcg led to a significant reduction of anxiety during an open 2-week trial. Six of the eight who did not improve had concurrent depressive symptoms [Svensson et al, 1978]. The authors concluded that clonidine was effective in the subgroup without depression.

The suppression of anxiety by clonidine in the opiate withdrawal syndrome may reflect a general anxiolytic effect of clonidine. Anxiety is often reported during opiate withdrawal and can progress to an extreme fear of dying. It has been suggested that this emotion may contribute to antisocial and even violent behavior, which is engaged in to obtain relief from the withdrawal state and to sustain the addiction. In the mind of the sufferer, this fear may also magnify the seriousness and intensity of the withdrawal syndrome beyond its true medical severity.

Clonidine reduces or eliminates this fear as well as self-rated nervousness and anxiety (Fig. 3). By itself, this effect might be expected to be a result of the overall amelioration of the withdrawal syndrome. Combined with the evidence reviewed above, however, it is another indication of a common neural basis for manifestations of fear and opiate withdrawal [Redmond et al, 1978]. One might also expect clonidine to alleviate other withdrawal syndromes prominently involving "anxiety" and anxiety-related physiological changes, such as withdrawal from tobacco, alcohol, barbiturates, and benzodiazepines — all of which affect NE systems in some way [Redmond and Huang, 1979]. However, if the action of clonidine on NE systems is responsible for its anxiolytic effect, the suppression of these other withdrawal syndromes would be less complete than suppression of opiate withdrawal symptoms, because the relation between these syndromes and NE activation is not as close. Moreover, alcohol, barbiturate, and benzodiazepine withdrawal syndromes are all likely to involve GABA-mediated effects that clonidine would not be expected to suppress. The results of one study, however, suggest that clonidine can indeed reduce the anxiety, tremor, hypertension, and sweating associated with alcohol withdrawal [Bjorkvist, 1975].

VII. OTHER POSSIBLE MEDICAL BENEFITS OF ANXIETY REDUCTION BY CLONIDINE

In addition to drug withdrawal syndromes and anxiety by itself, there are other psychiatric and medical conditions in which anxiety may contribute to dysfunction and morbidity and in which clonidine may have ameliorative effects. A therapeutically useful effect of clonidine on patients with Gilles de la Tourette's syndrome has been reported by some [Cohen et al, 1979] but not all investigators (Shapiro, personal communication). The improvement in this syndrome may be due either to the drug's interactions with the primary pathophysiologic features of the syndrome or to the relief of secondary anxiety, which exacerbates the symptoms and further limits social and motor function.

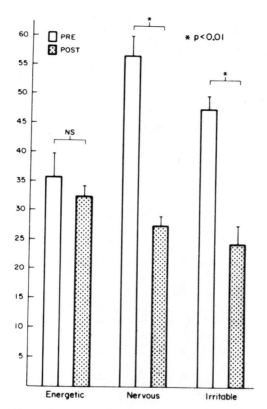

Fig. 3. Self-rated analog scales for "energetic," "nervous," and "irritable" in 11 patients during methadone withdrawal before and after clonidine. Maximum score 70. Means and SEM shown (from Gold et al, [1978]).

The usefulness of clonidine in the treatment of migraine headaches, too, may in part be a corollary of its action in reducing or preventing anxiety [Shafar et al, 1972; Anthony et al, 1972; Heathfield and Raiman, 1972; Brogden et al, 1975]. Beneficial effects in the phobic anxiety syndrome might also be predicted on the basis of a possible noradrenergic involvement in fear or anxiety. The commonly used benzodiazepine anxiolytics are relatively ineffective in this condition, whereas the more effective tricyclic antidepressants and monoamine oxidase inhibitors produce net effects on LC activity similar to those of clonidine [see Grant and Redmond, 1981]. Controlled, double-blind crossover studies of clonidine vs tricyclic antidepressants or benzodiazepines are needed to test this presumed noradrenergic involvement in phobic anxiety, and to assess the therapeutic usefulness of clonidine. Other conditions in which clonidine might prove beneficial include gastrointestinal conditions exacerbated by anxiety or stress, such as duodenal ulcer, ulcerative colitis, and the irritable colon syndrome [Engel, 1967; Rosenbaum, 1967], although other agents blocking NE effects such as β blockers may have more prolonged effects. The effect of clonidine on stress and anxiety in hypertensive patients should be evaluated as a possible beneficial side effect of its use for reduction of blood pressure. In view of the known contribution of stress to the pathophysiology of arteriosclerotic cardiovascular disease, an antihypertensive agent that relieves anxiety and stress may be doubly useful.

VIII. SUMMARY

One may conclude from this series of studies and the data of others reviewed at this symposium that NE systems are involved in fear or anxiety and in mediating the actions of opioids and endorphins. It is rational pharmacotherapy, therefore, to utilize anatomically and neurophysiologically characterized receptors to produce those desired specific effects on NE systems that are expected to reduce anxiety. These same receptor interactions could also be used to antagonize side effects or to reverse withdrawal syndromes via alternative receptor sites. This strategy of using different receptors to produce synergistic or antagonistic effects on a common neuronal pathway has benefited the treatment of pathological anxiety, pain, drug withdrawal symptoms, and other classical psychosomatic conditions. It should be emphasized, of course, that the LC-noradrenergic system has a much broader function than the mediation of fear or anxiety, and that the endorphins, opiates, and clonidine influence many other systems, as do their abstinence syndromes. Anatomical projections of the LC and similar central NE systems also produce the observed effects. Detailed studies are needed to discover precisely how the abnormalities observed in numerous biochemical systems [Eidelberg, 1976] are related to the alterations in NE function we have studied and discussed in this chapter. Finally, careful clinical studies are needed to determine, define, and delimit the potential therapeutic uses of clonidine in the areas suggested by the preliminary studies reviewed here.

IX. ACKNOWLEDGMENTS

Work reported in this chapter was supported by grants from the USPHS MH 31176, MH 25642, and DA 02321; by Yale University; by the State of Connecticut; and by the Harry Frank Guggenheim Foundation. The collaboration of Y.H. Huang, J.W. Maas, R.H. Roth, M. Davis, J.M. Baraban, D.R. Snyder, S.J. Grant, J. Baulu, M.S. Gold, H.D. Kleber, J.M. Stogin Jr., and D.J. Leahy are gratefully acknowledged. J.D. Elsworth, G.K. Aghajanian, and G.R. Heninger provided valuable advice and criticism, and Laura Fawcett provided editorial assistance.

X. REFERENCES

Aceto MD, Flora RE, Harris LS: The effects of naloxone and nalorphine during the development of morphine dependence in rhesus monkeys. Pharmacology 15:1–9, 1977.

Aghajanian GK, Cedarbaum JM, Wang RY: Evidence for norepinephrine-mediated collateral inhibition of locus coeruleus neurons. Brain Res 136:570–577, 1977.

Amery AK, Bossaert H, Fagard RH, Verstraete M: Clonidine versus methyldopa. Acta Cardiol (Brux) 27(1):82–99, 1972.

Anthony M, Lance JW, Somerville B: A comparative trial of prindolol, clonidine and carbamazepine in the interval therapy of migraine. Med J Aust 1(26):1343–1346, 1972.

Bertrand M: "The Behavioral Repertoire of the Stump Tail Macaque." New York: S. Karger, 1969, pp 95; 98–99; 175.

Bird SJ, Kuhar MJ: Iontophoretic applications of opiates to the locus coeruleus. Brain Res 122:523–533, 1977.

Bjorkqvist SE: Clonidine in alcohol withdrawal. Acta Psychiat Scand 52:256–263, 1975.

Blackly PH: Management of the opiate abstinence syndrome. Am J Psychiatry 122:743, 1966.

Bridges PK, Jones MT, Leak D: A comparative study of four physiological concomitants of anxiety. Arch Gen Psychiatry 19(2):141–145, 1968.

Brogden RN, Pinder RM, Sawyer PR, Speight TM, Avery GS: Low-dose clonidine: A review of its therapeutic efficacy in migraine prophylaxis. Drugs 10(5-6):357–365, 1975.

Bullock SA, Kruse H, Fielding S: The effect of clonidine on conflict behavior in rats: Is clonidine an anxiolytic agent? Pharmacologist 20:223, 1978.

Cedarbaum JM, Aghajanian GK: Catecholamine receptors on locus coeruleus neurons: Pharmacological characterization. Eur J Pharmacol 44:375–385, 1977.

Cedarbaum JM, Aghajanian GK: Noradrenergic neurons of the locus coeruleus: Inhibition by epinephrine and activation by the alpha-antagonist piperoxane. Brain Res 112:413–419, 1976.

Chi CC: The effect of amobarbital sodium on conditioned fear as measured by the potentiated startle response in rats. Psychopharmacologia 7:115–122, 1965.

Cohen DJ, Young JG, Nathanson JA, Shaywitz BA: Clonidine in Tourette's syndrome. Lancet 2:551–553, 1979.

Cook L, Davidson AB: Effects of behaviorally active drugs in a conflict-punishment procedure in rats. In Garattini S, Mussini E, Randall LO (eds): "The Benzodiazepines." New York: Raven Press, 1973, pp 327–345.

Cook L, Davidson AB: Behavioral pharmacology: Animal models involving aversive control of behavior. In Lipton MA, DiMascio A, Killam KF (eds): "Psychopharmacology: A Generation of Progress." New York: Raven Press, 1978, pp 563–567.

Cook L, Sepinwall J: Behavioral analysis of the effects and mechanisms of action of benzodiazepines. In Costa E, Greengard P (eds): "Mechanism of Action of Benzodiazepines." New York: Raven Press, 1975, pp 1–28.

Crowley TJ, Hydinger M, Stynes AJ, Feiger A: Monkey motor stimulation and altered social behaviour during chronic methadone administration. Psychopharmacologia (Berl) 43:135–144, 1975.

Darwin C: "The Expression of Emotions in Man and Animals." New York: Philosophical Library, 1872 (Reprint, 1955), p 134.

Davis M, Cedarbaum JM, Aghajanian GK, Gendelman DS: Effects of clonidine on habituation and sensitization of acoustic startle in normal, decerebrate, and locus coeruleus lesioned rats. Psychopharmacol 51:243–253, 1977.

Davis M, Astrachan DI: Conditioned fear and startle magnitude: Effects of different footshock or backshock intensities used in training. J. Exp Psychol 4:95–103, 1978.

Davis M, Redmond DE Jr, Baraban JM: Noradrenergic agonists and antagonists: Effects on conditioned fear as measured by the potentiated startle paradigm. Psychopharmacologia 65:111–118, 1979.

Eidelberg E: Possible actions of opiates upon synapses. Prog Neurobiol 6:81–102, 1976.

Eisenman AJ, Sloan JW, Martin WR: Catecholamine and 17 hydroxycort. Excretion during a cycle of morphine dependence in man. J Psychiatr Res 7:19–28, 1969.

Engel GL: Intestinal disorders. In Freedman AM, Kaplan HI (eds): "Comprehensive Textbook of Psychiatry." Baltimore: Williams and Wilkins, 1967, pp 1054–1059.

Feldman SS: Anxiety and orgasm. Psychoanal Q 20:528–549, 1951.

Fielding S, Wilker J, Hynes M, Szewczak M, Novick WJ Jr, Lal H: A comparison of clonidine with morphine for antinociceptive and antiwithdrawal actions. J Pharmacol Exp Ther 207:899:–905, 1978.

Friedhoff AJ (ed): "Catecholamines and Behavior." New York and London: Plenum Press, 1975, Vol 2.

Fuxe K, Lidbrink P, Hokfelt T, Bolme P, Goldstein M: Effects of piperoxane on sleep and waking in the rat. Evidence for increased waking by blocking inhibitory adrenaline receptors on the locus coeruleus. Acta Physiol Scand 91:566–567, 1974.

Geller I, Seifter J: The effects of meprobate, barbiturates, d-amphetamine and promazine on experimentally induced conflict in the rat. Psychopharmacologia 1:482–492, 1960.

Gianutsos G, Hynes MD, Lal H: Enhancement of morphine-withdrawal and apomorphine-induced aggression by clonidine. Psychopharmacol Commun 2(2):165–171, 1976.

Gold MS, Kleber HD: Clinical utility of clonidine in opiate withdrawal: The locus coeruleus connection. In Lal H, Fielding S (eds): "Psychopharmacology of Clonidine." New York: Alan R. Liss, Inc., 1981.

Gold MS, Redmond DE Jr, Kleber HD: Clonidine in opiate withdrawal. Lancet 1(8070):929–930, 1978a.

Gold MS, Redmond DE Jr, Kleber HD: Clonidine blocks acute opiate-withdrawal symptoms. Lancet 2(8090):599–602, 1978b.

Goldenberg M, Snyder CH, Aranow H Jr: New test for hypertension due to circulating epinephrine. JAMA 135:971–976, 1947.

Goldstein A: Heroin addiction and the role of methadone in its treatment. Arch Gen Psychiatry 26:291–297, 1972.

Grant SJ, Redmond DE Jr: The neuroanatomy and pharmacology of the nucleus locus coeruleus. In Lal H, Fielding S (eds): "Psychopharmacology of Clonidine." New York: Alan R. Liss, Inc., 1981, pp 5–27.

Hansson L, Hunyor SN, Julius S, Hoobler SW: Blood pressure crises following withdrawal of clonidine (Catapres, Catapresan), with special reference to arterial and urinary catecholamine levels, and suggestions for acute management. Am Heart J 85(5)605–610, 1973.

Healthfield KW, Raiman JD: The long-term management of migraine with clonidine. Practitioner 208(247):644–648, 1972.

Himmelsbach CK: The morphine abstinence syndrome, its nature and treatment. Am Int Med 15:829, 1941.

Himmelsbach CK: Studies of certain addiction characteristics of (a) dihydromorphine, (b) dihydrodesoxymorphine-d, (c) dihydrodesoxycodeine-d, (d) methyldihydromorphinone. J Pharmacol Exp Ther 67:239–242, 1939.

Holmberg G, Gershon S: Autonomic and psychic effects of yohimbine hydrochloride. Psychopharmacologia 2:93–106, 1961.

Hoobler SW, Sagastume E: Clonidine hydrochloride in the treatment of hypertension. Am J Cardiol 28(1):67–73, 1971.

Huang YH, Maas JW, Redmond DE Jr: Evidence for noradrenergic specificity of behavioral effects of electrical stimulation of the nucleus locus coeruleus. Neurosci Abstr 3:251, 1977.

Huang YH, Redmond DE Jr, Snyder DR, Maas JW: Loss of fear following bilateral lesions of the locus coeruleus in the monkey. Neurosci Abstr 2:573, 1976.

Huang YH, Redmond DE Jr, Snyder DR, Maas JW: In vivo location and destruction of the locus coeruleus in the stumptail macaque (Macaca arctoides). Brain Res 100:157–162, 1975.

Huff BB (ed): "Physicians' Desk Reference." Oradell, NJ: Medical Economics Co., 1975, pp 622, 1014.

Hughes J: Isolation of an endogenous compound from the brain with pharmacological properties similar to morphine. Brain Res 88:295–308, 1975.

Hunyor SN, Hansson L, Harrison TS, Hoobler SW: Effects of clonidine withdrawal: Possible mechanisms and suggestions for management. Br Med J 2(860):209–211, 1973.

Janisse MP: The relationship between pupil size and anxiety. A review. In Sarasan IG, Spielberger CD (eds): "Stress and Anxiety," Vol 3. New York: Wiley and Sons, 1976, pp 27–48.

Kellaway GS: Adverse drug reactions during treatment of hypertension. Drugs 11 (Suppl 1):91–99, 1976.

Kellett RJ, Hamilton M: The treatment of benign hypertension with clonidine. Scottish Med J 15:137–142, 1970.

Kielholz P (ed): "Beta-Blockers and the Central Nervous System." Baltimore, London, Tokyo: University Park Press, 1977.

Kleinlogel H, Scholtysik G, Sayers AC: Effects of clonidine and BS 100-141 on the EEG sleep pattern in rats. Eur J Pharmacol 33:159–163, 1975.

Kolb L, Himmelsbach CK: Clinical studies of drug addiction. III. A critical review of the withdrawal treatments with method of evaluating abstinence syndromes. Am J Psychiatry 94:759, 1938.

Korf J, Bunney BS, Aghajanian GK: Noradrenergic neurons: Morphine inhibition of spontaneous activity. Eur J Pharmacol 25:165–169, 1974.

Kruse H, Theurer KL, Dunn RW, Novick WJ Jr, Shearman GT: Attenuation of conflict-induced suppression by clonidine: Indication of anxiolytic activity. Drug Development Research 1:137–143, 1981.

Lader MH: Psychophysiological aspects of anxiety. In Lader MH (ed): "Studies of Anxiety." Ashford, Kent, England: World Psychiatric Association and Headley Brothers, 1973, Ch 8.

Lal H, Shearman GT: Psychotropic actions of clonidine. In Lal H, Fielding S (eds): "Psychopharmacology of Clonidine." New York: Alan R. Liss, Inc., 1981.

Lang WJ, Gershon S: Effects of psychoactive drugs on yohimbine induced responses in conscious dogs. A proposed screening procedure for anti-anxiety agents. Arch Int Pharmacodyn 142:446–457, 1963.

Leckman JF, Maas JW, Redmond DE Jr, Heninger GR: Effects of oral clonidine on plasma MHPG in man: Preliminary report. Life Sci 26:2179–2185, 1980.

Leverenz K, Redmond DE Jr, Huang YH: Suppression of feeding behavior in food deprived monkeys by locus coeruleus stimulation. Neurosci Abstr 4:177, 1978.

Lidbrink P: The effect of lesions of ascending noradrenaline pathways on sleep and waking in the rat. Brain Res 74:19–40, 1974.

Lief HI: Psychoneurotic disorders, I: Anxiety, conversion, dissociative, and phobic reactions. In Freedman AM, Kaplan HI (eds): "Comprehensive Textbook of Psychiatry." Baltimore: Williams and Wilkins, 1967, pp 857–870.

Lipman JJ, Spencer PSJ: Clonidine and opiate withdrawal. Lancet September 2, 1978, 2(8090)521.

Llorens C, Martres MP, Baudry M, Schwartz JC: Hypersensitivity to noradrenaline in cortex after chronic morphine: Relevance to tolerance and dependence. Nature 274:603–605, 1978.

Maas JW, Hattox SE, Landis DH, Roth RH: The determination of a brain arteriovenous difference for 3-methoxy-4-hydroxy-phenethylene glycol (MHPG). Brain Res 118:167–173, 1976.

Meyer DR, Sparber SB: Clonidine antagonizes body weight loss and other symptoms used to measure withdrawal in morphine pelleted rats given naloxone. Pharmacologist 18:236, 1976.

Mirin SM, Meyer RE, McNamee HB: Psychopathology and mood during heroin use. Arch Gen Psychiatry 33:1503–1508, 1976.

Montel H, Starke K, Taube HD: Morphine tolerance and dependence in noradrenaline neurons of the rat cortex. Naunyn Schmied Arch Pharmacol 288:415–426, 1975.

Nashold BS Jr, Wilson WP, Slaughter G: "Advances in Neurology," Vol IV. New York: Raven Press, 1974.

Onesti G, Schwartz AB, Kim KE, Paz-Matinez V, Schwartz C: Antihypertensive effects of clonidine. Circ Res 28(5) Suppl 2:53–69, 1971.

Paalzow L: Analgesia produced by clonidine in mice and rats. J Pharm Pharmacol 26(5):361–363, 1974.

Pasternak GW, Goodman R, Snyder SH: An endogenous morphine-like factor in mammalian brain. Life Sci 16:1765–1769, 1975.

Pert CB, Kuhar MJ, Snyder SH: Autoradiographic localization of the opiate receptor in rat brain. Life Sci 16:1849–1854, 1975.

Pettinger WA: Drug therapy: Clonidine, a new antihypertensive drug. N Engl J Med 293(23):1179–1180, 1975.

Pradhan SN, Dutta SN: Narcotic analgesics. In Pradhan SN, Dutta SN (eds): "Drug Abuse: Clinical and Basic Aspects." St. Louis: C.V. Mosby Co., 1977, pp 49–77.

Przuntek H, Phillippu A: Reduced pressor responses to stimulation of the locus coeruleus after lesion of the posterior hypothalamus. Naunyn-Schmiedeberg's Archives of Pharmacology 276:119–122, 1973.

Putzeys MR, Hoobler SW: Comparison of clonidine and methyldopa on blood pressure and side effects in hypertensive patients. Am Heart J 83(4):464–468, 1972.

Redmond DE Jr: New and old evidence for the involvement of a brain norepinephrine system in anxiety. In Fann WE et al (eds): "The Phenomenology and Treatment of Anxiety." New York: Spectrum, 1979a, pp 153–203.

Redmond DE Jr: The effects of destruction of the locus coeruleus on nonhuman primate behaviors. Psychopharmacol Bull 15:26–27, 1979b.

Redmond DE Jr: Alterations in the function of the nucleus locus coeruleus: A possible model for studies of anxiety. In Usdin E, Hanin I (eds): "Animal Models in Psychiatry and Neurology." Oxford and New York: Pergamon Press, 1977, pp 293–305.

Redmond DE Jr, Gold MS, Huang YH: Enkephalin acts to inhibit locus coeruleus mediated behaviors. Neurosci Abstr 4:413, 1978.

Redmond DE Jr, Hinrichs RL, Maas JW, Kling A: Behavior of free-ranging macaques after intraventricular 6-hydroxydopamine. Science 181:1256–1258, 1973.

Redmond DE Jr, Huang YH: New evidence for a locus coeruleus–norepinephrine connection with anxiety. Life Sci 25(26):2149–2162, 1979.

Redmond DE Jr, Huang YH, Baulu J, Gold MS: Evidence for the involvement of a brain norepinephrine system in anxiety. In Usdin E, Kopin I, Barchas J (eds): "Catecholamines: Basic and Clinical Frontiers," Vol 2. New York: Pergamon Press, 1979, 1693–1695.

Redmond DE Jr, Huang YH, Snyder DR, Baulu J, Maas JW: Behavioral changes following lesions of the locus coeruleus in M. arctoides. Neurosci Abstr 1:472, 1976a.

Redmond DE Jr, Huang YH, Snyder DR, Maas JW, Baulu J: Hyperphagia and hyperdipsia after locus coeruleus lesions in the stump-tailed monkey. Life Sci 20:1619–1628, 1977.

Redmond DE Jr, Huang YH, Snyder DR, Maas JW: Behavioral effects of stimulation of the locus coeruleus in the stumptail monkey (Macaca arctoides). Brain Res 116:502–510, 1976b.

Redmond DE Jr, Maas JW, Kling A, Graham CW, Dekirmenjian H: Social behavior of monkeys selectively depleted of monoamines. Science 174:428–431, 1971.

Rosenbaum M: Peptic ulcer. In Freedman AM, Kaplan HI (eds): "Comprehensive Textbook of Psychiatry." Baltimore: Williams and Wilkins, 1967, pp 1049–1054.

Samanin R, Bendotti C, Gradnik R, Miranda F: The effect of localized lesions of central monoaminergic neurons on morphine analgesia and physical dependence in rats. Proceedings of the Thirty-Seventh Annual Scientific Meeting, Committee on Problems of Drug Dependence, Inc., NIDA Research Monograph, 1975, pp 690–696.

Schalling D: Anxiety, pain, and coping. In Sarasan IG, Spielberger CD (eds): "Stress and Anxiety," Vol 3. New York: John Wiley and Sons, 1976 pp 49–71.

Scheel-Kruger J, Hasselager E: Studies of various amphetamines, apomorphine, and clonidine on body temperature and brain 5-hydroxytryptamine metabolism in rats. Psychopharmacologia 36:189–202, 1974.

Schildkraut JJ, Kety SS: Biogenic amines and emotion. Science 156:21–30, 1967.

Schlemmer RF, Casper RC, Narasimhachari N, Davis JM: Clonidine induced hyperphagia and weight gain in monkeys. Psychopharmacologia, 61(2):233–234, 1979.

Schmitt H, Schmitt H, Fenard S: Decrease in the sympatho-inhibitory action of clonidine after destruction of the sympatho-inhibitory area. Experientia 29:1247–1249, 1979.

Seedat YK, Vawda EI, Mitha S, Ramasar R: Clonidine in treatment of hypertension. Br Med J 1(739):47, 1971.

Seevers MH: Opiate addition in the monkey. J Pharmacol Exp Ther 56:147–156, 1936.

Shafar J, Tallet ER, Knowlson PA: Evaluation of clonidine in prophylaxis of migraine. Double-blind trial and follow-up. Lancet 1(747):403–407, 1972.

Simpson FO: Hypertension and depression and their treatment. Austr NZ J Psychiatry 7:133–137, 1973.

Snyder D, Huang YH, Redmond DE Jr: Contribution of locus coeruleus noradrenergic system to cardio-acceleration in nonhuman primates. Neurosci Abstr 3:261(828), 1977.

Soffer A: Reginine and benodaine in the diagnosis of pheochromocytoma. Med Clin N Am 38:375–384, 1954.

Starke K, Altman KP: Inhibition of adrenergic neurotransmission by clonidine: An action on prejunctional alpha-receptors. Neuropharmacology 12:339–347, 1973.

Starke K, Montel H: Involvement of alpha-receptors in clonidine induced inhibition of transmitter release from central monoamine neurons. Neuropharmacol 12:1073–1080, 1973.

Stokes GS: Drug-induced hypertension: Pathogenesis and management. Drugs 12(3):222–230, 1976.

Svensson TH, Bunney BS, Aghajanian GK: Inhibition of both noradrenergic and serotonergic neurons in brain by the alpha-adrenergic antagonist clonidine. Brain Res 92:291–306, 1975.

Svensson T, Persson R, Wallin L, Walinder J: Anxiolytic action of clonidine. Nordisk Psykiatrisk Tidskrift 32:439–441, 1978.

Svensson TH, Strombom U: Discontinuation of chronic clonidine treatment. Evidence for facilitated brain noradrenergic neurotransmission. Naunyn Schmied Arch Pharmacol 299:83–87, 1977.

Tatum AL, Seevers MH, Collins KK: Morphine addiction and its physiological interpretation based on experimental evidences. J Pharmacol Exp Ther 36:447–475, 1929.

Tseng LF, Loh HH, Wei ET: Effects of clonidine on morphine withdrawal signs in the rat. Eur J Pharmacol 30(1):93–99, 1975.

Tyrer PJ, Lader MH: Response to propranolol and diazepam in somatic and psychic anxiety. Br Med J 2(909):14–16, 1974.

Vetulani J, Bednarczyk B: Depression by clonidine of shaking behavior elicited by nolorphine in morphine-dependent rats. J Pharm Pharmacol 29:567–569, 1977.

Ward DG, Grizzle WE, Gann DS: Inhibitory and facilitatory areas of the rostral pons mediating ACTH release in the cat. Endocrinology 99:1220–1228, 1976.

Ward DG, Gunn DS: Locus coeruleus complex: Elicitation of a pressure response and a brain stem region necessary for its occurrence. Brain Res 107:401–406, 1976.

Washton AM, Resnick RB: The clinical use of clonidine in outpatient detoxification from opiates. In Lal H, Fielding S (eds): "Psychopharmacology of Clonidine." New York: Alan R. Liss, Inc., 1981.

Wikler A: Clinical and electroencephalographic studies on the effects of mescaline n-allylnormorphine and morphine in man. J Nerv Men Des 120:157–175, 1954.

Psychopharmacology of Clonidine, pages 165–175
© 1981 Alan R. Liss, Inc., 150 Fifth Avenue, New York, NY 10011

Clonidine: Antidepressant Potential?

Jeffrey B. Malick

I. INTRODUCTION

Clonidine (Catapres) is an α-adrenergic agonist that has been widely used in the treatment of hypertension [for review, see Pettinger, 1975]. Apparently its hypotensive activity is due to effects in the CNS: It most likely stimulates α-adrenergic receptors in the vasomotor center resulting in decreased sympathetic outflow [Kobinger and Walland, 1967].

Clonidine appears to act relatively selectively at noradrenergic sites: In man, it decreases urinary catecholamine excretion [Hokfelt et al, 1970] and produces significant decreases in cerebrospinal fluid (CSF) levels of 3-methoxy-4-hydroxyphenyl glycol (MHPG) [Bertilsson et al, 1977]. At low doses, clonidine appears to act preferentially as an agonist on α_2-adrenergic (autoreceptor) receptors, whereas at higher doses it also acts as an α_1 (postsynaptic) adrenergic agonist [Drew, 1976; Starke et al, 1975]. Clonidine has very slight effects on dopaminergic systems [Rochette and Bralet, 1975], although it does produce decreases in firing in 5-HT neurons and decreased 5-HT turnover [Svensson et al, 1975]; the latter effects on serotonergic systems in the CNS are believed to be secondary to actions at adrenergic receptors [Svensson et al, 1975].

In recent years, clonidine has been studied in a wide range of different clinical syndromes. It is now accepted as a valuable treatment in the suppression of the opiate abstinence syndrome and for opiate detoxification in man [Gold et al, 1978; Uhde et al, 1980; Washton and Resnick, 1980]. In fact, when compared to methadone-treated patients, clonidine produced significantly fewer withdrawal symptoms [Uhde et al, 1980]. Clonidine has been tested unsuccessfully in a limited number of schizophrenic patients, some of whom became more aggressive following clonidine [Jimerson et al, 1980]. However, clonidine exhibited "noteworthy antidepressant responses" in three of five depressed patients [Jimerson et al, 1980]; the responders were moderately to severely depressed women (two unipolar and one bipolar), and two of the patients exhibited an increase in depression scores upon clonidine withdrawal [Jimerson et al, 1980]. This finding of clinical antidepressant activity with clonidine prompted us to evaluate it in a range of preclinical animal models considered to be predictive of antidepressant activity.

II. ACTIVITY OF CLONIDINE IN LABORATORY TESTS CONSIDERED TO BE PREDICTIVE OF ANTIDEPRESSANT POTENTIAL

A. Antagonism of Tetrabenazine-Induced Ptosis in Mice

Since the discovery of the very first clinically effective antidepressants, pharmacologists have relied heavily on the ability of an agent to prevent or antagonize the sedative or hypothermic activities produced by amine depleting agents (eg, reserpine, tetrabenazine) as being predictive of antidepressant activity. Although we now know of several so-called "atypical" antidepressants (eg, mianserin, iprindole) that are either weak or inactive as inhibitors of amine reuptake mechanisms and are also not very active in such models, the use of these procedures has not diminished significantly through the years. Clonidine has been shown to antagonize RO-4-1284 (a benzoquinolizine derivative and an amine depleter) induced ptosis in mice [Niemegeers, 1975] and the ptosis and hypothermia (0.125–0.32 mg/kg, PO) produced in mice by reserpine [Gouret et al, 1977].

Thus, since clonidine had been shown to be an antagonist of the symptoms induced by amine depleters, we evaluated its activity in the Antagonism of Tetrabenazine-induced Ptosis Test in mice. In this laboratory, tetrabenazine is used rather than reserpine because it is more rapid in onset, and it affects the central nervous system more selectively (ie, it predominantly depletes catecholamines and serotonin in brain rather than in peripheral tissues) [Pletscher, 1957]. Ptosis was induced and scored by a modification of the method of Vernier and co-workers [1962]. Briefly, groups of six male Swiss-Webster mice (18–22 grams) were pretreated orally with either test drug or placebo 45 min prior to the intraperitoneal administration of tetrabenazine methanesulfonate (70 mg/kg). Immediately after tetrabenazine administration, mice were isolated and rated for ptosis (degree of eyelid closure) 30 min later. Imipramine, as expected, produced a dose-related antagonism of tetrabenazine-induced ptosis; its ED_{50} (ie, that dose of drug that would be expected to antagonize ptosis in 50% of the mice tested) was 9.4 mg/kg, PO. Clonidine was found to be an extremely potent antagonist (ED_{50} = 0.2 mg/kg, PO) of ptosis (see Table I).

Although clonidine was a very potent antagonist of ptosis, it was not clear from the results of this study whether its effects were due primarily to stimulation of the autoreceptors or to postsynaptic (α_1) stimulation. Tests were performed to assess the influence of clonidine on spontaneous locomotor activity in an attempt to determine whether the net effect, at doses that antagonized or prevented ptosis, were the result of α_1 or α_2 agonist activity. Since α_2 stimulation should inhibit NE release, locomotor activity should be suppressed by doses of clonidine with preferential activity at this site, whereas locomotor stimulation should be observed if the predominant effect were α_1 stimulation. Clonidine was tested over a wide range of doses (0.001 – 10 mg/kg, IP) and it only produced hypoactivity at all doses tested (mice grouped three per chamber during testing). Thus, in the motor activity studies, clonidine's net effect would appear to be α_2 agonist activity, which could account for the decrease in spontaneous activity that was observed at all doses tested. Although it did not appear to be the case, it would be more in harmony with the catecholamine hypothesis of depression if clonidine were acting via stimulation of postsynaptic noradrenergic receptors. Further studies need to be performed to determine the mechanism of action of clonidine in the tetrabenazine model. However, regardless of its mechanism of action, its potent activity in this procedure could be considered to be predictive of antidepressant potential.

TABLE I. Antagonism of Tetrabenazine-Induced Ptosis in Mice

Drug	Dose (mg/kg, PO)	N[a]	Antagonism of ptosis	
			% Blockade	ED_{50} (mg/kg, PO) (95% C.L.)[b]
Imipramine	3	30	13.3	9.4
	10	36	52.8	(6.9–12.6)
	17	24	70.8	
	31	12	91.7	
Clonidine	0.03	6	16.7	0.2
	0.1	12	25.0	(0.1–0.4)
	0.3	24	62.5	
	0.6	24	66.7	
	1.0	24	100.0	

[a]Number of mice tested.

[b]ED_{50} and 95% confidence limits calculated by the method of Litchfield and Wilcoxon [1949].

B. Mouse Learned Helplessness Swimming Test

Seligman [1972] and his collaborators have proposed that when exposed to a circumstance in which responses have no systematic outcomes, persons tend to become depressed, apathetic, and deficient in the learning of new responses. The motivational, affective, and learning manifestations of such an experience result in a generalization to other circumstances such that the individual exhibits a "learned helplessness" response; ie, he has failed previously under similar circumstances, and he generalizes to the new situation and feels he will fail again and is thus helpless in terms of controlling things in his environment.

This model has been tested in animals. For instance, if a rat is placed in a behavioral test chamber with a grid floor through which shocks can be introduced periodically, if there is no means of escaping the shock, the rat will quickly give up and simply huddle in the corner of the chamber and accept the shocks. If this rat, which has learned there is no way of escaping the shock, is then placed in a conventional situation where a normal, naive rat will quickly learn to terminate the shock or avoid it completely by making the appropriate response (eg, lever press), it will once again huddle in the corner and accept the shock rather than attempt to escape; the rat is exhibiting learned helplessness.

Recently, Porsolt and co-workers [1977] have described a swimming procedure in rodents that can be considered to be a learned helplessness model. Their initial test in rats, which required subacute drug treatment (three drug administrations in a 24-hour period between the first and second swimming tests), was reported to be sensitive to all known antidepressants (eg, iprindole, tricyclics, mianserin, MAOIs, electroconvulsive shock therapy). Subsequently, both we and Porsolt's group modified this procedure such that it could be performed in mice in a single day in order to facilitate its usefulness as a screen.

In what we refer to as the one-trial mouse learned helplessness swimming test or simply MLHS, drugs are typically administered intraperitoneally 1 hour before exposing them to an inescapable situation (a Plexiglas jar half-filled with water). During testing, a mouse is gently placed into the water and tested for a total of only 6 minutes as follows: During the first 2 minutes the animal quickly learns there is no escape and spends the vast majority of the last 4 minutes floating (tonic immobility). Nothing is recorded during the first 2 minutes (learning period), but the time (sec) spent in tonic immobility during the last 4 minutes of the session is recorded. Typically, controls average between 200 and 220 sec of the total 240 sec in tonic immobility. Control (vehicle-treated) groups are run each day, and drug-treated groups are compared to these via a Student's t-test.

The results of the MLHS test with imipramine and clonidine are summarized on Table II. Imipramine produced a dose-related decrease in tonic immobility scores and exhibited a minimal effective dose (MED; ie, the lowest

TABLE II. Effects of Imipramine and Clonidine in the Mouse Learned Helplessness Swimming Test

Treatment	Dose (mg/kg, IP)[a]	Change in immobility vs control (sec)[b]	P value [c]
Imipramine	2.5	0.0	NS[d]
	7.5	↓ 40.5	<0.01
	15.0	↓ 42.0	<0.05
	30.0	↓ 66.0	<0.01
	60.0	↓119.0	<0.001
Clonidine	0.01	↑ 13.5	NS
	0.1	↓ 14.0	NS
	0.3	↓ 14.5	NS
	0.6	↓ 18.0	NS
	0.6	↓ 42.5	<0.01
	1.0	↓ 47.0	<0.01
	1.0	↓ 24.5	NS
	1.0	↓ 37.5	<0.01
	3.0	↓ 43.0	<0.05
	3.0	↓ 71.0	<0.02
	10.0	↓ 82.5	<0.001[e]
	30.0	↓ 73.5	<0.001[e]

[a]N = 10 mice per group.

[b]Difference in tonic immobility scores between drug-treated and same-day vehicle-treated control groups.

[c]Drug-treated compared to control via Student's t-test.

[d]NS = not significant ($P > 0.05$).

[e]Tremors.

dose of drug producing a statistically significant effect) of 7.5 mg/kg, IP. Clonidine also produced a dose-related decrease in tonic immobility (Table II); the MED for clonidine was 1 mg/kg, IP (sizeable decreases in each of three separate trials although statistical significance was only reached in two of three trials).

Since, with very few exceptions (eg, stimulants, anticholinergics, antihistamines), only antidepressants will significantly reduce tonic immobility scores, clonidine exhibited an antidepressant-like profile in the MLHS test. In contrast to antidepressants, anxiolytic (eg, benzodiazepines) and antipsychotic (eg, clozapine, chlorpromazine) drugs produce increases in tonic immobility scores.

C. Antagonism of Muricidal (Mouse-Killing) Behavior

Mouse-killing behavior in rats is selectively (ie, at doses that do not produce concurrent neurological impairment) inhibited by all known clinically effective antidepressant drugs [Goldberg and Malick, 1980; Horovitz et al, 1966]. The use of the muricidal rat for the prediction of antidepressant activity is supported by the evidence that the site of action of these agents is in the amygdala [Horovitz et al, 1966], an area that appears to play a significant role in the control of emotional behavior, including muricide [Karli, 1956]. In addition, mouse killing is inhibited by lesions in the amygdala [Horovitz et al, 1966; Karli, 1956] and by direct infusion of imipramine, a tricyclic antidepressant, into the amygdala [Horovitz and Leaf, 1967].

The following is a brief description of the methods utilized for evaluating antimuricidal activity. Male Long-Evans hooded rats were tested for muricidal behavior, and only those that consistently killed mice within 5 min of presentation were used in this study. When utilized for drug testing, the rats were tested in the morning (same day control) and then given test drug or placebo in the afternoon and retested for killing 1 hour after drug administration. Any rat that failed to kill after placebo was discarded from the study. Immediately following the mouse-killing test, all rats were tested for neurological impairment (ataxia) on a 45° inclined screen. Subsequent drug administrations were at least 1 week apart.

The results of this study are presented on Table III. Imipramine produced a dose-related inhibition of muricidal behavior with a MED of 10 mg/kg, IP; this was a selective inhibition of the response in that no neuromuscular impairment (ataxia) was observed on the inclined screen at any dose tested (Table III). In fact, the MED for producing ataxia in another study was found to be 60 mg/kg, IP, for imipramine; therefore its therapeutic ratio (MED for neuromuscular impairment/MED for antimuricidal activity) was 6. Although clonidine produced a dose-related suppression of mouse-killing (MED = 0.3 mg/kg, IP), it also produced significant neuromuscular impairment over the same dose range (Table III). Thus clonidine failed to antagonize muricidal behavior selectively, a feature exhibited by all known clinically effective antidepressants [Goldberg and Malick, 1980; Horovitz et al, 1966]. The results obtained in this procedure would not lend themselves to

TABLE III. Effects of Clonidine and Imipramine on Mouse-Killing (Muricidal Behavior) by Rats

Treatment[a]	Dose (mg/kg, IP)	N[b]	% Blockade of mouse-killing	% Ataxia[c]
Clonidine	0.1	20	40.0	20.0
	0.3	20	75.0	50.0
	0.6	15	86.7	93.3
	1.0	10	90.0	100.0
Imipramine	6	5	20.0	0.0
	10	14	50.0	0.0
	17	10	80.0	0.0
	31	10	90.0	0.0

[a]Rats tested for mouse killing behavior 60 min post administration.
[b]Number of rats tested.
[c]Percent ataxia on a 45% inclined screen.

the prediction that clonidine would possess significant antidepressant activity in man.

In an earlier report, Nagaoka [1973] observed that spontaneously hypertensive rats (SHR) exhibited a much higher incidence of muricidal behavior than other strains, and that this activity seemed to increase as the hypertensive syndrome advanced; in SHR rats, in contrast to the results obtained in my laboratory, clonidine exhibited a "selective inhibitory action on muricide." Unfortunately, Nagaoka's report [1973] was only an abstract, and did not report the effective doses for clonidine; selectivity was assessed by comparing the antimuricidal dose to the dose that caused significant impairment of Rotarod performance. The selectivity observed in the SHR rat may be related to the apparent correlation between hypertension and mouse killing in these rats; thus the antihypertensive activity of clonidine, which occurs at very low doses, may have indirectly antagonized the killing response and accounted for the "selectivity" observed.

D. Yohimbine Potentiation in Mice

In 1963, Quinton reported that imipramine and representatives of several other classes of drugs increased the toxicity of yohimbine in mice [Quinton, 1963]. This procedure has been reevaluated recently in my laboratory, and has been found to be a useful test for the prediction of antidepressant potential [Malick, 1981]. The Potentiation of Yohimbine-induced Lethality Test in mice will detect the antidepressant potential of all known classes of clinically effective antidepressant drugs: tricyclics, atypicals (eg, mianserin, iprindole), MAO inhibitors. The only clinically effective treatment for depression that failed to potentiate yohimbine-induced toxicity was electroconvulsive shock therapy (ECT) [Malick, 1981]. Most other classes of psychoactive drugs (eg, anxiolytics, antipsychotics) were inactive, although antihistamines, anticholinergics, and stimulants were found to be active; these latter agents are frequently found active in antidepressant procedures (eg, muricide; mouse learned helplessness swimming).

Male Swiss-Webster mice, housed ten per cage, were treated orally with vehicle (HPMC) or test drug 60 min prior to yohimbine (30 mg/kg, SC). This dose of yohimbine very rarely produced any toxicity in vehicle-treated controls. The results of these studies are summarized on Table IV. In marked contrast to imipramine, which produced a dose-related potentiation of yohimbine-induced toxicity (MED = 10 mg/kg, PO), clonidine was inactive over a wide range of doses either orally (1–60 mg/kg) or intraperitoneally (0.01–30 mg/kg). Thus clonidine did not exhibit an antidepressant profile in this procedure.

E. Olfactory Bulbectomized Rat Model

The removal of the olfactory bulbs in rats produces a behavioral syndrome characterized by increased irritability and the induction of muricide

TABLE IV. Effects of Imipramine and Clonidine on Yohimbine Potentiation in Mice

Treatment	Dose (mg/kg, PO)	N[a]	% Lethality
Imipramine	3	10	0
	6	10	20
	10	10	60
	15	10	70
	30	20	75
Clonidine	1–60	60	Inactive
	0.01–30 IP	70	Inactive

[a]Number of mice tested.

[Malick, 1970], increased open field activity, and a decrease in the capacity to learn a passive avoidance task [Cairncross et al, 1978; van Riesen et al, 1977]; furthermore, such lesions cause a significant increase in plasma 11-hydroxycorticosteroids [Cairncross et al, 1978]. Malick [1976] reported that antidepressants selectively inhibited killing in both spontaneous and olfactory bulbectomy-induced muricidal rats. Antidepressants (eg, amitriptyline, viloxazine, mianserin), when given subacutely for 7 days, corrected the passive avoidance learning deficit, reduced the hyperirritability [Cairncross et al, 1978; van Riesen et al, 1977] and significantly decreased the elevated 11-hydroxycorticosteroid levels [Cairncross et al, 1978].

Broekkamp and co-workers [1980] recently studied the effects of serotonin-mimetic drugs (eg, fluoxetine, fenfluramine, quipazine) and clonidine in the olfactory bulbectomized rat model. As reported previously [Cairncross et al, 1978; van Riesen et al, 1977], the antidepressants reversed the passive avoidance deficit after subacute (5-day) but not after acute treatment. Although acute treatment with fluoxetine (a selective 5-HT reuptake inhibitor with clinical antidepressant activity), fenfluramine, and quipazine (also reported to possess antidepressant activity) [Rodriguez and Pardo, 1971] restored the capacity of olfactory bulbectomized rats to acquire the passive avoidance task, clonidine (0.1 and 0.5 mg/kg, IP) was ineffective [Broekkamp et al, 1980]. Unfortunately, clonidine was evaluated only after acute administration; thus, since most of the antidepressants are only active in this model after subacute treatment, further evaluations should be performed before it can be stated with certainty that it is inactive in this procedure.

F. Self-Stimulatory Behavior

In contrast to what would be expected, antidepressant drugs significantly suppress responding for reinforcing electrical stimulation of the brain (self-stimulation) [Goldstein and Malick, in press; Stein, 1962]. In fact, the only way to differentiate antidepressants from antipsychotics, which both suppress or inhibit self-stimulatory behavior, is by interacting these agents with amphetamine. Whereas antipsychotics antagonize the rate-enhancing effects of amphetamine, antidepressants enhance the stimulatory effects of amphetamine on self-stimulatory behavior [Goldstein and Malick, in press; Stein, 1962].

Clonidine has been shown to produce a dose-related inhibition of self-stimulatory responding [Hunt et al, 1978; Vetulani et al, 1977]. When interacted with amphetamine, clonidine antagonized the rate-enhancing effects of amphetamine on self-stimulation [Hunt et al, 1978; Vetulani et al, 1977]; thus, in this model, clonidine exhibited an antipsychotic-like profile rather than exhibiting antidepressant-like activity.

III. SUMMARY AND CONCLUSIONS

Although clonidine exhibited significant activity in two preclinical tests considered to be predictive of antidepressant activity (ie, antagonism of tetrabenazine-induced ptosis in mice, Mouse Learned Helplessness Swimming), it failed to exhibit an antidepressant-like profile in several other tests (eg, yohimbine potentiation in mice, antagonism of muricidal behavior, and self-stimulation in rats) that appear to be equally valid predictors of such activity.

In the clinic, as a result of a very preliminary double-blind placebo-controlled study, clonidine exhibited some antidepressant activity in three of the five depressed patients evaluated [Jimerson et al, 1980]. In this study by Jimerson and co-workers, the patients as a group showed no overall mood response to clonidine. However, three moderately to severely depressed women exhibited "noteworthy antidepressant responses," and two of these manifested increased depressive scores following clonidine withdrawal. In contrast, the two depressed men who received clonidine exhibited a slight increase in depressive symptoms following treatment. Although the results are extremely preliminary, clonidine may be more effective in treating depression in women than in men.

Simpson and Waal-Manning [1971] have reviewed the literature on the use of clonidine in the treatment of hypertension, and have noted that clonidine occasionally seems to produce depression. In their clinic, 4 of 39 patients who received clonidine for an average of 4 months exhibited symptoms of depression; other cases of what appears to be clonidine-induced depression have been reported [see Simpson and Waal-Manning, 1971, for review], and a high incidence of drowsiness and fatigue has also been observed. Simpson and Waal-Manning caution that "clonidine should be avoided in any patient who has a psychiatric history or who appears to be depressed or unstable."

Thus, as a result of evaluation in several laboratory animal models considered to be predictive of antidepressant potential, clonidine only mimicked the profile of the clinically effective antidepressants in a couple of models. In addition, the clinical reports are contradictory in that it was an effective antidepressant in a few patients, but it also appeared to precipitate depression in some patients being treated for hypertension. It appears that only careful and perhaps extensive clinical trials will answer the question of whether clonidine is effective in depression; it is possible that it may be an effective antidepressant in a specific subpopulation of depressives (eg, women).

IV. REFERENCES

Bertilsson L, Haglund R, Ostman J, Rawlins MD, Ringberger VA, Sjoqvist F: Monoamine metabolites in cerebrospinal fluid during clonidine or alprenolol. Eur J Clin Pharmacol 11:125, 1977.

Broekkamp CL, Garrigon D, Lloyd KG: Serotonin-mimetic and antidepressant drugs on passive avoidance learning by olfactory bulbectomised rats. Pharmacol Biochem Behav 13:643, 1980.

Cairncross KD, Cox B, Forster C, Wren AF: A new model for the detection of antidepressant drugs: Olfactory bulbectomy in the rat compared with existing models. J Pharmacol Meth 1:131, 1978.

Drew GM: Effects of α-adrenoceptor agonists and antagonists on pre- and postsynaptically located α-adrenoceptors. Eur J Pharmacol 36:313, 1976.

Gold MS, Redmond DE Jr, Kleber HD: Clonidine in opiate withdrawal. Lancet 1:929, 1978.

Goldberg ME, Malick JB: Predatory aggression: Its influence by antidepressants and other psychotropic agents. Proc CINP Congress, Goteborg, Sweden, 1980.

Goldstein JM, Malick JB: An automated descending rate-intensity self-stimulation paradigm: Usefulness for distinguishing antidepressants from neuroleptics. Pharmacol Biochem Behav (in press).

Gouret G, Mocquet G, Coston A, Raynaud G: Interaction de divers psychotropes avec cinq effets de la reserpine chez la souris et chez le chat. J Pharmacol 8:333, 1977.

Hokfelt B, Hedeland H, Dymling JF: Studies on catecholamines, renin and aldosterone following catepresan (2-(2,6-dichloro-phenylamine)-2-imidazoline hydrochloride) in hypertensive patients. J Pharmacol 10:389, 1970.

Horovitz ZP: The relationship of the amygdala to the mechanism of action of two types of antidepressants. In Wortis J (ed): "Recent Advances in Biological Psychiatry." New York: Plenum Press, 1966, pp 21–31.

Horovitz ZP, Leaf RC: The effects of direct injections of psychotropic drugs on the amygdala of rats and the relationship to antidepressant site of action. In Brill H et al (eds): "Excerpta Medica International Congress Series," No. 129. Amsterdam: Excerpta Medica Foundation, 1967, p 1042.

Horovitz ZP, Piala JJ, High JP, Burke JC, Leaf RC: Effects of drugs on the mouse-killing (muricide) test and its relationship to amygdaloid function. Int J Neuropharmacol 5:405, 1966.

Hunt GE, Atrens DM, Becker FT, Paxinos G: α-Adrenergic modulation of hypothalamic self-stimulation: Effects of phenoxybenzamine, yohimbine, dexamphetamine and their interactions with clonidine. Eur J Pharmacol 53:1, 1978.

Jimerson DC, Post RM, Stoddard FJ, Gillin JC Bunney WE Jr: Preliminary trials of the noradrenergic agonist clonidine in psychiatric patients. Biol Psychiatry 15:45, 1980.

Karli P: The Norway rat's killing response to the white mouse: An experimental analysis. Behavior 10:81, 1956.

Kobinger W, Walland A: Investigation into the hypotensive effect of 2-(2,6-dichlorophenylamino)-2-imidazoline-HCl. Eur J Pharmacol 2:155, 1967.

Litchfield JT Jr, Wilcoxon F: A simplified method of evaluating dose-effect experiments. J Pharmacol Exp Ther 96:99, 1949.

Malick JB: A behavioral comparison of three lesion-induced models of aggression in the rat. Physiol Behav 5:679, 1970.

Malick JB: Pharmacological antagonism of mouse-killing behavior in the olfactory bulb lesion-induced killer rat. Aggressive Behav 2:123, 1976.

Malick JB: Yohimbine potentiation as a predictor of antidepressant action. In Enna SJ, Malick JB, Richelson E (eds): "Antidepressants: Neurochemical, Behavioral and Clinical Perspectives." New York: Raven Press, 1981, pp 141–155.

Nagaoka A: Pharmacological studies on mechanism of muricidal response in the spontaneously hypertensive rat. Jpn J Pharmacol 23(Suppl):67, 1973.

Niemegeers CJE: Antagonism of reserpine-like activity. In Fielding S, Lal H (eds): "Antidepressants." Mount Kisco, New York: Futura Publishing, 1975, pp 73–98.

Pettinger WA: Clonidine, a new antihypertensive drug. N Engl J Med 293:1179, 1975.

Pletscher A: Release of 5-HT by benzoquinolizine derivatives with sedative action. Science 126:507, 1957.

Porsolt RD, Bertin A, Jalfre M: Behavioral despair in mice: A primary screen for antidepressants. Arch Intern Pharmacodyn Ther 229:327, 1977.

Quinton RM: The increase in toxicity of yohimbine induced by imipramine and other drugs in mice. Br J Pharmacol 21:51, 1963.

Rochette L, Bralet J: Effect of clonidine on the synthesis of cerebral dopamine. Biochem Pharmacol 24:307, 1975.

Rodriguez R, Pardo EG: Quipazine: A new type of antidepressant agent. Psychopharmacologia (Berl) 21:89, 1971.

Selgman MEP: Learned helplessness. Ann Rev Med 23:407, 1972.

Simpson FO, Waal-Manning HJ: Hypertension and depression: Interrelated problems in therapy. J R Coll Physicians (Lond) 6:14, 1971.

Starke K, Endo T, Taube HD: Pre- and postsynaptic components in effect of drugs with α-adrenoceptor affinity. Nature 254:440, 1975.

Stein L: Effects of interactions of imipramine, chlorpromazine, reserpine and amphetamine on self-stimulation: Possible neurophysiological basis of depression. In Wortes J (ed): "Recent Advances in Biological Psychiatry." New York: Plenum Press, 1962, p 288.

Svensson TH, Bunney BS, Aghajanian GK: Inhibition of both noradrenergic and serotonergic neurons in brain by the α-adrenergic agonist clonidine. Brain Res 92:291, 1975.

Uhde TW, Redmond DE, Kleber HD: Clonidine suppresses the opioid abstinence syndrome without clonidine-withdrawal symptoms: A blind inpatient study. Psychiatry Res 2:37, 1980.

van Riezen H, Schnieden H, Wren AF: Olfactory bulb ablation in the rat: Behavioral changes and their reversal by antidepressant drugs. Br J Pharmacol 60:521, 1977.

Vernier VG, Hanson HM, Stone CA: The pharmocodynamics of amitriptyline. In Nodine JH, Moyer JH (eds): "Psychosomatic Medicine." Philadelphia: Lea & Fibiger, 1962, pp 683–690.

Vetulani J, Leith NJ, Stawarz RJ, Sulser F: Effect of clonidine on the noradrenergic cyclic AMP generating system in the limbic forebrain and on medial forebrain bundle self-stimulation. Experientia 33:1490, 1977.

Washton AM, Resnick RB: Clonidine for opiate detoxification: Outpatient clinical trials. Am J Psychiatry 137:1129, 1980.

Psychopharmacology of Clonidine, pages 177–196

Brain Reinforcement Mechanisms: Alpha-Adrenergic and Dopaminergic Agonists and Antagonists

A. Wauquier, G. Clincke, and J. Fransen

I. INTRODUCTION

In 1954, Olds and Milner [1954] reported that rats would learn to press a lever that triggered electrical stimulation via implanted electrodes in lateral hypothalamic and septal sites in the brain. This and many experiments thereafter demonstrated that the activation of specific neurons in the brain produced a strong behavioral reinforcement [Wauquier and Rolls, 1976].

Originally mapping of self-stimulation sites was carried out in search of an anatomical substrate of the brain-stimulation reward. The sites where intracranial self-stimulation (ICS) could be elicited overlapped with the medial forebrain bundle (MFB) fiber course. This suggested that the anatomical substrate of ICS was the MFB. Because high-intensity ICS was found in or near the lateral hypothalamus, it was thought that the center of reward was the lateral hypothalamus.

Dresse [1966] was the first to demonstrate that ICS had a biochemical substrate. He related the ICS sites to the sites where cell bodies of what he thought were noradrenaline-containing neurons were localized as visualized using the histofluorescence technique. His suggestion was that self-stimulation in the ventral tegmental area was mediated through an activation of noradrenergic neurons. His findings corroborated the previously reported pharmacological results by Stein [1964a, b], specifically the amphetamine effects. Dresse's results were in line with the growing knowledge that drugs elicited their effects by interfering with brain neurotransmitters.

The finding that ICS sites were localized along noradrenergic and dopaminergic fibers suggested that ICS was mediated by an activation of these transmitters. These ideas culminated in the formulation of the so-called catecholamine (CA) hypothesis by Crow [1972]. Mapping of ICS sites in the cell bodies of origin of the catecholamines and extensive pharmacological studies gave support to the hypothesis. In spite of many criticisms, the CA hypothesis is still able to frame most of the existing data. That DA is involved in ICS is well supported by pharmacological studies and somewhat less by the anatomical studies. That NA is involved in ICS is reasonably well supported by the anatomical data, but very weakly by the pharmacological data.

Defining the functional role of these transmitter systems, however, goes hand in hand with methodological problems. For a long time and even today, lever pressing has been the method of choice in studying the rewarding effects of ICS. Originally, this technique was introduced to quantify the reinforcement strength. It has become clear that the quantity of lever pressing does not necessarily reflect the quality of the reward. A more general problem is the use of behavioral measures to infer psychological constructs such as motivation. Many factors such as motor activity, memory processing, and arousal jointly determine the behavior. Specific experimental setups and comparative studies are required to separate the various factors involved.

A further complicating factor is that brain-stimulation reward is looked upon as a unitary concept. "Noradrenergic" ICS and "dopaminergic" ICS appear to be quite different; forebrain self-stimulation versus posterior brain self-stimulation appears different; the fact that self-stimulation is still found after massive forebrain lesions [Huston and Borbély, 1973] further demonstrates that various levels of reward exist.

The present study is a pharmacological study, but it does not attempt to review the pharmacological data with respect to the CA hypothesis, which has been done previously [Crow and Deakin, 1966; Wauquier, 1976, 1978, 1979, 1980]. We deliberately restricted the number of compounds, but tested them in a variety of situations that would allow us to comment on the pharmacological evidences related to the CA hypothesis. The main selected compounds were: the DA-antagonist spiperone, the DA-agonist apomorphine, the α-antagonist phenoxybenzamine and the α-agonist clonidine.

II. THE CLASSICAL LEVER-PRESSING SITUATION

A. Electrical Parameter Variation

Over the past decades an exponentially increasing number of drugs have been tested on ICS, using lever pressing as the required behavior to obtain brain stimulation. The assessment of drugs is clearly dependent on the baseline rates of responding. The technique usually applied was to lower the intensity of the stimulation so as to have low to moderate rates of responding, enabling enhancement to be shown; conversely, high rates of responding by applying high intensity stimulation were used, allowing inhibitory drug effects to be demonstrated.

In our pharmacological studies [Wauquier and Niemegeers, 1972; Wauquier, 1976, 1979], we adopted a system in which different baseline rates of responding were achieved within one session and within the same rats by selecting six different combinations of electrical stimulation parameters (SPC), as based on our stimulus parameter study [Wauquier et al, 1972]. Each session consisted of six 10-minute periods during which a different SPC was selected each time. Of the six SPCs chosen, two elicited low lever-pressing rates, two high lever-pressing rates, and two intermediate lever-pressing rates; the pairs were constituted each time by a combination of a relatively low-intensity or a relatively low-frequency stimulation. The SPCs were given to groups of rats in a randomized sequence, but the particular sequence given to a rat remained constant. The design and analysis of control values was previously described in detail [Wauquier, 1979]. Rats were implanted in the lateral hypothalamus and drug-treated once a week after training and stabilization.

Hereafter follow a description and interpretation of the effects of spiperone, apomorphine, phenoxybenzamine, and clonidine as tested in the above-described procedure.

1. Spiperone. The DA-antagonist spiperone dose-relatedly inhibited ICS, its ED_{50} being 0.019 mg/kg (Fig. 1). As such, it does not differ from any other neuroleptic, but it is so far the most potent neuroleptic known. Characteristically, the inhibition is inversely related to the baseline rates of responding; that is, a high inhibition is obtained on low SPCs and vice versa. This suggests that the inhibitory effects depend on the stimulation strength, and that a strong stimulation is able to overcome the suppressing neuroleptic effect in a similar way as cataleptic rats will overcome their catalepsy when subjected to strong stimuli (eg, being dropped into water).

The inhibition appears, however, not to be due to a direct motor inhibition, since the pattern of responding following neuroleptic treatment follows an extinction pattern [Fouriezos and Wise, 1976].

The extinction curve seen suggests a direct effect on the reinforcing value of the stimulation. An alternative interpretation is that neuroleptic rats are unable to sustain responding. In this respect it is worthwhile to consider that physical debilitation is not necessarily an all-or-none effect, but rather a gradual phenomenon.

Since negatively reinforced behavior in a similar dose range is dose-relatedly inhibited by spiperone or other neuroleptics [eg, Niemegeers et al 1972; Wauquier and Niemegeers, 1972], it appears that interfering with the DA system in general disrupts operant behavior. The question could then be posed whether DA is a reward transmitter or rather a transmitter within the chain of systems supporting reinforcement in general. As formulated earlier [Wauquier and Niemegeers, 1972], DA appears an essential final link in the behavioral output, with the restriction that it is concerned with complex behavior. Interfering with the DA system by neuroleptics disrupts the stimulus–response contingency.

2. Apomorphine. Drugs enhancing DA transmission, such as amphetamine, are known to enhance low baseline rates of responding; however, depression of high baseline rates of responding is seen at high-doses [Wauquier and Niemegeers, 1974a, b].

Apomorphine also enhances low baseline rates of responding and dose-relatedly depresses high baseline rates of responding [Wauquier and Niemegeers, 1973]. That rats press the lever at almost equal rates independent of the baseline, and that extinction is delayed, suggests that the effects of apomorphine cannot be attributed to an increased reinforcement, but rather to a response-facilitating effect. Dopamine agonists lacking locomotor-facilitating properties indeed do not facilitate ICS, but again dose-relatedly inhibit the high baseline rates of responding [Wauquier, 1978]. Facilitation is more pronounced with drugs that do not induce stereotype behavior (such as with subcutaneously given cocaine) or release DA, than

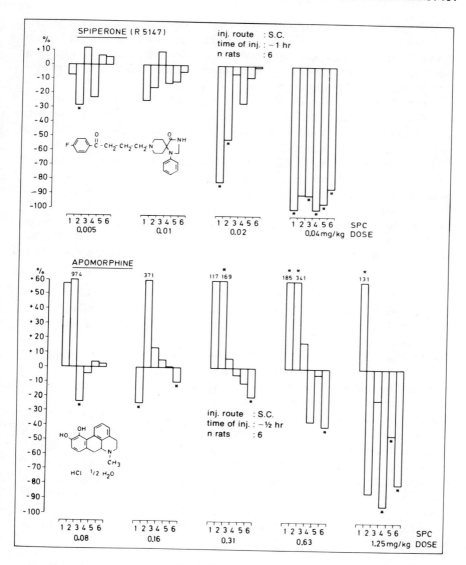

Fig. 1. Self-stimulation response rates (all rats combined) in percentages of the respective control response rates, obtained with different doses (mg/kg) and for each stimulus parameter combination (SPC) with spiperone (top) and apomorphine (bottom). Asterisks indicate significant difference (p ≤ 0.05) as compared to control (Wilcoxon's matched-pairs signed ranks test, one-tailed probability).

with drugs, such as apomorphine, which stimulate DA receptors in a non-stimulus-contingent way. That response enhancement is nevertheless seen is thus most probably due to locomotor facilitation, which results in a higher amount of lever pressing since, in the learned situation, lever pressing has the highest response probability.

The delayed extinction and the response enhancement again demonstrate that activation of the DA system mediates response facilitation; in a noncontingent way, it leads to response inhibition, which might be due to a competition between stereotype behavior and the learned task.

These findings do not totally exclude that apomorphine has additional rewarding effects on its own. In as far as threshold reduction is a measure of enhanced reward, apomorphine might enhance reward through its threshold reducing effect. It has further been shown by Yokel and Wise [1975] that rats self-administer more amphetamine when treated with low doses of the DA blocker pimozide. Thus it cannot be ruled out that response enhancement is a joint effect of locomotor facilitation and inherent rewarding effects.

3. Phenoxybenzamine. In general drugs depleting CA, such as reserpine or alphamethylparatyrosine, produce a strong inhibition of ICS. DA-β-hydroxylase inhibitors, causing a fall in NA, but not in DA, in general do not suppress ICS. Disulfiram, however, also produced an inhibition of ICS, though Roll [1970] reported that this was due to a nonspecific sedation, since arousing the rats made them self-stimulate again.

With phenoxybenzamine (Fig. 2), only a small reduction of ICS was found. Another α-adrenergic antagonist, phentolamine, is more active, causing a nearly 50% reduction of ICS at the very high dose of 40 mg/kg. This effect is also due to a nonspecific sedative action of the compound. A failure of these drugs to effect ICS obtained in the lateral hypothalamus might suggest that other amines are capable of maintaining ICS. This would imply that NA is not important at least for certain self-stimulation sites. One of the only positive experiments in this respect is reported by Wise and Stein [1969]. In their experiments, intraventricular injections of NA reversed the inhibition of ICS produced by disulfiram and diethyldithiocarbamate.

4. Clonidine. The α-agonist clonidine produced a dose-related inhibition of ICS, its calculated ED_{50} value being 0.042 mg/kg. Since clonidine is an α-agonist decreasing the firing rate of NA neurons in the locus coeruleus, it might be suggested that clonidine exerts its effects on ICS by interfering with NA [Schmitt et al, 1979]. However, DA release might also be reduced at the doses inhibiting ICS [Schmitt et al, 1979]. Further, the

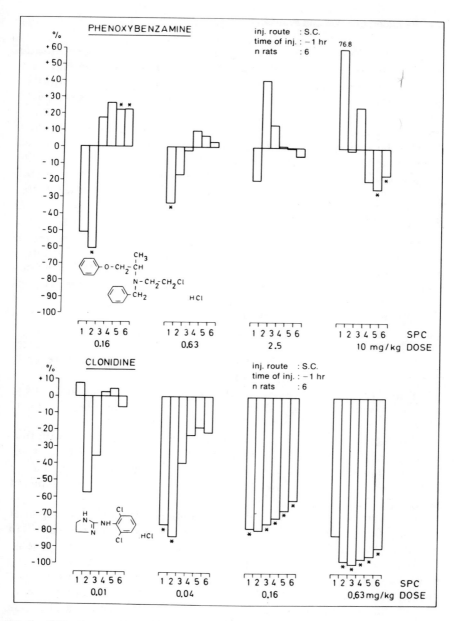

Fig. 2. Self-stimulation response rates (all rats combined) in percentages of the respective control response rates, obtained with different doses (mg/kg) and for each stimulus parameter combination (SPC) with phenoxybenzamine (top) and clonidine (bottom). Asterisks indicate significant difference ($p \leq 0.05$) as compared to control (Wilcoxon's matched-pairs signed ranks test, one-tailed probability).

sedative effects are clearly visible in the behavior so that a nonspecific action is probably involved in the inhibitory effects of clonidine on ICS.

At lower doses, low SPCs are more sensitive toward the inhibitory effects of clonidine. This is in line with the report by Vetulani et al [1977]. They argued, however, that this proves that the decreased responding is not due to a general physical debilitation of the animals. Indeed the animals do press the lever when the stimulation intensity is higher. Again it is logical to conceive that the weak stimulation resulting in low ICS is more sensitive toward behavioral depressant effects, whereas higher stimulation intensities associated with high ICS might antagonize the depressant drug effects.

B. Implantation Site and Species Differences

With neuroleptics site-related effects are reported, but there are as many other reports in which no differences were found in the inhibitory properties of neuroleptics. As discussed before [Wauquier, 1979], the discrepancies found in the literature are possibly due to methodological differences rather than real differences. Important is the fact that independent of the self-stimulation site DA blockers do suppress self-stimulation in all sites tested, although the actual degree of the suppression may differ. These findings strongly support the idea that DA is a necessary transmitter in ICS, even when the electrodes are localized in pure noradrenergic structures such as the locus coeruleus.

In dogs too, ICS is dose-relatedly suppressed by neuroleptics, but at high doses motor inhibitory effects may play an important role [Wauquier, 1979].

With α blockers large discrepancies are found. For instance, with thymoxamine, an α blocker, Herberg et al [1976] reported a suppressing effect on self-stimulation in the locus coeruleus, substantia nigra, and lateral hypothalamus, but others failed to demonstrate inhibitory effects [Lippa et al, 1973].

In dogs trained to respond during a conditioned stimulus [Wauquier et al, 1978] (Fig. 3), the α agonist clonidine dose-relatedly suppressed ICS in the lateral hypothalamus, lateral preoptic region, and nucleus accumbens. On one nucleus accumbens, electrode self-stimulation appeared more sensitive toward the suppressing effects. However, at the dose of 0.04 mg/kg, clonidine exerted variable effects, which are apparently independent of the localization of the electrode. A complete inhibition of ICS is found at the dose of 0.16 mg/kg, which is exclusively due to the strong sedative properties of the compound. The fall in blood pressure at this dose might be involved in the nonspecific suppressing effects.

A differential site-related effect with clonidine was reported by Spencer and Revzin [1976]. In the squirrel monkey, clonidine at the dose of 0.1

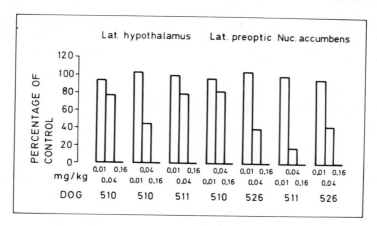

Fig. 3. Self-stimulation response rates in percentages of the respective control response rates obtained with different doses (mg/kg) of clonidine and for three different electrodes in dogs. Dogs were trained to press a lever during a conditioned stimulus (tone of 1,000 Hz) (method described in Wauquier et al [1978]).

mg/kg inhibited lateral hypothalamus ICS but less ICS in the caudate nucleus. This might suggest a more specific effect with the low dose of clonidine. At 0.25 mg/kg, ICS in both sites was suppressed, again because of the sedative effects.

C. Conclusion

Whereas the pharmacological evidence that DA is a necessary transmitter in ICS is strong, the pharmacological evidence that NA is involved in ICS is weak. Independent of the site of stimulation or the species tested, drugs blocking DA transmission do inhibit ICS. Since other positively motivated behavior as well as negatively motivated behavior is suppressed, it is suggested that DA is involved in all operant behavior. Even more, DA appears to be a necessary transmitter for all forms of complex behavior.

Drugs blocking the NA transmission in most cases do not suppress or weakly antagonize ICS, even with electrodes in the cell bodies of the NA dorsal bundle. The α agonist clonidine does suppress ICS in different sites and in the different species tested. Its effects are more pronounced and more reliable than with the α blockers.

Though an indirect action on DA release by clonidine is not excluded, these effects might point toward a more specific action. However, as soon as inhibiting effects become pronounced, nonspecific sedative effects are not ruled out. This would lead to the parsimonious conclusion that the NA system maintains a general arousal level, not specifically related to operant behavior. That ICS can be obtained in the pure noradrenergic locus coeruleus is not sufficiently convincing proof that NA is a necessary transmitter in ICS.

III. ALTERED LEVER-PRESSING SITUATION

Since at certain high dose levels drugs may exert their effect by interfering with the motor system, we thought that this could be made evident in a situation where the work load involved in lever pressing is altered to various degrees. Two different situations were used: Rats were trained to press a lever in 20-minute sessions during which the lever was either positioned low (5 cm above the grid floor) or high (17 cm above the grid floor); other rats were trained to press either a light lever (10-gram force) or a heavy lever (40-gram force). The alteration of the low (L) and high (H) or light and heavy lever was as follows: first week, LHHLH; second week, LLHHL; third week, as in the first week; etc. After training, groups of at least six rats with a mean lever-pressing rate of around 1,000 per 20-minute session were treated with various doses of apomorphine, spiperone, the preferentially NA and serotonergic blocking neuroleptic pipamperone and clonidine, as shown in Figure 4. At least two sessions separated drug treatment, but such that each dose was tested in each of the conditions.

In general, during control sessions there was no significant difference between the lever-pressing rate on the high or low and on the light or heavy lever. This seemed a necessary condition for the present experiments, since different baseline rates of responding would otherwise be a confounding factor for the interpretation of the results.

A. Apomorphine

With apomorphine a dose-related inhibition of lever pressing was found in all conditions. This confirms previous results that showed that high rates of responding are dose-relatedly inhibited by DA agonists [Wauquier, 1978; Wauquier and Niemegeers, 1973] (see above).

The inhibition obtained is similar for the light and the heavy lever situation, but in the low versus high lever situation there are some differences. At the two highest doses tested (0.63 and 2.5 mg/kg), apomorphine significantly depressed more lever pressing when the lever was positioned low. Since at these doses stereotype behavior emerges [Wauquier and Niemegeers, 1973], the present differentiation could be expected. In fact, apomorphine at stereotype doses does facilitate behavior in a horizontal plane such as forward locomotion and sniffing (gnawing only occurs at higher doses), and does not promote rearing. This again demonstrates that

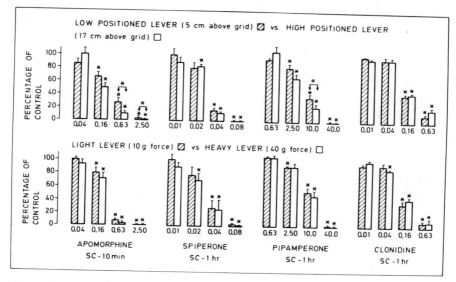

Fig. 4.   Self-stimulation response rates in percentages of the control response rates obtained with different doses of apomorphine, spiperone, pipamperone, and clonidine. Rats pressed either a low (▨) or a high (□) positioned lever (in top) or a light (▨) or a heavy (□) lever (bottom). Asterisks indicate significant difference (p ≤ 0.05) as compared to control (Wilcoxon's matched-pairs signed ranks test, two-tailed probability).

under apomorphine there is a competition between the learned response and the components of the behavior facilitated by apomorphine.

B. Spiperone

With spiperone a dose-related inhibition of lever pressing occurred in the various conditions tested. There was, however, no significant difference between the inhibition on the low vs the high lever situation, nor on the light vs the heavy lever situation. This reinforces the idea that a specific neuroleptic predominantly interferes with stimulus-response contingency, and that the working load involved is not a crucial determinant factor.

C. Pipamperone

With pipamperone a dose-related inhibition of lever pressing occurred in the various conditions tested. This confirms the previously described inhibition of ICS using the classical lever-pressing situation [Wauquier, 1979; Wauquier and Niemegeers, 1972].

There was only a significantly larger inhibition on pressing the high lever than on pressing the low lever at the dose of 10 mg/kg of pipamperone. The inhibition was similar for the other doses and in the other conditions of ICS. Though pipamperone is a sedative neuroleptic, its effects are obvious only at higher doses. At lower doses it also specifically blocks DA receptors, and as such it behaves as spiperone in the present situations.

The significant difference found at one dose might suggest that the sedative properties are more rapidly demonstrated when the rats have to rear up. The difference is, however, small.

D. Clonidine

With clonidine there was a dose-related inhibition of lever pressing on all the conditions tested. The only difference with the other compounds is that the inhibition curve is somewhat more steep in that up to 0.04 mg/kg almost no inhibition is seen, whereas higher doses severely suppress self-stimulation. Because sedation is an important factor in the inhibition of ICS obtained with clonidine, it appears that this nonspecific action is expressed whatever the working load involved. It also demonstrates, however, that the presently used variations may still not be subtle enough to allow a differentiation to be made.

E. Conclusion

In the present experiments, the lever-pressing situation was altered with the aim of allowing a differentiation to be made between a specific effect and a nonspecific effect on the performance capability of the animal. Apart from the effects obtained with apomorphine, no such differentiation could be found with the other drugs. The reason might be that the situation still deals with the very same response leading to the reinforcing brain stimulation.

In a previously described experiment [Wauquier and Niemegeers, 1979] it was found that neuroleptics do suppress self-stimulation more when the required task to obtain brain stimulation was licking than when it was lever pressing. It was then argued that the link task-reinforcer codetermined by the specific task leading to the stimulation was the crucial factor determining the sensitivity toward the neuroleptics. The fact that in the present experiments no differentiation was found indicates that the suppressing effects are rather independent of the working load. Further enhancing the difference in the working load would result in altered baseline rates of responding, which then are known to be differentially sensitive and confound the aim of the present experiment.

IV. RATE-FREE MEASURE OF REWARD

Valenstein [1964] discussed at length various problems related to the interpretation of brain-stimulation reward, since in the normally used lever-pressing situation it appears difficult to separate effects on reward reinforcement from, for instance, performance effects. Valenstein and Meyers [1964] then proposed a rate-independent task. Basically, in this test situation rats are taught to turn on and off brain stimulation by crossing forth and back in a shuttle box. In this test rats learn to initiate ICS by a locomotor response. The latency to initiate ICS (length of time before the rats go to stimulation compartment) is considered an operational definition of reward, whereas the latency to escape ICS (length of time that the brain stimulation is left on) is considered an index of aversion. Atrens and Becker [1975] suggested that both measures are independent of each other. They and other authors [Levitt et al, 1978] suggested that in this shuttle box situation, specific reward effects can be dissociated from nonspecific performance effects.

In our experiments rats were trained to obtain brain stimulation in one part of a two-compartment shuttle box and to turn it off by going to the other part of the cage. The side where brain stimulation could be obtained was randomly varied each minute during 16-minute sessions. The sequence of the left (L)–right (R) part of the cage was as follows: LRRLR, RRLLR, LRRLR, RRLLR.

Rats were implanted in the lateral hypothalamus and trained for approximately 3 weeks in the shuttle box until the responding stabilized. Thereafter they were treated with various doses of haloperidol or clonidine, as shown in Figures 5 and 6.

Two sessions separated each drug treatment or more if responding did not return to the control level. The parameters recorded were: latencies to initiate ICS, latencies to escape ICS, the number of crossings, and the total amount of brain stimulation obtained.

A. Haloperidol

Haloperidol produced a dose-related increase in the latency to initiate ICS, and the latency to escape slightly decreased at the lowest dose (0.01 mg/kg) and was increased to an equal extent with the other doses tested (Fig. 5). The total amount of the stimulation decreased at the two highest doses and the total crossings dose-relatedly decreased.

An increase in the latency to initiate ICS would indicate that the rewarding effect of the stimulation decreased, but since the latency to escape is also increased, together with a decreased total time of stimulation and a decreased number of crossings, a specific effect on reward can be stated only for the lowest dose (0.01 and 0.02 mg/kg). The effects seen at the two highest doses do not allow us to interpret the data in terms of an effect on reward, but rather they point to an effect on the performance.

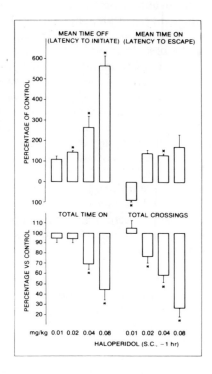

Fig. 5.   Percentage of control obtained with different doses of haloperidol on mean (± SEM) response latencies to initiate and escape hypothalamic brain stimulation, mean (± SEM) total time of stimulation obtained and on mean (±SEM) total number of crossings in a two-way shuttle box. Asterisks indicate significant difference (p ≤ 0.05) as compared to control (Wilcoxon's matched-pairs signed ranks test, one-tailed probability).

B. Clonidine

With clonidine a dose-related increase in the latency to initiate brain stimulation occurred and except for the lowest dose tested, the latency to escape increased, but not dose-relatedly (Fig. 6). The total time of stimulation as well as the number of crossings dose-relatedly decreased. Again the increased latencies to initiate would indicate that the reward is decreased, but because the latency to escape is also increased and both total time and crossings decreased, an interpretation in terms of a specific effect seems

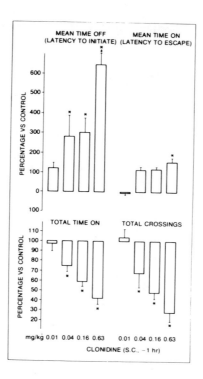

Fig. 6.   Percentage of control obtained with different doses of clonidine on mean (± SEM) response latencies to initiate and escape hypothalamic brain stimulation, mean (± SEM) total time of stimulation obtained and on mean (± SEM) total number of crossings in a two-way shuttle box. Asterisks indicate significant difference (p ≤ 0.05) as compared to control (Wilcoxon's matched-pairs signed ranks test, one-tailed probability).

not warranted. Except for the lowest dose tested, clonidine appears to exert a nonspecific effect, again probably because of its general sedating properties.

C. Discussion

The data from Atrens et al [1976] on haloperidol and those of Hunt et al [1976, 1978] on clonidine corroborate reasonably well with the present results in that, at low doses, both compounds mainly increase the latency to initiate brain stimulation, indicating that the reward is decreased and that higher doses inhibit ICS in a nonspecific way (that is, not directly related to the rewarding properties of the brain stimulation). In the case of haloperidol, cataleptogenic properties, and, in the case of clonidine, sedative properties cannot be eliminated as possible codeterminants or causes of the deficits.

The major differences between the studies of the former authors and our present study are the dose range tested. Atrens et al [1975] even at the lowest dose of 0.025 mg/kg, given IP, obtained an increase in the latency to escape and to initiate brain stimulation. In our experiments, haloperidol at the dose of 0.01 mg/kg, given SC, increased the latency to initiate and decreased the latency to escape brain stimulation. Hunt et al [1976] found specific effects with clonidine with doses ranging from 0.0039 to 0.0625 mg/kg, given IP. The doses we consider to elicit specific effects (between 0.01 and 0.04 mg/kg, given SC) are in the range of their lower doses; higher doses in any case produce a nonspecific sedative effect in a similar way as they obtained with 0.0625 mg/kg given IP.

The nonspecific effect on the performance was demonstrated in another way. The locomotor activity of naive rats was measured in a Doppler motility test system [Vanuytven et al, 1979] during 1 hour after treatment with different doses of clonidine, given SC 1 hour before. The percentage activity versus control, equalized at 100%, is displayed in Figure 7. As seen, a dose-related decrease of the motility was observed, which perfectly paral-

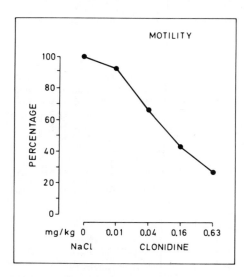

Fig. 7. Percentage activity versus control as measured in the Doppler Motility test [Vanuytven et al, 1979] after different doses of clonidine.

leled the decreased crossings in the rate-free measure of self-stimulation described above.

Though in the shuttle box situation the latency to initiate ICS is a reasonable measure of reward, independent of the locomotor performance, it appears that measuring specific drug effects is rather limited to a very narrow range of doses at the lower end. As soon as the crossings are influenced, it appears that effects on the latencies are seen as well, though the reverse is not necessarily true, at least at very low doses of the drugs tested. Even in a rate-free situation, the required performance to obtain brain stimulation can be a confounding variable, especially with drugs that effect behavior. As such, the rate-free measure of reward currently used has limits in delineating out drug effects on reward.

There appears further a semantic confusing as to what constitutes the reward reinforcement in the rate-free situation. Whereas the time off—that is, the latency to initiate ICS—is considered as an operational definition of reward, some authors consider the opposite as an index of the reward. Crow and Deakin [1966] interpreted the increased stimulation time produced by amphetamine (from the Liebman and Butcher [1974] experiment) as indicating a specific effect on reward. Levitt et al [1978] consider the increase in average on-times produced by morphine as an index of the reinforcement enhancement. Both effects would rather point to a lessened aversion than to an increased reward, since the time on (latency to escape brain stimulation) is a rate independent measure of aversion [Atrens and Becker, 1975]. In the light of other results [Atrens et al, 1974], amphetamine, again at lower doses, would selectively decrease the latency to initiate ICS. That haloperidol at doses that specifically block DA receptors and clonidine as a presynaptic α-adrenergic agonist elicit the same effects poses again the question of which transmitter is specifically involved in brain stimulation reward.

In the experiments by Hunt et al [1978] using the rate-free measure, phenoxybenzamine did not effect ICS, but largely potentiated the inhibition produced by clonidine. Here again, a nonspecific sedative effect was not ruled out. The slight increase in the latency to initiate ICS obtained with clonidine would suggest that there is some specific effect; however, these effects are so small that the validity of the conclusion is doubtful especially when these effects are not proved statistically [Hunt et al, 1976].

Herberg et al [1976] also found that clonidine, irrespective of the self-stimulation site, produced inhibition. In light of these experiments they reached the conclusion that noradrenergic ICS transsynaptically requires a dopaminergic activation. Again one is left with the conclusion that the DA transmission is necessary, whereas the effects on the noradrenergic system would be responsible for a nonspecific sedative effect.

V. ACKNOWLEDGMENT

We sincerely thank David Ashton for his help in the preparation of this paper.

VI. REFERENCES

Atrens DM, Becker FT: Assessing the aversiveness of intracranial stimulation. Psychopharmacologia 44:159–163, 1975.

Atrens DM, Ljundberg T, Ungerstedt U: Modulation of reward and aversion processes in the rat diencephalon by neuroleptics: Differential effects of clozapine and haloperidol. Psychopharmacologia 49:97–100, 1976.

Atrens DM, Von Vietinghoff-Riesch F, Der Karabetian H, Masliyah E: Modulation of reward and aversion processes in the rat diencephalon by amphetamine. Am J Physiol 226:874–880, 1974.

Crow TJ: Catecholamine-containing neurones and electrical self-stimulation. Part 1 (a review of some data). Psychol Med 2:414–421, 1972.

Crow TJ, Deakin JFW: Brain reinforcement centers and psychoactive drugs. In Israel Y, Glaser FB, Kalant H (eds): "Research Advances in Alcohol and Drug Problems," Vol. 2. New York: Plenum, 1966, pp 25–76.

Dresse A: Importance du système mésencéphalo-télencéphalique noradrénergique comme substratum anatomique du comportement d'autostimulation. Life Sci 5:1003–1004, 1966.

Fouriezos G, Wise RA: Pimozide-induced extinction of intracranial self-stimulation response patterns rule out motor or performance deficits. Brain Res 103:377–380, 1976.

Herberg LJ, Stephens DN, Franklin KBJ: Catecholamines and self-stimulation: Evidence suggesting a reinforcing role for noradrenaline and a motivating role for dopamine. Pharmacol Biochem Behav 4:575–582, 1976.

Hunt GE, Atrens DM, Chesher G, Becker FT: α-Noradrenergic modulation of hypothalamic self-stimulation: Studies employing clonidine, 1-phenylephrine and α-methyl-p-tyrosine. Eur J Pharmacol 37:105–111, 1976.

Hunt GE, Atrens DM, Becker FT, Paxinos G: α-Adrenergic modulation of hypothalamic self-stimulation: Effects of phenoxybenzamine, yokumbine, dexamphatamine and their interactions with clonidine. Eur J Pharmacol 53:1–8, 1978.

Huston JR, Borbély AA: Operant conditioning in forebrain ablurted rats by use of rewarding hypothalamic stimulation. Brain Res 50:467–472, 1973.

Levitt RA, Stilwell DJ, Evers TM: Morphine and shuttle box self-stimulation in the rat: Tolerance studies. Pharmacol Biochem Behav 9:567–569, 1978.

Liebman JM, Butcher LL: Comparative involvement of dopamine and noradrenaline in rate-free self-stimulation in substantia nigra, lateral hypothalamus and mesencephalic central gray. Naunyn-Schmiedeberg's Arch Pharmacol 284:167–194, 1974.

Lippa AS, Antelman SM, Fisher AE, Canfield DR: Neurochemical mediation of reward: A significant role for dopamine. Pharmacol Biochem Behav 1:23–28, 1973.

Niemegeers CJE, Verbruggen FJ, Wauquier A, Janssen PAJ: The influence of haloperidol and amphetamine on two different noise-escape situations in rats. Psychopharmacologia 25:22–31, 1972.

Olds J, Milner P: Positive reinforcement produced by electrical stimulation of septal area and other regions of the rat brain. J Comp Physiol Psychol 47:419–427, 1954.

Roll SK: Intracranial self-stimulation and wakefulness: Effects of manipulating ambient brain catecholamines. Science 168:1370–1372, 1970.

Schmitt H, Schmitt-Jubeau H, Daskalopoulos NT: Central mechanisms of clonidine. TIPS, November, 71–73, 1979.

Spencer J, Revzin A: Amphetamine, chlorpromazine and clonidine effects on self-stimulation in caudate or hypothalamus of the squirrel monkey. Pharmacol Biochem Behav 5:149–156, 1976.

Stein L: Self-stimulation of the brain and the central stimulant action of amphetamine. Fed Proc 23:836–850, 1964a.

Stein L: Reciprocal actions of reward and punishment mechanisms. In Heath RG (ed): "The Role of Pleasure in Behavior." New York: Harper and Row, 1964b, pp 113–119.

Valenstein ES: Problems of measurement and interpretation with reinforcing brain-stimulation. Psychol Rev 71:415–437, 1964.

Valenstein ES, Meyers WJ: Rate-independent test of reinforcing consequences of brain-stimulation. J Comp Physiol Psychol 57:52–60, 1964.

Vanuytven M, Vermeire J, Niemegeers CJE: A new motility meter based on the Doppler principle. Psychopharmacologia 64:333–336, 1979.

Vetulani J, Leith NJ, Stawarz RJ, Sulser F: Effects of clonidine on the noradrenergic cyclic AMP generating system in the limbic forebrain and on medial forebrain bundle self-stimulation behavior. Experientia 33:1490–1491, 1977.

Wauquier A: The influence of psychoactive drugs on brain self-stimulation: A review. In Wauquier A, Rolls ET (eds): "Brain-Stimulation Reward." Amsterdam: North-Holland, 1976, pp 123–170.

Wauquier A: Differential actions of dopamine agonists on brain self-stimulation behavior in rats. Arch Int Pharmacodyn Ther 236:325–328, 1978.

Wauquier A: Neuroleptics and brain self-stimulation behavior. Int Rev Neurobiol 21:335–403, 1979.

Wauquier A: The pharmacology of catecholamine involvement in the neural mechanisms of reward. Acta Neurobiol Exp 40:665–686, 1980.

Wauquier A, Niemegeers CJE: Intracranial self-stimulation in rats as a function of various stimulus parameters. II. The influence of haloperidol, pimozide and pipamperone on medial forebrain bundle stimulation with monopolar electrodes. Psychopharmacologia 27:191–202, 1972.

Wauquier A, Niemegeers CJE: Intracranial self-stimulation in rats as a function of various stimulus parameters. III. The influence of apomorphine on medial forebrain bundle stimulation with monopolar electrodes. Psychopharmacologia 30:163–172, 1973.

Wauquier A, Niemegeers CJE: Intracranial self-stimulation in rats as a function of various stimulus parameters. IV. The influence of amphetamine on medial forebrain bundle stimulation with monopolar electrodes. Psychopharmacologia 34:265–274, 1974a.

Wauquier A, Niemegeers CJE: Intracranial self-stimulation in rats as a function of various stimulus parameters. V. The influence of cocaine on medial forebrain bundle stimulation with monopolar electrodes. Psychopharmacologia 38:201–210, 1974b.

Wauquier A, Niemegeers CJE: A comparison between lick- or lever-pressing contingent reward and the effects of neuroleptics thereon. Arch Int Pharmacodyn Ther 239:230–240, 1979.

Wauquier A, Rolls ET (eds): "Brain-Stimulation Reward." Amsterdam: North-Holland, 1976, pp 622.

Wauquier A, Niemegeers CJE, Geivers HA: Intracranial self-stimulation in rats as a function of various stimuli parameters. I. An empirical study with monopolar electrodes in the medial forebrain bundle. Psychopharmacologia 23:238–260, 1972.

Wauquier A, Melis W, Niemegeers CJE, Janssen PAJ: A putative multipartite model of haloperidol interaction in apomorphine, disturbed behavior in the dog. Psychopharmacologia 59:255–258, 1978.

Wise RA, Stein L: Facilitation of brain self-stimulation by central administration of norepinephrine. Science 163:299–301, 1969.

Yokel RA, Wise RA: Increased lever-pressing for amphetamine after pimozide in rats: Implications for a dopamine theory of reward. Science 187:547–549, 1975.

Psychopharmacology of Clonidine, pages 197–210

Hyperphagia and Weight Gain in Monkeys Treated With Clonidine

R. Francis Schlemmer, Jr., Regina C. Casper, Janice K. Elder, and John M. Davis

Acute or chronic administration of clonidine has been shown to affect a number of physiological and behavioral parameters, but few studies have been concerned with the effect of clonidine on feeding. This is somewhat surprising since central noradrenergic systems have long been implicated in the regulation of hunger and eating behavior [Grossman, 1975; Hoebel, 1977]. To date, the effect of clonidine on eating has been formally studied in only four species — rats, dogs, rabbits, and, in the present study, monkeys.

We will describe a series of experiments that explored the effect of clonidine on the feeding and drinking of stump-tailed macaque monkeys and the pharmacologic mechanisms regulating this effect.

I. METHODS AND RESULTS

A. Experiment 1: Dose-Dependent Effects of Clonidine on Eating Behavior of Monkeys

The pronounced effect of clonidine on the eating behavior of stump-tailed macaques was initially discovered during an experimental study of the effect of clonidine on the social and solitary behavior of primates. In the study, two selected members of a stable social colony of four adult stump-tailed macaques (Macaca arctoides) were acutely treated with six doses of clonidine. After these monkeys had received each of the six clonidine doses, the two previously untreated monkeys received a similar clonidine treatment in a crossover design. The clonidine doses range from 0.003 to 1.0 mg/kg (all doses refer to the HCl salt) and were given intramuscularly. Only one clonidine dose was given per day, and 48 hours separated each clonidine dosing of the same animal. Saline was administered IM to all four animals before the initiation of drug treatment to establish baseline levels. Also, those monkeys that did not receive the drug on a given day were given a saline injection at the same time as the other animals received their clonidine injection.

A behavioral observation of 1 hour began 15 minutes after the saline or drug injection. During this time, an experienced primate observer who was unaware of the drug treatment schedule quantified and recorded the behavior of all animals in the colony with reference to a checklist of 48 social, solitary, and abnormal types of behavior of this species, using the focal sampling technique. Each monkey in the colony was observed in rotation for a 30-second period every 5 minutes during 1 hour.

The colony received a generous supply of food (Purina Monkey Chow) each morning approximately 2 hours prior to treatment so that they had completed their morning feeding before the observation session, with an abundant supply of food remaining available during observation. Water was continuously available for 24 hours a day throughout the study. All data were statistically analyzed by a three-way partially crossed analysis of variance (ANOVA) and by the least-significant-difference method for comparing means.

As the clonidine dose was increased, the treated animals became engrossed in eating in preference to interaction with other members of the colony. The dose-dependent effect of clonidine on eating can be seen in the "chew food" category (Fig. 1). Clonidine-treated monkeys showed a significant increase above baseline levels in the number of 30-second periods in which they were observed chewing food in doses of 0.01–1.0 mg/kg. It appeared that clonidine increased the food intake. Clonidine also caused a significant increase in another food-related category, "handle food." Surprisingly, drinking was *not* increased.

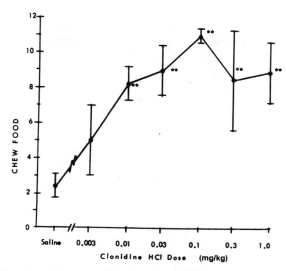

Fig. 1. Dose-dependent effect of clonidine on eating behavior of monkeys. Each point represents the mean ± standard error of the mean (SEM) for chew food for four monkeys at each dose. A monkey received a score of 1 for each 30-second scoring period in the 1-hour observation period during which the observer found the animal chewing food. A statistically significant difference from saline is indicated as ** = P < 0.01.

The activity of clonidine-treated monkeys primarily centered around eating, which resulted in significant changes in several other behavioral categories. In general, social interaction was decreased from baseline levels as exemplified by a significant decrease in total initiated social activity by treated monkeys during clonidine administration. Clonidine significantly increased vocalizations at doses greater than 0.01 mg/kg. These were primarily the high-pitched "food cries" typical of this species. In addition, ptosis was noted in all clonidine-treated monkeys at doses of 0.1–1.0 mg/kg.

B. Experiment 2: Effect of Clonidine on Food Intake and Weight of Individually Caged Monkeys

To verify the impression gained in the first experiment, we performed Experiment 2 to examine the effect of repeated clonidine administration on individually housed adult stump-tailed macaques whose daily food intake could be measured and for each of which an equal access to food was assured.

Ten monkeys (six females, four males), none of which had been subjects in Experiment 1, were divided into two groups of two males and three females each for the experiment. Each monkey was housed in a Harford cage (0.5 m × 1.0 m × 1.0 m), which had a continuous water supply. The animals received food from a standard feeder attached to the outside of each cage.

Each monkey was weighed daily at 8 a.m., beginning 3 days before the treatment (baseline) and throughout the saline and drug treatment periods. After the weighing, each monkey received a continuous supply of food (Purina Monkey Chow biscuits) throughout the day. The food was offered in 250-gm rations, beginning immediately after weighing (about 8:30 a.m.), the last ration being offered at 4 p.m. Any biscuits remaining in the cage or feeder the next morning were weighed and discarded at the morning weighing. This weight was then subtracted from the weight of the biscuits offered during the previous day to obtain the total food intake for that day. Since the biscuits were much larger than the mesh openings of the cage, floor spillage was negligible.

The experiment was divided into two 7-day treatment periods. During the first 7 days, Group I received saline, 0.05 cc/kg, and Group II received clonidine HCl, 0.1 mg/kg, once daily at 10:30 a.m. The, during the second week, Group I received clonidine and Group II received saline for 7 days in a crossover design. Saline and clonidine were both administered intramuscularly. A three-way partially crossed ANOVA and the least-significant-difference method were used to determine the statistical significance of all data.

Clonidine induced a significant increase in daily food intake in both groups when compared with their respective saline treatment periods (Table I). Note that all ten monkeys increased their food consumption while on clonidine. Typically, clonidine-treated monkeys began eating approximately 10 minutes after the drug injection. In most cases, these animals stuffed their pouches to maximum capacity (Fig. 2) and continued to eat for approximately 2 hours. By contrast, saline-treated monkeys showed only a casual interest in eating, if any, after injection. Interestingly, from day 2 through day 7, monkeys undergoing clonidine treatment were notably less interested in eating immediately after the initial morning feeding (8:30 a.m.) than saline-treated animals, which consumed the majority of their food intake at this time.

The clonidine-induced increase in food intake resulted in weight gain in eight of the ten monkeys by the end of the 7-day treatment period (Table II). Seven of these eight monkeys had an increase in body weight of at least 0.5 kg. Placed in perspective, this represents a 5-16% weight gain in only 1 week.

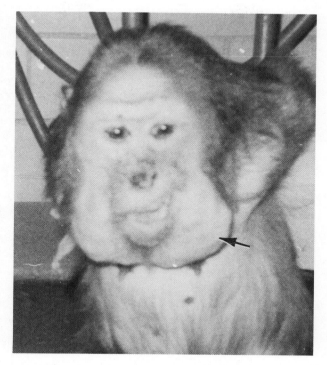

Fig. 2. A stump-tailed macaque female 30 minutes after injection of clonidine HCl, 0.1 mg/kg. Note that her pouches are filled to capacity with monkey biscuits (arrow).

C. Experiment 3: Effect of Clonidine on Water Intake in Monkeys

Although Experiment 1 suggested that clonidine treatment does not alter drinking behavior, a quantitative measurement of water intake could not be made in Experiment 2, and therefore the contribution of water intake to the weight gain seen in the previous experiment remained unknown. So the effect of clonidine on drinking was assessed at a later time in three of the monkeys (one male, #1862; two females, #823 and #1295) that had gained more than 0.5 kg during clonidine administration in Experiment 2. For this experiment, each monkey was individually housed in slightly larger cages equipped with an outside feeder and water bottles with standard spouts to allow measurement of water intake.

Table I. Effect of Clonidine on Food Intake in Monkeys

Monkeys	Week 1	Week 2
Group I	Saline	Clonidine
1,513 ♀	120.71 ± 18.97 gm/day	259.29 ± 16.56 gm/day
823 ♀	490.00 ± 60.91	561.43 ± 56.80
3,531 ♀	249.29 ± 18.40	348.57 ± 17.92
1,504 ♂	271.43 ± 26.04	481.43 ± 52.89
1,862 ♂	424.29 ± 62.71	519.29 ± 50.34
Group I	311.14 ± 28.76 gm/day	434.00 ± 26.40 gm/day**
Group II	Clonidine	Saline
3,428 ♀	370.00 ± 33.09 gm/day	28.57 ± 6.70 gm/day
1,295 ♀	530.00 ± 69.73	120.00 ± 13.45
3,535 ♀	495.71 ± 42.53	208.57 ± 30.03
3,513 ♂	341.43 ± 55.01	172.86 ± 18.74
716 ♂	301.43 ± 50.40	231.43 ± 18.57
Group II	407.71 ± 26.55 gm/day**	152.29 ± 14.78 gm/day

Total Group: Saline, 231.72 ± 18.68 gm/day
Clonidine, 420.86 ± 18.65 gm/day**

Each value represents the mean daily food intake ± SEM during each week of Experiment 2.
** = $P < 0.01$ vs respective saline treatment.

Because monkey biscuits are dry and salty, the increased food intake induced by clonidine could conceivably lead to a secondary increase in water intake. In order to investigate this possibility, the experiment was run both with and without food restriction. Each monkey received acutely three injections of clonidine, 0.1 mg/kg, both with and without food restriction. Each animal also received an equal number of sham injections of saline under each experimental condition. During the *food restriction* part of the experiment, each monkey was offered 250 gm of monkey biscuits at 8:30 a.m. At 10:30 a.m., any remaining biscuits were removed from the feeders and the cages and discarded. No food was given to these animals until 8:30 the next morning. Immediately after removal of the food, all three monkeys received an intramuscular injection of clonidine or saline. During the *food ad lib* part of the experiment, the monkeys had continuous access to food as described in Experiment 2. As before, each animal received an injection of clonidine or saline at 10:30 a.m.

All monkeys had continuous access to water throughout both parts of the experiment. The water intake was measured and recorded, and the water bottles were refilled at 8:30 a.m., 10:30 a.m., and 3 p.m. daily. The results

Table II. Weight Change After Clonidine Treatment

	Monkeys	Weight change	% Change
Females	1,513	+0.20 kg	2.4%
	823	+0.60	6.4%
	3,531	+0.95	11.5%
	3,428	+0.53	5.6%
	1,295	+0.80	10.4%
	3,535	+1.25	15.4%
Males	1,504	+1.20	9.0%
	1,862	+1.80	15.8%
	3,513	+0.03	0.3%
	716	-0.23	1.9%

were analyzed by two-way ANOVA and the least-significant-difference method.

The effect of clonidine on water intake is show in Figure 3. The results are shown as the effect of clonidine on 24-hour water intake, which has direct relevance to Experiment 2, and also as the effect during the first 4½ hours (10:30 a.m. − 3 p.m.) after clonidine injection, which is a slightly longer period than the duration of clonidine-induced eating. With continuous access to food, clonidine induced a nonsignificant decrease in the mean 24-hour water intake, verifying the impression gained from Experiment 1. With food restriction, clonidine significantly decreased the 24-hour water intake. The clonidine-induced reduction in drinking is even more evident from the water intake during the first 4½ hours after injection, when their water intake was decreased with and without food restriction. Since the duration of action of clonidine on food intake was comprised within this period, it is assumed that the direct effect of clonidine on water intake is represented by these latter results. It may be inferred from the 24-hour water intake data that water intake did not contribute to the weight gain seen with clonidine in Experiment 2.

D. Experiment 4: Evidence for α_2-Noradrenergic Receptor Mediation of Clonidine Hyperphagia

Although clonidine-induced hyperphagia is presumably mediated by α-noradrenergic receptors, the effect could be mediated by either postsynaptic facilitation or presynaptic inhibition of noradrenergic

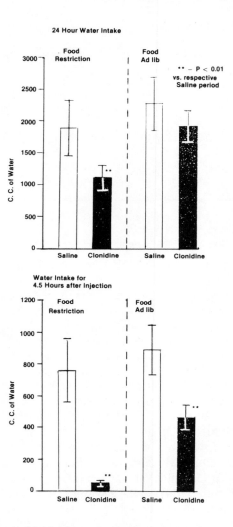

Fig. 3. Effect of clonidine on drinking in monkeys with and without food restriction. Each bar represents the mean ± SEM water intake in three monkeys that received saline or clonidine HCl, 0.1 mg/kg, with food either restricted to 250 gm/day food restriction or allowed ad lib. Each monkey acutely received three injections of drug and saline under each condition. The top graph depicts the 24-hour water intake, and the bottom graph the water intake during the first 4½ hours after injection. A statistically significant difference from the respective saline treatment is shown as ** = P < 0.01.

transmission [Anden et al, 1976; Cedarbaum and Aghajanian, 1977; Starke, 1977]. In the next experiment we attempted to elucidate this mechanism. We tested two α-adrenergic antagonists, prazosin and yohimbine, for their effect on clonidine-induced hyperphagia. Prazosin is believed to block α_1-receptors preferentially [Cambridge et al, 1977; Doxey et al, 1977; U'Prichard et al, 1978] and yohimbine is thought to block α_2-receptors preferentially [Starke et al, 1975; Anden et al, 1976].

The methods used for housing, feeding, and weighing the monkeys were identical to those used in Experiment 2. However, in this experiment, 12 adult stump-tailed macaques (four males, eight females) served as subjects. The study comprised six 1-week periods in each of which all monkeys received drug or saline treatment on Monday, Tuesday, and Wednesday, with the remaining four days serving as drug "washout" days. On the treatment days each monkey received either saline, yohimbine, or prazosin at 10:15 a.m., followed by saline or clonidine at 10:30 a.m. Saline and all drugs were administered intramuscularly in the following doses: clonidine 0.1 mg/kg, yohimbine 5 mg/kg, and prazosin 0.1 mg/kg. All drug doses refer to the hydrochlorides. Yohimbine and prazosin doses were determined in pilot studies with other monkeys. The experiment began with two monkeys from the group receiving one of the six treatment combinations (saline + saline, saline + clonidine, yohimbine + saline, yohimbine + clonidine, prazosin + saline, prazosin + clonidine) during the first week. The animals were then rotated through the six treatment combinations during the 6-week period so that by the end of the experiment all the monkeys had received each of the different treatments. However, treatment was discontinued in one female before the completion of the experiment on the advice of a primate veterinarian because of infection unrelated to the study. All data from this animal were disregarded. The 11 remaining monkeys did successfully complete the experiment. All data from these animals were analyzed by a two-way ANOVA (monkey × treatment periods) and the least-significant-difference method for comparing means.

As before, clonidine treatment (saline + clonidine) led to a significant increase in food intake over baseline levels (saline + saline) (Table III). Prazosin *failed* to antagonize the clonidine effect, but yohimbine significantly antagonized the increase in food intake after clonidine. Neither prazosin alone nor yohimbine alone significantly changed the food intake as compared with baseline levels.

The changes in body weight noted at the completion of each treatment were consistent with the changes in food intake that were associated with treatments. As expected, clonidine induced a significant weight gain (Fig. 4). Yohimbine prevented the weight gain otherwise induced by clonidine;

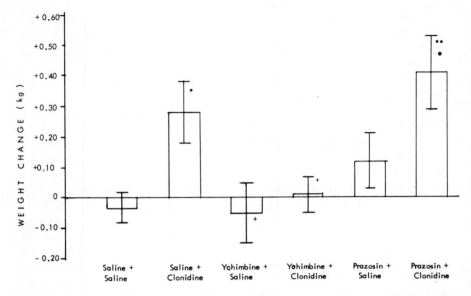

Fig. 4. Change in body weight of monkeys after treatment with selected alpha-adrenergic agents for 3 days. Each bar represents the mean ± SEM change in body weight in kilograms for 11 adult stump-tailed macaques that completed all six drug treatments. Weight change was determined by subtracting the weight of each individual animal immediately before each treatment period from the weight of the animal after the third treatment day. Statistical significance of the difference from saline + saline (baseline) is shown as * = P< 0.05 or ** = P < 0.01; for the comparison with saline + clonidine, + = P < 0.05; and • = P < 0.05 for comparison with prazosin + saline.

Table III. Effect of α-Noradrenergic Antagonists and Clonidine on Food Intake in Monkeys

Treatment	Daily food intake
Saline + saline	235.76 ± 27.61 gm/day
Saline + clonidine	322.58 ± 35.52[a]
Yohimbine + saline	182.7 ± 22.37[b]
Yohimbine + clonidine	182.12 ± 21.70[b]
Prazosin + saline	218.18 ± 24.24[b]
Prazosin + clonidine	335.45 ± 25.04[a,c]

[a]P < 0.01 when compared with saline + saline.
[b]P < 0.01 when compared with saline + clonidine.
[c]P < 0.01 when compared with prazosin + saline.

prazosin did not. The weight gain with prazosin + clonidine was also significantly greater than the weight change after prazosin alone. Yohimbine alone did not alter body weight significantly.

II. DISCUSSION

The results of this study have shown that the α-noradrenergic agonist clonidine induces a dose-dependent increase in food intake in primates. The hyperphagia induced by clonidine subsequently resulted in a substantial weight gain of short duration in most of the treated monkeys. These findings are consistent with those reported for lower species. Most investigators found clonidine to increase food intake in satiated rats when administered intracerebrally [Broekkamp and van Rossum, 1972; Ritter et al, 1975] or peripherally [Pfister et al, 1978; Mauron et al, 1980]. However, LeDouarec et al [1972] found a reduction in food intake after oral administration of clonidine. The same investigators reported a dose-dependent biphasic effect of oral clonidine on eating in dogs with lower doses (0.05–0.75 mg/kg) increasing and higher doses (1–4 mg/kg) decreasing food intake [LeDouarec et al, 1972]. In rabbits, clonidine stimulated feeding immediately after injection [Waller and O'Donnell, submitted for publication]. Thus clonidine (in doses lower than 1 mg/kg) has been shown to increase food intake in several species. Unfortunately, systematic studies of the effect of clonidine on eating humans are lacking.

Since clonidine did not increase water intake and in some cases decreased it, it is unlikely that fluid intake could account for the weight gain seen with clonidine treatment. This finding is in agreement with the results of LeDouarec et al [1971], who found that clonidine reduced water intake in water-deprived rats. It is indeed unusual to find a drug that increases food intake, induces diuresis, and decreases salivation, yet at the same time reduces water intake. This suggests that clonidine exerts a strong central inhibitory effect on drinking.

Central noradrenergic systems are known to play an important role in the mediation of feeding behavior. This mediation appears to be a complex process [Grossman, 1975; Hoebel, 1977; Garattini and Samanin, 1978]. Both inhibition [Redmond et al, 1977a] and facilitation [Liebowitz, 1978] of noradrenergic transmission have been implicated in the stimulation of feeding. Since clonidine can act to inhibit or facilitate noradrenergic transmission, either mechanism could be responsible for the hyperphagia seen in monkeys. Inasmuch as yohimbine, a selective α_2-receptor-blocking agent, totally antagonized both clonidine-induced hyperphagia and weight gain, whereas prazosin, a selective α_1-receptor blocker, did not, α_2-noradrenergic receptors are involved in the mediation of both effects [Schlemmer et al, 1981]. It may be argued that the yohimbine dose used in this study (5 mg (salt)/kg) could cause α_1-blockade in addition to α_2-receptor blockade. This is unlikely, however. Gold et al [1979] found that 2.5 mg/kg of yohimbine given intravenously produced a rapid and significant increase in serum prolactin levels in male stump-tailed macaques. The investigators proposed antagonism of α_2-noradrenergic receptors as a possible explanation for this effect since similar results were obtained with piperoxan (2.5 mg/kg), another preferential α_2-antagonist. A lower dose of yohimbine (1 mg/kg) failed to elicit this response, suggesting that 2.5 mg/kg may be the minimally effective yohimbine dose for central α_2-noradrenergic receptor blockade in this species. In pilot studies for Experiment 4, yohimbine doses of 1 mg/kg and lower were also ineffective in antagonizing clonidine-induced eating. The difference between the 2.5 mg/kg dose in the Gold et al [1979] study and the 5 mg/kg dose in our study could be attributed to the different routes of administration in the two studies — intravenous and intramuscular.

The results of Experiment 4 may be further confounded by sedative effects of the agents used. Could synergistic or additive sedative effects of a particular combination of antagonist + clonidine lead to a reduction in eating? Clearly, at the doses used in the study, prazosin and clonidine caused the most sedation. Yet the animals ate more (Table III) and gained the most weight (Fig. 4) during prazosin + clonidine treatment. Moreover, the treated monkeys showed no significant reduction in food intake and no significant weight loss during any of the treatment periods. The nonsignificant decrease in food intake seen with yohimbine alone and yohimbine + clonidine may reflect a slight nonspecific sedative effect, but it could just as easily be explained as the result of α_2-receptor blockade by yohimbine, which facilitates the release of norepinephrine [Anden et al, 1976].

Stimulation of α_2-receptors by agonists such as clonidine is believed to lead to an inhibition of norepinephrine release [Starke, 1977]. Biochemical [Braestrup, 1974; Anden et al, 1976; Maas et al, 1976] and electrophysiological [Svensson et al, 1975; Cedarbaum and Agnajanian, 1977; Huang et al, 1977] evidence from this and other species suggests that clonidine is a potent α_2-agonist inhibiting noradrenergic transmission. The results of experiment 4 clearly point to decreased noradrenergic transmission as the mechanism responsible for the hyperphagia in clonidine-treated monkyes.

Additional evidence for α_2-receptor mediation of clonidine hyperphagia comes from other primate studies in which hyperphagia resulted from anatomical disruption of noradrenergic pathways. Discrete bilateral lesions of the locus coeruleus caused profound hyperphagia and weight gain in this species [Redmond et al, 1977b;]. Furthermore, the weight gain correlated significantly with a reduction in cerebral mantle levels of 3-methoxy-4-hydroxy-phenylethylene glycol (MHPG), a major CNS metabolite of norepinephrine. Hyperphagia has also been reported in rhesus monkeys (Macaca mulatta) following disconnection of the ventral medial hypothalamus (VMH) regions by knife cut [McHugh et al, 1975]. A disruption of catecholamine function was also involved in this last study, for these monkeys were more resistant to the anorexic effects of amphetamine than the controls, which had not had this operation.

Aside from the theoretical implications of the present study, the results may be of clinical interest as well. The appetite-stimulating effect of clonidine may be of therapeutic benefit in the treatment of eating disorders. Conversely, a difference in eating response to clonidine between normal controls and patients with eating disorders could conceivably provide important clues to a neurochemical dysfunction underlying such disorders.

III. ACKNOWLEDGMENTS

This work was conducted at the University of Illinois Biologic Resources Laboratory, Chicago. The authors thank Mr. Wonnie Jones, Mr. Willie Sanford, and Frank Z. Beluhan, DVM, for their valuable technical assistance throughout the study; Boehringer-Ingelheim, Ltd, Elmsford, New York, and Pfizer, Inc, Groton, Connecticut, for the generous supplies of clonidine and prazosin powders, respectively.

IV. REFERENCES

Anden NE, Grabowska M, Strombom U: Different alpha-adrenoceptors in the central nervous system mediating biochemical and functional effects of clonidine and receptor blocking agents. Naunyn-Schmiedeberg's Arch Pharmacol 292:43–52, 1976.

Braestrup C: Effects of phenoxybenzamine, aceperone, and clonidine on the level of 3-methoxy-4-hydroxyphenylglycol (MOPEC) in rat brain. J Pharm Pharmacol 26:139–141, 1974.

Broekkamp C, van Rossum JM: Clonidine induced intrahypothalamic stimulation of eating in rats. Psychopharmacologia 25:162–68, 1972.

Cambridge D, Davey MJ, Massingham R: Prazosin, a selective antagonist of post-synaptic alpha-adrenoceptors. Br J Pharmacol 59:514P–515P, 1977.

Cedarbaum JM, Aghajanian GK: Catecholamine receptors on locus coeruleus neurons: Pharmacological characterization. Eur J Pharmacol 44:375–385, 1977.

Doxey JC, Smith CFC, Walker JM: Selectivity of blocking agents for pre- and post-synaptic alpha-adrenoceptors. Br J Pharmacol 60:91–96, 1977.

Garattini S, Samanin R: Central mechanisms of anorectic drugs. New York: Raven Press, 1978.

Gold MS, Donabedian RK, Redmond DE Jr: Further evidence for alpha-2 adrenergic receptor mediated inhibition of prolactin secretion: The effect of yohimbine. Psychoneuroendocrinology 3:253–260, 1979.

Grossman SP: Role of the hypothalamus in the regulation of food and water intake. Psychol Rev 82:200–224, 1975.

Hoebel BG: The psychopharmacology of feeding. In Iversen LL, Iversen SD, Snyder SH (eds):"Handbook of Psychopharmacology," Vol. 8. New York: Plenum Press, 1977, pp 55–129.

Huang YH, Maas JW, Redmond DE Jr: Evidence for noradrenergic specificity of behavioral effects of electrical stimulation of the nucleus locus coeruleus. Neurosci, Abstr 3:251, 1977.

LeDouarec JC, Schmitt H, Lucet B: Effect of clonidine and alpha-sympathomimetics on water intake in rats deprived of water. J Pharmacol (Paris) 2:435–444, 1971.

LeDouarec JC, Schmitt H, Lucet B: Effects of clonidine and of alpha-sympathomimetic agents of food intake. Antagonism by adrenolytics. J Pharmacol (Paris) 3:187–198, 1972.

Leibowitz SF: Paraventricular nucleus: A primary site mediating adrenergic stimulation of feeding and drinking. Pharmacol Biochem Behav 8:163–175, 1978.

Maas JW, Hattox SE, Landis DH, Roth RH: The determination of a brain arteriovenous difference for 3-methoxy-4-hydroxyphenethyleneglycol (MHPG). Brian Res 118:167–173, 1976.

Mauron C, Wurtman JJ, Wurtman RJ: Clonidine increases food and protein consumption in rats. Life Sci 27:781–791, 1980.

McHugh PR, Gibbs J, Falasco JD, Moran T, Smith GP: Inhibitions on feeding examined in rhesus monkeys with hypothalamic disconnexions. Brain 98:441–454, 1975.

Pfister WR, Yau ET, Mennear JH, Yim GKW: Comparison of appetite stimulation by chlordiazepoxide, chlordimeform, clonidine, and cyproheptadine in rats. Fed Proc 37:860, 1978.

Redmond DE Jr, Huang YH, Baulu J, Snyder DR, Maas JW: Norepinephrine and satiety in monkeys. In Vigersky RA (ed): "Anorexia Nervosa." New York: Raven Press, 1977b, pp 81–96.

Redmond DE Jr, Huang YH, Snyder DR, Maas JW: Hyperphagia and hyperdipsia after locus coeruleus lesions in ten stump-tailed monkeys. Life Sci 20:1619–1628, 1977a.

Ritter S, Wise CD, Stein L: Neurochemical regulation of feeding in the rat: Facilitation by α-noradrenergic, but not dopaminergic, receptor stimulants. J Comp Physiol Psych 88:778–784, 1975.

Schlemmer RF Jr, Elder JK, Casper RC, Davis JM: Clonidine-induced hyperphagia in monkeys: Evidence for α_2-noradrenergic receptor mediation. Psychopharmacology 73:99–100, 1981.

Starke K: Regulation of noradrenaline release by presynaptic recepetor systems. Rev Physiol Biochem Pharmacol 77:2–124, 1977.

Starke K, Borowski E, Endo T: Preferential blockade or presynaptic alpha-adrenoceptors by yohimbine. Eur J Pharmacol 34:385, 1975.

Svensson TH, Bunney BS, Aghajanian GK: Inhibition of both noradrenergic and serotonergic neurons in brain by the alpha-adrenergic agonist clonidine. Brian Res 92:291–306, 1975.

U'Prichard DC, Charness ME, Robertson D, Snyder SH: Prazosin: Differential affinities for two populations of alpha-noradrenergic receptor binding sites. Eur J Pharmacol 50:87–89, 1978.

Waller DP, O'Donnell A: Clonidine induced hyperphagia in rabbits. Submitted for publication, 1980.

Psychopharmacology of Clonidine, pages 211–223

Clonidine in Korsakoff Disease: Pathophysiologic and Therapeutic Implications

William J. McEntee, Robert G. Mair, and Philip J. Langlais

I. INTRODUCTION

Investigations into the biologic derangements underlying human memory disorders are often hampered by the progressive and variable nature of the illness and other associated cognitive and intellectual impairments. An evaluation of potential therapeutic agents for alleviation of the memory disorder is complicated by the same factors. Patients afflicted with the characteristic memory disorder of the Wernicke-Korsakoff syndrome provide a human model of disordered memory that is relatively stable in its course after chronicity is established, homogeneous in its clinical pattern, varying only in severity, and not significantly complicated by the presence of other impaired higher cortical functions [Talland, 1965; Victor et al, 1971]. This does not mean that the underlying cause of this amnesic state is common to other human memory ailments; it does mean that the Korsakoff patient provides an opportunity to study a relatively "pure" memory disorder.

The Wernicke-Korsakoff syndrome typically occurs in nutritionally depleted chronic alcoholic individuals. The acute phase of the illness, Wernicke's encephalopathy, is characterized clinically by disordered ocular motility, ataxia, and global confusion, and has long been attributed to thiamine deficiency. After adequate treatment with thiamine, the acute illness usually subsides gradually, and as the confused state clears, the typical amnesic syndrome of the chronic phase, Korsakoff disease,* becomes evident. The relationship between thiamine deficiency and/or chronic alcohol consumption and Korsakoff disease is not clear. Blass and Gibson [1977] reported a defect in transketolase, a thiamine-dependent enzyme, in cell cultures from four patients with the Korsakoff syndrome; nevertheless, the neurologic basis for the memory deficit seen in this illness is not understood.

Korsakoff disease is manifested by two principal features: 1) an inability to recall information acquired in the months or years before onset of the illness (retrograde amnesia); and 2) an inability to acquire new information (anterograde amnesia). As parallel changes have been observed in the severity of retrograde and anterograde components, it has been suggested that both result from the same pathologic mechanism [Victor et al, 1971]. Perceptual impairments have also been observed quite consistently in patients with Korsakoff psychosis, but these deficits are minor in relation to the striking degree of memory disturbance.

II. PATHOLOGIC LESIONS IN KORSAKOFF DISEASE: RELATIONSHIP TO AMNESIA

The pathologic anatomy of the Wernicke-Korsakoff syndrome has been thoroughly described. The fact that lesions in postmortem brain specimens from patients who have died in the acute or chronic phase of the illness are similar in topography accounts for the hyphenated designation. Small necrotic and/or hemorrhagic lesions forming a symmetrical pattern are consistently found in the brainstem and diencephalon near the third and fourth ventricles and the Sylvian aqueduct. While the number and specific locations of lesions vary from case to case, the mammillary bodies and the medial dorsal thalamic nuclei are involved in a high percentage of cases [Malamud and Skillicorn, 1956; Victor et al, 1971]. The relationship between these lesions and the symptoms of Korsakoff psychosis is not certain. A number of pathologically involved brain structures have been implicated as the underlying anatomic substrate of the amnesia of this illness, but attention has focused most on the consistently observed mammillary body injury [Gamper, 1928; Delay and Brion 1954; Hecaen and De Ajuriaguerra, 1956; Delay et al, 1958]. The hypothesis of its causative role is particularly attractive in view of

---

*The terms Korsakoff disease, Korsakoff psychosis, Korsakoff syndrome, and Korsakoff amnesia are used interchangeably in the text.

the apparent direct connection between mammillary bodies and the hippocampus, a structure that has traditionally been associated with memory function, by way of the fornix. However, animal experiments with the use of autoradiographic techniques [Swanson and Cowan, 1975] have shown that fornical fibers terminating in the hypothalamus that were thought to arise in the hippocampus do not in fact originate in the hippocampus proper, but derive from the adjacent subiculum, a relatively poorly understood and unexplored region of the cerebral cortex. The traditional perspective of the role of the hippocampal-fornix-mammillary body circuit in regard to memory function may therefore have to be revised. Other investigators of the Wernicke-Korsakoff syndrome have sought to identify the lesions found in the medial dorsal nuclei of the thalamus along the walls of the third ventrical as the pathoanatomic basis for the memory impairment in this disease [Malamud and Skillicorn, 1956; Victor et al, 1971]. Victor and associates [1971] are the strongest advocates of this position. Their conclusions are based on an extensive neuropathological study of the Wernicke-Korsakoff syndrome in which they found lesions of the medial dorsal thalamic nuclei in each of those cases in which amnesia was documented. However, there were five patients who had recovered from the acute phase of the syndrome, Wernicke encephalopathy, without evidence of memory impairment, and in all of these there was evidence of extensive mammillary body pathology, but no thalamic lesions. As mammillary body injury was discovered in all of their cases, Victor and co-workers [1971] could not entirely dismiss this finding as a contributing cause of the Korsakoff syndrome. More recently, McEntee et al [1976] reported a case of a severely amnesic patient whose brain at postmortem examination showed bilateral thalamic tumor invasion and mammillary bodies free of disease. These findings tend to support the contention of Victor et al [1971] that thalamic lesions can be associated with amnesia in the absence of mammillary body damage. McEntee et al [1976] also reviewed the subject of tumors in the region of the third ventricle that cause amnesia. They concluded that the dorsomedial thalamus was probably not involved in all such reported cases, and that apparently no single structure or known interrelated group of structures acts as the mandatory substrate for amnesia in lesions of the mesodiencephalic region; it seemed more likely that small lesions at a number of different sites, the anatomical relationship of which is not yet entirely clear, can produce remarkably similar, profound memory disturbances. Horel [1978] gave further support to the position of Victor et al [1971] by presenting experimental evidence that the temporal stem, which contains fibers connecting the temporal cortex to the medial dorsal thalamic nucleus, rather than the hippocampus, is the anatomic structure in the temporal lobe that produces amnesia when injured. Mair et al [1979] carry the controversy one step further by suggesting that Korsakoff amnesia results from combined lesions of the mammillary bodies and medial thalamus, avoiding implication of any specific thalamic nucleus. These conflicting views illustrate the difficulties that have been encountered in attempts to correlate human memory disturbances with specific anatomic lesions.

Besides the controversy that has surrounded the anatomical basis of Korsakoff amnesia, it is still unclear why such small lesions deep in the substance of the brain produce such a profound global amnesia. One explanation may be that the brain damage that has been demonstrated in this disease interrupts a neuronal system(s) which has connections over a large portion of the central nervous system. It is of particular interest in this regard that the characteristic brainstem and diencephalic lesions found in the Wernicke-Korsakoff syndrome post-mortem were located in brain regions containing heavy concentrations of ascending monoamine-containing neurons, which have been traced in experimental animals by histochemical methods [Nobin and Bjorklund, 1973; Olson et al, 1973; Lindvall and Bjorklund, 1974]. These neurons, which contain the putative neurotransmitters norepinephrine (NE), dopamine (DA), and serotonin(5-HT), arise in clusters of cell bodies located mainly in the brainstem, from which their axons ascend and, to a lesser extent, descend to innervate wide areas of the CNS. The localization and mapping of these extensive neurochemical neuronal networks, which began in the mid-1960s, has stimulated considerable research efforts to relate them to specific neurological and behavioral functions. It has been hypothesized that the monoamines contained in these neuronal pathways, particularly NE, play important roles in memory and learning [Kety, 1970, 1972; German and Bowden, 1974; Stein, 1975; Hall et al, 1976; Fibiger, 1978; Mason and Iversen, 1979].

If the memory deficit of Korsakoff psychosis is related to damaged CNS monoamine systems, one might expect to find changes in the CSF concentrations of one or more of the brain metabolites of these reputed neurotransmitters, namely, 3-methoxy 4-hydroxyphenylglycol (MHPG) and vanillylmandelic acid (VMA), homovanillic acid (HVA), and 5-hydroxyindoleacetic acid (5-HIAA), which are central metabolic products of NE, DA and 5-HT, respectively. If measurements should show a significant alteration from normal concentrations, it might be possible to correlate the data with clinical features of the disease and to attempt restoration of the memory function in the Korsakoff patient by pharmacological manipulation. Using this experimental approach, we have completed a number of studies with Korsakoff patients [McEntee and Mair, 1978, 1980a, b], a review of which follows.

III. CSF LEVELS OF MONOAMINE METABOLITES IN KORSAKOFF DISEASE

We examined the cerebrospinal fluid (CSF) of nine patients with Korsakoff psychosis. The patients ranged in age from 40 to 57 years. All fulfilled the criteria for Korsakoff disease as described by Victor et al [1971] and all had a history of chronic alcoholism. All the patients moved freely about the hospital and had received no drugs for at least 2 weeks prior to the lumbar puncture except for one patient who was on long-term Dilantin therapy for a seizure disorder. Lumbar puncture was performed between 10 and 11 a.m. and CSF samples were obtained and processed according to the method described by Gordon and Oliver [1971]. The CSF was analyzed for MHPG, VMA, and HVA by the gas chromatographic-mass fragmentography method of Gordon et al [1974], and the concentration of 5-HIAA was determined by the fluorometric method of Ashcroft and Sharman [1962].

The results of the CSF monoamine metabolite measurements showed that the concentration of MHPG, considered the primary brain metabolite of NE, was significantly lower than in a control group of patients with a variety of psychiatric illnesses (t = 2.74, P < 0.01). The mean concentrations of the other monoamine metabolites were not significantly different from those of the control population.

All patients in whom the CSF monoamine metabolites were measured had their memory tested before the lumbar puncture by comparing the memory quotient (MQ) derived from the Wechsler Memory Scale (WMS), a standardized battery of subtests measuring a number of functions related to amnesia [Wechsler, 1917], with the full-scale intelligence quotient (IQ) derived from the Wechsler Adult Intelligence Scale. In normal persons the IQ and corrected MQ scores should be about the same, whereas in patients with Korsakoff disease the MQ falls disproportionately in comparison with the IQ. When the IQ-MQ difference was compared with the CSF metabolite levels, a strong correlation was found between the degree of memory impairment (IQ minus MQ) and the extent to which CSF levels of MHPG were reduced (r = −0.83, P < 0.005). No like correlation was found with the other CSF monoamine metabolite values.

Mair et al [1979] have argued that several subtests of the WMS do not accurately measure amnesia, and that the CSF MHPG-memory impairment correlation reported by McEntee and Mair [1978] may not be valid. They maintained that only two of the subtests of the WMS, viz memory passages and visual reproduction, can be used as a measure of amnesia. If these arguments are accepted and those two subtests are used alone, the correlation between CSF MHPG and the severity of memory impairment is still significant (r = 0.71); when the standard WMS age corrections were added to the raw scores for memory passages and visual reproduction, an even stronger correlation was found between the CSF MHPG levels and the degree of memory impairment (r = 0.88) than by use of the IQ-MQ difference.

That a relation should be found between the memory impairment observed in patients with Korsakoff disease and diminished central noradrenergic activity is not surprising. More direct evidence of pathologic involvement of the NE-containing neurons has been provided by Victor et al [1971], who detected, by light microscopy, lesions of the locus coeruleus in 68% of their autopsied cases in which this structure was specifically examined. Numerous studies have demonstrated that the locus coeruleus is the origin of a highly diffuse noradrenergic system that innervates nearly all levels of the central nervous system [Ungerstedt, 1971; Olson et al, 1973; Kobayashi et al, 1974; Pickel et al, 1974; Nobin and Bjorklund, 1973; Jones and Moore, 1977; Jones et al, 1977]. Victor et al [1971] were unable to detect lesions of the fiber tracts in the medial forebrain bundle, a major pathway for ascending locus coeruleus axons, but the conventional silver stains and light-microscopic examinations used in their studies could not be expected to reveal structural changes in these small unmyelinated nerve fibers.

IV. DRUG TREATMENT OF KORSAKOFF DISEASE

If the amnesia of Korsakoff disease is related to diminished central NE activity, then treatment with NE-agonists might lessen the severity of these symptoms. To test this hypothesis and learn whether Korsakoff amnesia would respond to pharmacological treatment, we treated a group of Korsakoff patients with preparations that exercise NE-agonist activity through distinct pharmacologic mechanisms. The drugs selected for study were clonidine, d-amphetamine, and methysergide. Clonidine, a putative α-adrenoceptor agonist, is believed to stimulate directly both postsynaptic receptors and presynaptic autoreceptors [Anden et al, 1970, 1976; Schmitt and Schmitt, 1970; Starke and Montel, 1973; Starke et al, 1974]. d-Amphetamine presumably enhances the release and blocks the reuptake of NE, DA, and 5-HT [Fuxe and Ungerstedt, 1970]. Methysergide, considered to be a 5-HT blocker, was chosen for this experiment because of a suggested reciprocal relationship between the effects of NE and 5-HT on learning [Katz and Carroll, 1977; Redgrave, 1978].

In intact animals, the action of clonidine has been associated with decreased response to intracranial self-stimulation and impaired conditioned avoidance learning, and these effects are diminished by the presynaptic α adrenoceptor-blocking agent piperoxan [Laverty and Taylor, 1969; Herberg et al, 1976; Drew et al, 1977; Franklin and Herberg, 1977; Robson et al, 1978]. The results of these experiments suggest that clonidine interferes with learning in intact animals by lowering the rate of release of NE from presynaptic terminals through its activation of presynaptic autoreceptors. The experiments also indicate that clonidine may preferentially activate presynaptic α adrenoceptors in opposition to its own postsynaptic activation effects. Therefore, if Korsakoff disease is associated with diminished NE activity as suggested by the CSF metabolite measurements, the presynaptic inhibitory effects of clonidine may be bypassed by postsynaptic activation, so that central NE activity is increased and the memory function in these patients is possibly improved. This view is supported by recent animal experiments in which clonidine (but not d-amphetamine) reversed the amnesia associated with reduced NE activity due to dopamine β-hydroxylase inhibition [Freedman et al, 1979]. However, there is experimental evidence that d-amphetamine facilitates the performance of learning tasks in animals by its presynaptic facilitation of NE and DA activity [McGaugh, 1973; Stein, 1975; Fibiger, 1978]. The extent to which d-amphetamine facilitates learning and memory in Korsakoff patients may thus depend on the extent of combined damage to presynaptic NE and DA elements in individual patients. The rational for including methysergide was the assumption that the 5-HT-antagonistic effect of this drug might indirectly enhance brain NE activity by a disinhibiting mechanism.

Eight patients with Korsakoff disease were given each of the following four treatments twice daily, at 12-hour intervals: 0.3 mg of clonidine, 10 mg of d-amphetamine, 4 mg of methysergide, and placebo. Each test preparation was given for a period of 2 weeks to allow attainment of steady-state conditions, and a 2-week washout was interposed between treatment trials. The order of treatments was randomized among the subjects; the personnel testing memory functions and the subjects were kept blind to their assigned order of treatments. The subjects were given a battery of neuropsychological tests before treatment and on the last day of each treatment trial. This neuropsychological test battery required performance of a number of tasks similar or identical to those that Korsakoff patients have been reported to perform significantly worse than controls. They included the Wechsler Memory Scale (WMS), a standardized battery of subtests measuring a number of functions related to amnesia [Wechsler, 1917; Talland, 1965]; multiple-choice retrograde memory tests measuring recall of events occurring from the 1920s through the 1970s [Seltzer and Benson, 1974; Albert et al, 1979]; the Consonant Trigrams Test (CCC), which measures short-term recall of verbal information by the method of Peterson and Peterson [1959] as modified by Butters and Cermak [1975]; the Face-Face Test measuring short-term recognition of human faces using a multiple choice format [Dricker et al, 1978]; Witkin Children's Embedded Figures Test, measuring the ability to perceive simple geometric shapes embedded in more complex figures [Glosser et al, 1977]; the Digit-Symbol Subtest from the Wechsler Adult Intelligence Scale, which is sensitive to deficits in new learning and visuoperceptive abilities [Butters et al, 1977; Glosser et al, 1977]; and the Carey Faces Test measuring perceptual recognition of human faces obscured by superficial distracting stimuli [Carey and Diamond, 1977; Diamond and Carey, 1977; Dricker et al, 1978].

The results reflected significant changes across drug trials in two of the psychometric tests, the WMS and the CCC. Analysis of variance with repeated measures indicated an overall drug treatment effect on WMS performance (F(4,28) = 12.29, P < 0.01). Subsequent analysis by Scheffe's test showed that the patients performed significantly better after treatment with clonidine than after placebo (P < 0.01). Treatment with *d*-amphetamine and methysergide did not cause any significant mean change in WMS performance as compared with placebo, but some individuals did show substantial improvements after treatment with these drugs.

The WMS includes subtests that measure a wide range of cognitive functions. To what extent do the results of the drug study reflect improvement of memory rather than of related functions also measured by the WMS? The overall improvement in MQ observed after treatment with clonidine as compared with placebo is apparent in only three of the WMS subtests, namely, digit span, memory passages, and visual reproduction. An analysis of variance with repeated measures indicates a significant overall effect in only two of these subsets, memory passages (F(4,28) = 24.00, P < 0.01) and visual reproduction (F(4,28) = 5.33, P < 0.01). Subsequent analysis with Scheffe's test for the memory passages subtest showed a significant difference between clonidine and placebo (P < 0.01), but not between the other active preparations and placebo. For the visual reproduction subtest, Scheffe's test demonstrated a significant difference between clonidine and placebo (P < 0.01), *d*-amphetamine and placebo (P < 0.05), and methysergide and placebo (P < 0.05). The finding that only the memory passages and visual reproduction subtests improved significantly after clonidine treatment is interesting for several reasons. First, they are generally considered to be the WMS subtests that most directly measure memory [Mair et al, 1979]. Second, performance was measured in modified versions of these subtests in which a 10-minute interval was interposed between presentation of stimulus information and recall testing. The results of these modified subtests were consistent with those of the regular subtests in demonstrating significant improvement after treatment with clonidine. Thus, the improvement apparent in the standard subtests was maintained over a moderate retention interval. Third, post-hoc analysis revealed a significant correlation between the CSF MHPG levels and the raw scores for performance in these two subtests (r = 0.71). In sum, performance in the two WMS subtests considered to be most directly related to memory correlated significantly with the CSF MHPG levels, improving significantly after treatment with clonidine, and the improvement persisted after a 10-minute interval.

The WMS results suggest that clonidine improves performance in tests measuring the recall of recently presented information. Of the tests in the neuropsychological test battery, only the CCC test directly measures similar capabilities. The results of the CCC test were generally consistent with the WMS results. Analysis of variance with repeated measures showed that CCC performance varied significantly with different drugs (F(4,28) = 4.43, P <

0.01). Subsequent analysis by Scheffe's test, however, demonstrated a significant difference only for the clonidine baseline comparison. Although no significant differences were found between performance after drugs and placebo in general, a more consistent pattern of improvement in the CCC test was apparent with clonidine than with the other active preparations, five of eight patients showing substantial improvement as compared to placebo. No significant mean improvement was noted with any of the medications in tasks measuring retrograde memory (using a multiple-choice format), recognition memory for complex stimuli, or visuoperceptive abilities.

As mentioned previously, some patients showed substantial improvement although the mean changes were not statistically significant after treatment with d-amphetamine. Post-hoc analysis demonstrated a significant correlation between CSF HVA levels and the extent to which d-amphetamine treatment improved performance on the WMS ($r^2 = 0.85$). This result suggests that the effectiveness of d-amphetamine as a treatment for Korsakoff amnesia may be limited by the degree of DA activity in individual patients as determined by the CSF concentration of HVA. No correlation was found between the effectiveness of methysergide and the CSF levels of monoamine metabolites.

In sum, WMS performance among the Korsakoff patients was generally improved after 2 weeks of subacute treatment with 0.3 mg of clonidine b.i.d. and improvement after treatment with d-amphetamine at a dose of 10 mg b.i.d. given for 2 weeks was limited to patients with normal CSF levels of HVA. The results of the drug studies as well as the CSF metabolite data suggest that Korsakoff disease may be associated with consistent lesions of brain NE pathways and variable impairment of brain DA pathways. Thus, our experiments in patients with Korsakoff disease parallel animal experiments indicating that the effectiveness of clonidine in improving memory function depends on the extent to which its presynaptic inhibitory effects are overridden by its postsynaptic excitatory effects. The drug studies support the hypothesis, based on results of the CSF studies, that presynaptic elements of NE-containing neurons are damaged in patients with Korsakoff psychosis. This damage, which is reflected in reduced CSF MHPG levels, allows the preferential presynaptic effects of clonidine to be overridden, with the result that postsynaptic adrenoceptors are activated, and certain psychometric measures of memory function subsequently improve. This interpretation is consistent with the observation that other effects of clonidine generally attributed to its presynaptic actions, namely hypotension and sedation, were not apparent at the doses used in this study. In contrast to clonidine, d-amphetamine requires intact presynaptic elements in order to exercise its NE and DA agonist activity. Therefore, damage to presynaptic NE elements in all patients and to presynaptic DA elements in patients with low CSF HVA levels may account for the limited effectiveness of d-amphetamine in the Korsakoff patients tested.

It appears, then, that the dose of clonidine employed in this drug study can improve the recall of recently presented information, but does not lead to a significant reduction of other deficits associated with this disease. Consequently, the suggestion that central NE systems are impaired in Korsakoff psychosis does not necessarily imply that such damage accounts for all of the symptoms of this disease. Ascending noradrenergic pathways follow classically demonstrated nonadrenergic pathways [Lindvall and Bjorklund, 1974] so that the pathologic lesions found in postmortem brain specimens of patients with Korsakoff disease may also involve other fiber systems that course in close proximity. This possibility is heightened by the failure of perceptually demanding tasks to improve in response to the dosage of clonidine used in our studies. On the other hand, the limited effectiveness of clonidine we observed could be related to a restricted scope of action of the drug on CNS adrenoceptors.

If the effectiveness of clonidine is related to postsynaptic activation of NE receptors overriding its presumably preferential presynaptic inhibitory effect, then it seems possible that the drug's beneficial effects could be enhanced by use of larger doses. This conjecture is supported by the work of Freedman et al [1979], who showed that the amnesia produced by dopamine β-hydroxylase inhibition can be reversed by clonidine, and that the degree of this reversal is dose-related, increasing with increasing doses of clonidine. Studies of the effect of larger doses of clonidine on memory function in patients with Korsakoff psychosis are currently under way in our laboratory. Whatever the outcome of these studies, it appears that the memory function of patients with Korsakoff disease can be improved by pharmacological intervention with a putative α-adrenoceptor agonist. Although substantial improvements were observed in response to clonidine in some of the subjects of our drug trials, none approached normal levels of memory functioning. Clonidine may eventually not prove suitable for the treatment of Korsakoff amnesia or other human memory disorders related to deficient functioning of CNS noradrenergic systems, but it is hoped that the studies described above will at least provide the impetus to a more intensive search for other NE agonists that may qualify as therapeutic agents for Korsakoff disease.

V. ACKNOWLEDGMENT

This study was supported by Veterans Administration research funds.

VI. REFERENCES

Albert MS, Butters N, Levin J: Temporal gradients in the retrograde amnesia of patients with alcoholic Korsakoff's disease. Arch Neurol 36:211–216, 1979.

Anden NE, Corrodi H, Fuxe K, Hokfelt B, Hokfelt T, Rydin C, Svensson T: Evidence for a central noradrenaline receptor stimulation by clonidine. Life Sci 9:513–523, 1970.

Anden NE, Corrodi H, Fuxe K, et al: Different alpha-adrenoceptors in the central nervous system mediating biochemical and functional effects of clonidine and receptor blocking agent. Naunym Schmeilberg's Arch Pharmacol 292:43–52, 1976.

Aschroft GW, Sharman DF: Drug induced changes in the concentration of 5-OH indolyl compounds in cerebrospinal fluid and caudate nucleus. Br J Pharmacol 19:153–160, 1962.

Blass JP, Gibson GE: Abnormality of a thiamine-requiring enzyme in patients with Wernicke-Korsakoff syndrome. N Engl J Med 297:1367–1370, 1977.

Butters N, Cermak LS: Some analyses of amnesia syndromes in brain damaged patients. In Isaacon RL, Pribram KH (eds): "The Hippocampus," Vol. 2. New York: Plenum Press, 1975.

Butters N, Cermak LS, Montgomery K, Adinolfi A: Some comparison of the memory and visuoperceptive deficits of chronic alcoholics and patients with Korsakoff's disease. Alcoholism 1:73–80, 1977.

Carey S, Diamond R: From piecemeal to configurational representation of faces. Science 195:312–314, 1977.

Delay J, Bordin G, Brion S, Barbizet J: Etude anatamo-clinique de huit encephalopathies alcooliques. Encephale 47:99–142, 1958.

Delay J, Brion S: Syndrome de Korsakoff et corps mamillaires. Encephale 43:193–200, 1954.

Diamond R, Carey S: Developmental changes in the representation of faces. J Exp Child Psychol 23:1–22, 1977.

Drew GM, Gower AJ, Mariott AS: Pharmacological characterization of alpha-adrenoceptors which mediate clonidine induced sedation. Br J Pharmacol 61:468P, 1977.

Dricker J, Butters N, Berman G, Samuels I, Carey S: The recognition and encoding of faces by alcoholic Korsakoff patients and right hemisphere patients. Neuropsychologia 16:683–695, 1978.

Fibiger HC: Drugs and reinforcement mechanisms: A critical review of the catecholamine theory. Ann Rev Pharmacol Toxicol 19:37–56, 1978.

Franklin KBJ, Herberg LJ: Presynaptic alpha adrenoceptors: The depression of self stimulation by clonidine and its restoration by piperoxane but not by phentolamine or phenoxybenzamine. Eur J Pharmacol 43:33–38, 1977.

Freedman LS, Backman MZ, Quartermain D: Clonidine reverses the amnesia induced by dopamine beta hydroxylase inhibition. Pharmacol Biochem Behav 11:259–263, 1979.

Fuxe K, Ungerstedt U: Histochemical, biochemical and functional studies on central monoamine neurons after acute and chronic amphetamine administration. In Costa E, Grattini S (eds): "Amphetamine and Related Compounds." New York: Raven Press, 1970, pp 257–288.

Gamper E: Zur frage der polinoencephalitis haemorrhagica der chronischen alkoholiker: Anatomische befund beim akoholischen Korsakow und ihre beziehungen zum klinischen bild. Deutsche Ztschr Nervenh 102:122–129, 1928.

German DE, Bowden DM: Catecholamine systems as the neural substrate for intracranial self-stimulation: A hypothesis. Brain Res 73:381–419, 1974.

Glosser G, Butters N, Kaplan E: Visuoperceptual process in brain damaged patients on the digit symbol substitution test. Int J Neurosci 7:59–66, 1977.

Gordon EK, Oliver J: 3-Methoxy-4-hydroxyphenylethylene glycol in human cerebrospinal fluid. Clin Chem Acta 35:145-150, 1971.

Gordon EK, Oliver J, Black K, Kopin IJ: Simultaneous assay by mass fragmentography of vanillylmandelic acid, homovanillic acid and 3-methoxy-4-hydroxyphenylethylene glycol in cerebrospinal fluid and urine. Biochem Med 11:32-40, 1974.

Hall RD, Bloom FE, Olds J: Neuronal and neurochemical substrates of reinforcement. Neurosci Res Prog Bull 15:136-313, 1976.

Hecaen MH, De Ajuriaguerra J: Les encephalopathies alcooliques subaiguees et chroniques. Rev Neurol 94:528-555, 1956.

Herberg LJ, Stephens DN, Franklin KBJ: Catecholamines and self-stimulation: Evidence suggesting a reinforcing role for noradrenaline and motivating role for dopamine. Pharmacol Biochem Behav 4:575-582, 1976.

Horel JA: The neuroanatomy of amnesia- A critique of the hippocampal memory hypothesis. Brain 101:403-445, 1978.

Jones BE, Halaris AE, McIlhany M, Moore RY: Ascending projections of the locus coeruleus in the rat. I. Axonal transport in central noradrenaline neurons. Brain Res 127:1-21, 1977.

Jones BE, More RY: Ascending projections of the locus coeruleus in the rat. II. Autoradiographic study. Brain Res 127:23-53, 1977.

Katz RJ, Carroll BJ: Intracranial reward after Lilly 110140 (Fluoxetine HCL): Evidence for an inhibitory role for serotonin. Psychopharmacology 51:189-193, 1977.

Kety SS: The biogenic amines in the central nervous system: Their possible roles in arousal, emotion, and learning. In Schmitt FO (ed): "The Neurosciences. A Second Study Program." New York: Rockefeller University Press, 1970.

Kety SS: The possible role of the adrenergic systems of the cortex in learning. In Kopin IJ (ed): "Neurotransmitters." Baltimore: Williams and Wilkins, 1972.

Kobayashi RM, Palkovits M, Kopin IJ, Jacobowitz DM: Biochemical mapping of noradrenergic nerves arising from the rat locus coeruleus. Brain Res 77:269-279, 1974.

Laverty R, Taylor KM: Behavioral and biochemical effect of 2-(2,6)-dichlorophenylamino-2 imidazoline hydrochloride (ST 155) on the central nervous system. Br J Pharmacol Chemother 35:253-264, 1969.

Lindvall O, Bjorklund A: The organization of the ascending catecholamine neuron systems in the rat brain as revealed by the glyoxylic acid fluorescence method. Acta Physiol, Scand, Suppl 412:1-48, 1974.

Mair WPG, Warrington EK, Weiskrantz L: Memory disorder in Korsakoff's psychosis: A neuropathological and neuropsychological investigation of two cases. Brain 102:749-785, 1979.

Malamud N, Skillicorn SA: Relationship between the Wernicke and Korsakoff syndrome: A clinicopathologic study of seventy cases. A M A Arch Neurol Psychiat 76:575-596, 1956.

Mason ST, Iversen S: Theories of the dorsal bundle extinction effect. Brain Res Rev 1:107-137, 1979.

McEntee WJ, Biber MP, Perl DP, Benson DF: Diencephalic amnesia: A reappraisal. J Neurol Neurosurg Psychiat 39:436-441, 1976.

McEntee WJ, Mair RG: Memory impairment in Korsakoff's psychosis: A correlation with brain noradrenergic activity. Science 202:905-907, 1978.

McEntee WJ, Mair RG: Korsakoff's amnesia: A noradrenergic hypothesis. Psychopharmacol Bull 16:22-24, 1980.

McEntee WJ, Mair RG: Memory enhancement in Korsakoff's psychosis by clonidine: Further evidence for a noradrenergic deficit. Ann Neurol 7:466-470, 1980.

McGaugh JL: Drug facilitation of learning and memory. Ann Rev Pharmacol 13:299-241, 1973.

Nobin A, Bjorklund A: Topography of the monoamine neuron system in the human brain as revealed in fetuses. Acta Physiol Scand Suppl 388:1-40, 1973.

Olson L, Boreus LO, Seiger A: Histochemical demonstration and mapping of 5-hydroxytrypta-mine and catecholamine containing neuron systems in the human fetal brain. Z Anat Entwickl Qesch 139:259–282, 1973.

Peterson LR, Peterson MJ: Short-term retention of individual verbal items. J Exp Psychol 58:193–198, 1959.

Pickel VM, Segal M, Bloom FE: A radioautographic study of the efferent pathways of the lo-cus coeruleus. J Comp Neurol 155:15–42, 1974.

Redgrave P: Modulation of intracranial self- stimulation behavior by local perfusions of dopa-mine, noradrenaline, and serotonin within the caudate nucleus and the nucleus accumbens. Brain Res 155:277–295, 1978.

Robson RD, Antonaccio MJ, Saelens JK, Leibman J: Antagonism by mianserin and classical alpha adrenoceptor blocking drugs of some cardiovascular and behavioral effects of cloni-dine. Eur J Pharmacol 47:431–442, 1978.

Schmitt H, Schmitt H: Interactions between 2-6,6-dichlorophenylamino-2-imidazoline hydro-chloride (Catapresan) and alpha adrenergic blocking drugs. Eur J Pharmacol 9:7–13, 1970.

Seltzer B, Benson DF: The temporal pattern of retrograde amnesia in Korsakoff's disease. Neurology (Minneap) 24:527–530, 1974.

Starke K, Montel H: Involvement of alpha receptors in clonidine induced inhibition of transmit-ter release from central monoamine neurones. Neuropharmacology 12:1073–1080, 1973.

Starke K, Montel H, Gayk W, Merker R: Comparison of the effects of clonidine on pre- and postsynaptic adrenoceptors in the rabbit pulmonary artery. Naunyn Schmeideberg's Arch Pharmacol 285:133–150, 1974.

Stein L: Norepinephrine reward pathways: Role in self-stimulation, memory consolidation, and schizophrenia. Nebr Symp Motiv 22:113–159, 1975.

Swanson LW, Cowan WM: Hippocampo- hypothalamic connections: Origin in subicular cor-tex, not Ammon's horn. Science 189:303–304, 1975.

Talland GA: "Deranged Memory." New York: Academic Press, 1965.

Ungerstedt U: Stereotaxic mapping of the monoamine pathways in the rat brain. Acta Physiol Scand Suppl 367:1–48, 1971.

Victor M, Adams RD, Collins GH: "The Wernicke-Korsakoff Syndrome." Philadelphia: Davis, 1971.

Wechsler D: A study of retention in Korsakoff psychosis. Psychiatr Bull NY State Hosp 2:403–451, 1917.

Psychopharmacology of Clonidine, pages 225–242
© 1981 Alan R. Liss, Inc., 150 Fifth Avenue, New York, NY 10011

Antinociceptive Actions of Clonidine

Stuart Fielding, Theodore C. Spaulding, and Harbans Lal

Neurochemical modulation has been associated with the transmission of nociceptive information and the alteration of responses to analgesic agents. Reviews have been published on the involvement of a variety of biogenic amines and peptides in antinociceptive activity [Pepeu, 1976; Frederickson, 1977; Greenberg and Palmer, 1978] and in the expression of opiate-induced analgesia [Takemori, 1976].

Clonidine has been shown to produce antinociceptive effects in several different procedures believed to induce pain in laboratory animals (Table I). These tests include the inhibition of writhing provoked by phenyl-p-benzoquinone [Fielding et al, 1978]; acetic acid and acetylcholine [Bentley et al, 1977]; tail flick response to radiant heat [Fielding et al, 1978; Spaulding et al, 1979a,b]; tail withdrawal from hot water [Sewell and Spencer, 1976; Fielding et al, 1978]; electrical stimulation of the tail [Paalzow, 1974; Schmitt et al, 1974; Paalzow and Paalzow, 1976]; shock titration [Yaksh and Reddy, 1980]; skin twitch [Reddy and Yaksh, 1980]; pressure applied to an inflamed paw [Fielding et al, 1978]; and hot plate (56°C) [Schmitt et al, 1974]. The analgesic effectiveness of clonidine has been studied in relation to its interaction with noradrenergic mechanisms and its activity in morphine-sensitive systems.

The processing of noxious inputs and the associated responses have been studied at the spinal and supraspinal levels. Anatomical localizations of morphine-sensitive areas associated with a decrease in pain responding have been reviewed [Kerr, 1975; Yaksh and Rudy, 1978]. The postulation that clonidine acts to reduce nociceptive responding through an α-adrenergic mechanism in association with morphine-sensitive sites is based on ascending and descending projections in pain-associated pathways. These noradrenergically sensitive sites have been localized in the locus coeruleus

TABLE I. Antinociceptive Activity of Clonidine

Test	Species	Reference
Writhing		
Phenylquinone	Mouse	Fielding et al, 1978
		Aceto et al, 1979
Acetic acid, ACh	Mouse	Bentley et al, 1977
Tail flick	Mouse	Fielding et al, 1978
		Spaulding et al, 1979
		Aceto et al, 1979
	Rat	Zemlan et al, 1980
Tail immersion	Mouse	Lipman and Spencer, 1979
	Rat	Fielding et al, 1978
Electrical stimulated tail	Rat	Schmitt et al, 1974
		Paalzow and Paalzow, 1976
Shock titration	Monkey	Yaksh and Reddy (in preparation)
Skin twitch	Cat	Maderdrut et al, 1980
Inflamed paw press	Rat	Fielding et al, 1978
Hot plate	Mouse	Schmitt et al, 1974

[Price and Fibiger, 1975; Redmond, 1977], nucleus raphe magnus [Lobatz et al, 1976], and the bulbospinal n. reticularis gigantocellularis [Takagi et al, 1976, 1979].

Stimulation experiments by Margalit and Segal [1979] provided further evidence for an adrenergic component in analgesia. Direct stimulation of the locus coeruleus resulted in an analgesic response (hot plate) that was attenuated by naloxone, an opiate antagonist, cyproheptadine, a serotonin antagonist, and an α-adrenergic antagonist, WB-4101. These observations indicate that there are morphinergic, serotonergic, and α-adrenergic components to stimulation-induced analgesia at this site. In addition, adrenergic projections from the locus coeruleus have been found in the hippocampus, cortex, and spinal cord [Ader et al, 1979] areas implicated in analgesia.

In addition to clonidine, other imidazolines such as xylazine, tetrazaline, and oxymetazoline have been shown to induce analgesia when injected intracerebroventricularly [Handley and Spencer, 1969; Schmitt et al, 1974]. The analgesia activity of these compounds after systemic administration depends on the lipid-solubility of the agent, hence, its capacity to pass the blood brain barrier [Schmitt et al, 1974; Timmermans et al, 1977; Lipman and Spencer, 1979]. Apparently, clonidine is the best in this class.

The studies of the antinociceptive activity of clonidine reported below were designed 1) to determine its activity after noxious stimulation by chemical, thermal, or mechanical methods; 2) to differentiate between receptor for morphine and clonidine; 3) to test for synergistic interaction between morphine and clonidine; and 4) to explore the spinal activity of clonidine.

I. METHODS

Male hooded rats of the Long Evans strain weighing 250–300 gm, female Wistar rats weighing 130–175 gm, and male Swiss albino mice of the CD-1 COBS strain weighing 22–28 gm were used. All drugs were dissolved in saline or suspended in carboxymethylcellulose.

A. Measurement of Analgesia

1. Phenylquinone writhing in mice. This test measures the ability of a drug to alter the writhing induced by 1.25 mg/kg of intraperitoneally administered phenylquinone. It was carried out according to Siegmund et al [1957].

Writhing is defined as an inward rotation of one or several feet with twisting and turning of the trunk, drawing in of the abdominal wall, and arching of the back (lordosis). A drug is considered to produce analgesia in this test if the number of writhes induced by the clinical agent is significantly decreased.

2. Tail withdrawal in rats. Analgesia in rats was measured by inhibition of tail withdrawal [Janssen et al, 1963] as described recently by Miksic and Lal [1977]. Each rat received the drug or vehicle (0.9% saline) by injection and was placed in a specially constructed rat holder with its tail protruding and hanging freely. Thirty minutes after morphine or naloxone administration and 60 minutes after clonidine administration, the distal end of the tail was immersed to a depth of 5 cm in a beaker of water kept at 55°C. The tail withdrawal latency was the time interval at which the tail was clearly withdrawn from the water.

3. Randall-Selitto test in rats. The Randall-Selitto test measures the ability of drugs to alter the reaction to pressure applied to a yeast-inflamed paw by an analgesia meter. The pain response was defined as either a struggle or turning to bite. A drug is considered to produce analgesia if the amount of pressure required to induce a reaction is significantly increased.

4. Tail flick test in mice. Antinociceptive testing was performed by the radiant heat method (tail flick test) of D'Amour and Smith [1941] in nonfasting male Swiss Webster CD-1 mice weighing 18–28 gm. Each mouse was secured so that its tail rested in a grooved block and shielded the aperture of a photocell from the light of a heat lamp. Activation of the lamp simultaneously started a timer, and when the mouse flicked its tail light deactivated the timer. The control tail flick latencies averaged approximately 2 seconds. Analgesia was considered to have been produced if the latency of the tail flick after treatment was greater than the mean + 2 standard deviations of the corresponding control time. Drugs and vehicle were administered subcutaneously (SC), and all analyses were performed at the time of the peak antinociceptive effect, which was 15 minutes for clonidine and 30 minutes for morphine. In this and in other studies to follow, statistical analyses and calculations of ED_{50}, slope function, and potency ratio were performed according to Litchfield and Wilcoxon [1949].

B. Interaction Studies

1. Clonidine + naloxone. In order to ascertain whether or not clonidine interacts with opiate receptors, changes in the mouse tail flick latency were determined with clonidine in the presence or absence of naloxone. Naloxone was administered simultaneously with clonidine in a dose of 10 mg/kg.

2. Clonidine + yohimbine. In order to ascertain whether or not clonidine interacts with α-presynaptic adrenergic receptors, changes in the mouse tail flick latency were determined with clonidine in the presence or absence of yohimbine.

3. Clonidine + phenoxybenzamine. In order to ascertain whether or not clonidine interacts with postsynaptic α-adrenoreceptors, changes in the mouse tail flick latency were determined with clonidine in the presence or absence of phenoxybenzamine.

4. Morphine pretreatment + clonidine in tail flick test. Dose-response curves for clonidine were plotted after pretreatment with morphine doses of 0.04, 0.16, or 0.64 mg/kg. To show the receptor specificity of morphine in the interaction with clonidine, a naloxone dose of 10 mg/kg was administered SC 10 minutes prior to testing.

5. Clonidine pretreatment + morphine activity in tail flick test. Since morphine potentiated clonidine activity in the tail flick test, we sought to determine whether or not clonidine potentiates morphine activity at doses that did not affect tail flick latency. We plotted dose-response curves for morphine in the presence of 16 or 32 mg/kg of clonidine administered 15 minutes before testing.

6. Cross-tolerance in morphine-pelleted mice. In addition to demonstrating naloxone-insensitive analgesia in the tail flick test, we conducted studies to confirm the lack of a direct interaction with opiate receptors or opiate systems. For this purpose we studied a possible cross-tolerance for clonidine in morphine-tolerant mice, using the tail flick test. The mice were rendered tolerant to morphine by subcutaneous implantation of a morphine-base pellet containing 50 mg of morphine. A placebo pellet was implanted in control mice. Dose-response curves for morphine and clonidine were obtained 96 hours after implantation; the pellets were not removed before testing.

7. Pithing. In addition to receptor-site differentiation in the actions of morphine and clonidine, we tried to determine if there is a gross anatomical distinction between the compounds in terms of spinal versus supraspinal activity. In our experiments, mice were pithed under pentobarbital anesthesia between the sixth and eighth thoracic vertebrae. Twenty-four or 72 hours later, dose-response curves for morphine and clonidine were generated. At these times there was no difference in the tail flick latencies between sham-operated and spinally transected mice.

II. RESULTS

A. Measurement of Analgesia

1. Phenylquinone writhing in mice. As illustrated in Figure 1, writhing induced by phenylquinone was blocked by both morphine and clonidine to a dose-dependent degree. Clonidine (ED_{50} = 0.03 mg/kg SC) was 17 times more potent than morphine (ED_{50} = 0.5 mg/kg SC). The effect of naloxone on the antiwrithing effects of morphine and clonidine is shown in Table II. Morphine-induced inhibition of writhing was antagonized by naloxone, a specific narcotic antagonist, as expected. However, the antiwrithing action of clonidine was not antagonized by naloxone.

2. Tail withdrawal in rats. Clonidine and morphine were also effective in blocking tail withdrawal from hot water in rats (Table III). In this test, the effective dose of clonidine was in a range similar to that of morphine. Again, while the activity of morphine was antagonized by naloxone, the action of clonidine was not.

3. Randall-Selitto test in rats. In the modified Randall-Selitto test, clonidine significantly inhibits the pain response in both inflamed and noninflamed paws (Table IV). Comparing clonidine and morphine in the inflamed paw model, we see that clonidine (200% increase at 1 mg/kg SC)

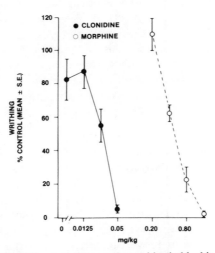

Fig. 1. Comparison of effects of clonidine and morphine in blocking phenylquinone-induced abdominal constriction in mice. In saline-pretreated mice an injection of phenylquinone caused a mean of 41 (± SE, 4.77) constrictions. The number of constrictions produced after test drug in each mouse was divided by the saline mean to obtain the data plotted on the Y axis.

TABLE II. Effects of Morphine, Clonidine, and Naloxone on Phenylquinone-Induced (1.25 mg/kg IP) Writhing in Mice

Treatment	Dose (mg/kg SC)	Mean writhes (± SE)	% Inhibition of Writhing
Vehicle	—	36.9 ± 1.9	—
Morphine	2.0	0.4 ± 0.2	99
Clonidine	0.05	1.3 ± 0.4	96
Naloxone	1.0	33.3 ± 3.2	6
Morphine + Naloxone	2.0 1.0	26.5 ± 4.7	20
Clonidine + Naloxone	0.05 1.0	1.5 ± 1.5	96

TABLE III. Inhibition of Tail Withdrawal Response to Warm Water Treatment

Drug	Dose mg/kg SC	N	% Showing inhibition of tail withdrawal*
Saline solution	5.0	20	0
Naloxone	5.0	10	0
Clonidine	2.5	12	85
	10.0	12	75
Morphine	2.5	12	75
	5.0	12	75
	10.0	12	92
Naloxone ± Morphine	5.0 10.0	10	0
Naloxone ± Clonidine	5.0 2.5	6	75

*Percentage of animals showing tail withdrawal latency greater than sum of mean and 2 SD obtained in saline-treated rats.

was approximately four times as potent as morphine (238% increase at 4 mg/kg SC) in preventing the pain response. The data collected on the noninflamed paw model for clonidine show clonidine to be effective at 1 mg/kg SC in inhibiting the pain response. Published data on morphine show that morphine is also effective in this model [Randall and Selitto, 1957].

TABLE IV. Effects of Morphine and Clonidine on Randall-Selitto Pain Response

Drug	Dose mg/kg SC	Before drug[a,b]	After drug[a] gm	% Change[c]
Morphine	0.0	67 ± 5	80 ± 12	19
Inflamed	0.5	78 ± 4	80 ± 10	3
Paw	1.0	77 ± 5	140 ± 30	82**
	2.0	77 ± 4	145 ± 33	88*
	4.0	77 ± 6	264 ± 52	238**
Clonidine	0.0	52 ± 4	46 ± 2	− 12
Inflamed	0.125	48 ± 2	62 ± 6	29
Paw	0.25	46 ± 4	72 ± 6	56*
	0.5	48 ± 4	84 ± 10	75*
	1.0	50 ± 4	150 ± 10	200*
Clonidine	0.0	74 ± 6	66 ± 4	− 11
Non-Inflamed	0.125	48 ± 4	74 ± 10	54*
Paw	0.25	56 ± 8	62 ± 8	11
	0.5	58 ± 4	66 ± 8	14
	1.0	66 ± 8	98 ± 10	48*

*$P < 0.05$ calculated by paired t-test compared to predrug values.
**$P < 0.01$ calculated by paired t-test compared to predrug values.
[a]Data are mean ± SE grams of pressure applied to elicit pain response. Mean is based on ten rats in each group.
[b]All predrug controls were compared, and no significant variance was shown according to F-maximum test for homogeneity of variances.
[c]Percent change from predrug controls.

4. Tail flick test in mice. Clonidine and morphine also inhibited the tail flick response of mice to radiant heat, to a dose-dependent degree, at $ED_{50}s$ of 0.7 mg/kg SC and 3.8 mg/kg SC, respectively (Fig. 2).

B. Interaction Studies

1. Clonidine + naloxone. Clonidine was effective in increasing the latency of the tail flick response to a dose-dependent degree up to 4 mg/kg (Fig. 3). Naloxone at 10 mg/kg did not significantly alter the increase in reaction time after clonidine administration. This dose caused an increase in the ED_{50} for subcutaneously administered morphine from 1.0 mg/kg to 15.7 mg/kg (unpublished observations). The mean control and test tail flick latencies ± standard error were 1.92 ± 0.06 and 1.83 ± 0.08 seconds, respectively, after H_2O–H_2O administration and 1.88 ± 0.05 and 1.83 ± 0.06 seconds, respectively, for a naloxone–H_2O combination.

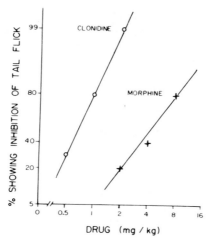

Fig. 2. Comparison of effects of clonidine and morphine in blocking heat-induced tail flick response in mice. Increase in latency greater than 2 SD was taken as a positive analgesic response. The mean tail withdrawal latency of all mice before they were treated with a drug was 1.78 sec.

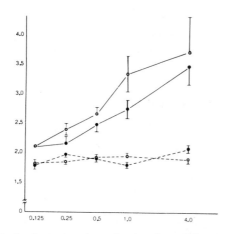

Fig. 3. The effect of naloxone on the antinociceptive activity of clonidine in the mouse tail flick assay. The dashed lines repeat preinjection control latencies, and the solid lines postinjection latencies. Clonidine HCl was administered simultaneously with H_2O (○) or 10 mg/kg of naloxone hydrochloride (●). There was no significant change in tail flick latencies after H_2O or naloxone given alone. Ordinate: tail flick latency. Abscissa: clonidine (mg/kg).

2. Clonidine + yohimbine. Clonidine activity at the high dose was reduced approximately 30 times, by both doses of yohimbine. These data, displayed in Table V, suggest a direct competition between yohimbine and clonidine. Interestingly, at the higher dose (2.5 mg/kg) yohimbine reduced the analgesic response to morphine approximately 4 times. This could mean some weak direct competition with morphine or a competitive effect on a final common pathway of analgesia.

3. Clonidine + phenoxybenzamine. The presynaptic nature of the antinociception induced by clonidine via an α-adrenergic site was confirmed by the observation that a 10 mg/kg dose of phenoxybenzamine, a postsynaptic α blocker, did not alter the effect of clonidine in the tail flick test (Table VI).

Although the activities of morphine and clonidine are not channelled through a common receptor, we investigated the interaction of these compounds in the mouse tail flick test.

4. Morphine pretreatment + clonidine in tail flick test. The $ED_{50}s$ of clonidine in the presence of morphine are presented in Table VII. Pretreatment with morphine, 0.04 mg/kg, decreased the clonidine ED_{50} slightly, to 0.084 mg/kg, and a morphine dose of 0.16 mg/kg, which did not increase tail flick latency, maximally potentiated the clonidine activity, decreasing the ED_{50} from 0.10 mg/kg to 0.025 mg/kg. Although the antinociceptive response to clonidine was not further increased after 0.64 mg/kg of morphine, the potency ratio was significantly different from that of the H_2O controls. The slope functions of the individual curves are not significantly different, reflecting a parallel shift of the dose-response curve. The margin between ineffective and maximally potentiating doses of morphine is

TABLE V. Effect of Yohimbine on Antinociceptive Activity of Morphine and Clonidine in Mouse Tail Flick Test

Treatment	Dose yohimbine mg/kg SC	ED_{50}(95% CL) mg/kg SC	Potency[a] ratio
Morphine	H_2O	1.1 (0.6–2.2)	—
Morphine	0.625	2.0 (1.3–3.1)	1.8
Morphine	2.50	4.5 (4.3–4.7)	4.1[b]
Clonidine	H_2O	0.09 (0.04–0.21)	—
Clonidine	0.625	0.47 (0.29–0.76)	5.2[b]
Clonidine	2.50	2.52 (2.22–2.92)	27.8[b]

[a]Potency ratio = $\dfrac{ED_{50} \text{ treatment + yohimbine}}{ED_{50} \text{ treatment + } H_2O}$.

[b]Significantly different from H_2O controls [Litchfield and Wilcoxon, 1949].

TABLE VI. Effects of Morphine and Clonidine on Tail Flick Response

Drug	Dose mg/kg SC	N	% Inhibition of tail flick[a]
Vehicle		20	0
Morphine	8.0	20	80
Clonidine	1.0	20	80
Phenoxybenzamine	10.0	10	20
Naloxone	1.0	20	0
Morphine +	8.0		
Naloxone	1.0	20	30
Clonidine +	1.0		
Naloxone	1.0	20	80
Clonidine	1.0		
Phenoxybenzamine	10.0	20	80

[a]Increase of response latency greater than 2 SD.

TABLE VII. Effect of Morphine Pretreatment on the Antinociceptive Activity of Clonidine in Mouse Tail Flick Test

Morphine dose[a] mg/kg, SC	Clonidine HCl ED_{50}[b] (95% CL) mg/kg, SC	Slope function (95% CL)	Potency ratio
H_2O	0.100 (0.056–0.179)	2.56 (1.28–5.12)	1.0
0.040	0.084 (0.055–0.128)	1.98 (1.33–2.95)	1.2
0.160	0.025 (0.016–0.040)	2.15 (1.28–3.60)	4.0[c]
0.640	0.32　(0.020–0.052)	2.58 (0.89–3.60)	3.1[c]

[a]Morphine was administered 30 min and clonidine 15 min before testing.
[b]Cutoff times for ED_{50} determinations ranged between 2.6 and 3.0 sec.
[c]Potency differs significantly when compared to clonidine $= 1$.

narrow. A dose of 0.105 mg/kg was necessary to double the potency of clonidine (estimated by graphic analysis).

The potentiating effect of morphine (0.16 mg/kg) was reversed by naloxone (10 mg/kg) administered 10 minutes before testing (Fig. 4). The resulting clonidine ED_{50} was 0.150 (0.104–0.190) mg/kg with a slope function of 1.61 (1.16–2.23). The potency ratio of 1.5 and the comparative slopes did not differ significantly when compared with an ED_{50} of 0.100 (0.056–0.179) and a slope function of 2.56 (1.28–5.12) for clonidine alone.

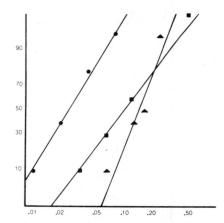

Fig. 4. The effect of naloxone on potentiation of the antinociceptive effect of clonidine by morphine in the mouse tail flick assay. Clonidine HCl alone (■) had an ED_{50} of 0.10 mg/kg. Tail flick activity of clonidine was potentiated (ED_{50} = 0.025 mg/kg) by morphine 0.16 mg/kg (•). Administration of naloxone reversed the potentiating effect of morphine on clonidine (ED_{50} = 0.150 mg/kg) activity (▲). Ordinate: % analgesia. Abscissa: clonidine HCl (mg/kg).

5. Clonidine pretreatment + morphine activity in tail flick test. A reciprocal relationship between clonidine and morphine was established by the finding that clonidine effectively reduced the analgesic ED_{50} of morphine. A clonidine dose of 0.016 mg/kg (ED_{50} = 0.10 mg/kg) was no more effective in potentiating the activity of morphine than the higher dose of 0.032 mg/kg (Table VIII). The slope functions of the dose-response curves do not differ statistically from parallelism.

6. Cross-tolerance in morphine-pelleted mice. Tolerance to morphine in morphine pellet (50 mg base) implanted mice was ten-fold 4 days after implantation (Table IX). There was no cross-tolerance to the antinociceptive effect of clonidine during this time. Although there was an increase in control tail flick latencies between placebo-implanted and morphine pellet-implanted mice (Table IX, footnote d), this did not seem to diminish the increase in the number of animals responding with an increase in dose of either morphine or clonidine. The curves generated from the antinociceptive effects on placebo-treated and morphine-implanted mice did not show a significant difference from parallelism. Furthermore, the lack of effect of either placebo or morphine pellet treatment on clonidine activity (ED_{50} = 0.10 mg/kg SC) was confirmed in this study.

TABLE VIII. Effect of Clonidine on the Antinociceptive Response of Mice to Morphine in the Tail Flick Test

Pretreatment	Dose (mg/kg)	Morphine ED_{50} (95% limits)		
		(mg/kg)	Slope function	Potency ratio[a]
H_2O	—	1.25 (0.93–1.68)[b]	1.81 (1.24– 2.64)	1
Clonidine HCl	0.016	0.26 (0.06–1.12)	4.28 (1.16–15.75)	4.8[c]
Clonidine HCl	0.032	0.41 (0.23–0.73)	3.69 (1.25–10.92)	3.0[c]

[a]95% confidence limits are in parentheses (n = 10 mice per dose and 3 doses/ED_{50} determination).
[b]Potency differs significantly when compared to morphine = 1.
[c]H_2O: clonidine.

7. Pithing. The differences between the antinociceptive activities of morphine and clonidine after pithing are shown in Table X. The ED_{50} of morphine was significantly decreased, viz 4–7 lower, 1 or 3 days after pithing, whereas clonidine activity was not significantly changed when compared with the controls. The dose-response curves for morphine did not differ from parallelism.

These data point to a distinct difference between the main sites of activity of morphine and clonidine in the tail flick test. The spinal and supraspinal levels of morphine activity were reconfirmed inasmuch as spinal transection partially suppressed the morphine-induced analgesia. On the other hand, the major portion of the clonidine-induced analgesia appears to involve the spinal reflex with no input from supraspinal structures. Furthermore, the spinal cord may contain opiate receptor-independent site(s) associated with the potentiation of morphine activity in the tail flick test [Spaulding et al, 1979a]. Further clarification of the sites of antinociceptive action will require direct application of clonidine to various supraspinal areas associated with analgesic activity.

III. DISCUSSION

The present studies have shown that clonidine produces a dose-dependent analgesia that is greater than or equal to that caused by morphine in a variety of tests known to induce pain in laboratory animals. It is apparent that α-adrenergically mediated analgesia is not due to an opiate receptor interaction, since naloxone failed to antagonize the action of clonidine in all

TABLE IX. Antinociceptive Effects of Clonidine and Morphine on Placebo and Morphine Pellet-Implanted Mice in the Tail Flick Test

Drug	Placebo pellet[a]		Morphine pellet[a]	
	ED_{50} (mg/kg SC)	Slope function	ED_{50} (mg/kg SC)	Slope function
Morphine	1.09[d] (0.74–1.61)[b]	1.88 (1.27–2.78)	9.99[c,d] (8.39–11.89)	1.40 (1.12–1.75)
Clonidine HCl	0.108[d] (0.075–0.155)	1.80 (0.92–3.29)	0.105[d] (0.054–0.204)	3.73 (0.23–61.5)

[a]Pellets were implanted 96 hours before test and were not removed prior to test.

[b]95% confidence limits are in parentheses.

[c]Significantly different from placebo-implanted control.

[d]Mean control times ± SD in placebo-implanted mice for morphine and clonidine-treated mice were 2.31 ± 0.27 sec and 2.24 ± 0.31 sec, respectively. In morphine pellet-implanted mice, times were 2.90 ± 0.32 sec and 2.96 ± 0.14 sec, respectively.

TABLE X. Antinociceptive Activity of Morphine and Clonidine After T_6–T_8 Spinal Transectomy in Mice

Treatment	ED_{50} (mg/kg SC)	
	Morphine	Clonidine HCl
Intact	1.28	0.11
	(0.80–2.10)	(0.07–0.16)
Spinal	6.65[a]	0.07[b]
(24 hours)	(3.44–12.87)	(0.04–0.12)
Spinal	4.65[a]	0.07[b]
(72 hours)	(1.06–4.43)	(0.05–0.11)

N = 10 mice per dose and 3–4 doses per ED_{50} determination. Values are expressed as ED_{50} with 95% confidence limits in parentheses. 24 and 72 hours = times after spinal transectomy.
[a]Significantly different from intact controls.
[b]Not significantly different from intact controls.

instances. The inhibitory effect that clonidine has on noradrenergic neurons appears to result from presynaptic activation of α receptors [Anden et al, 1970; Starke, 1972; Svensson et al, 1975]. Our data support this finding since phenoxybenzamine, a postsynaptic α-adrenoreceptor blocker, did not antagonize the effect of clonidine in the tail flick test. On the other hand, pretreatment with yohimbine, a presynaptic α-adrenoreceptor antagonist, did inhibit the activity of clonidine. Anden et al [1976] have suggested that yohimbine is more effective as an antagonist of presynaptic than of postsynaptic biochemical events.

Our data further suggest that clonidine and morphine act to produce analgesia along a common neuronal pathway. This was shown by the fact that clonidine and morphine increased each other's antinociceptive activity. The possibility that clonidine and morphine act at a common site (locus coeruleus) to produce the same effect through independent receptors has been suggested by Redmond [1977]. However, in contrast to narcotic analgesia, cross-tolerance was not observed in morphine-dependent mice.

Zemlan et al [1980] have hypothesized that clonidine acts at one synapse "downstream" from a narcotic-sensitive receptor site. This could account for the observed lack of cross-tolerance to clonidine in morphine-tolerant mice [Spaulding et al, 1979b] and the cross-tolerance to morphine in clonidine-tolerant mice [Paalzow, 1978]. Although these observations may have an anatomical basis, differences in testing procedure with different endpoints (tail flick vs vocalization) may also account for the discrepant results.

The antinociceptive effects of clonidine appear to be mediated centrally

[Schmitt et al, 1974; Lipman and Spencer, 1979]. It was shown by Schmitt et al [1974] that other α-sympathomimetics of the imadazoline series that do not cross the blood brain barrier have analgesic activity only when administered intracerebroventricularly. The experiments by Dr. Spaulding using the tail flick test show a distinct difference between the major action sites of morphine and clonidine. Spinal transection partially suppressed morphine analgesia, confirming the spinal and supraspinal levels of its activity.

On the other hand, the antinociceptive effect of clonidine was largely unaffected by thoracic spinal transection. These observations suggest that either the primary site of clonidine activity is at the segmental level or that supraspinal and spinal sites are equisensitive to clonidine-induced antinociception in the tail flick test.

Finally, the effect of clonidine in the phenylquinone writhing test may be due to its stimulating effect on α adrenoreceptors at the periphery, since Bentley et al [1977] have shown that other α agonists that do not cross the blood brain barrier are also active against writhing.

In summary, these studies show that the antinociceptive activities of clonidine and morphine are distinct. However, the total manifestation of analgesic activity in a variety of tests discloses common features between the two drugs. Whether a modification of common systems or clarification of their independent sites of activity is sufficient for the clinical efficacy of clonidine in a variety of pain states remains to be critically appraised.

IV. REFERENCES

Ader JP, Postema F, Korf J: Contribution of the locus coeruleus to the adrenergic innervation of the rat spinal cord: A biochemical study. J Neural Transmission 44:159–173, 1979.

Anden NE, Corrodi H, Fuxe K, Hokfelt B, Hokfelt T, Rydin C, Svensson T: Evidence for a central noradrenaline receptor stimulation by clonidine. Life Sci 9:513–523, 1970.

Anden NE, Grabowska M, Strombom U: Different alpha-adrenoceptors in the central nervous system mediating biochemical and functional effects of clonidine receptor blocking agents. Naunyn Schmiedeberg's Arch Pharmacol 292:43–52, 1976.

Bentley GA, Copeland IW, Starr J: The actions of some α-adrenoreceptor agonists and antagonists in an antinociceptive test in mice. Clin Exp Pharmacol Physiol 4:405–419, 1977.

D'Amour FE, Smith DL: A method for determining loss of pain sensation. J Pharmacol Exp Ther 72:74–79, 1941.

Fielding S, Wilker J, Hynes M, Szewczak M, Novick WJ, Lal H: A comparison of clonidine with morphine for antinociceptive and antiwithdrawal actions. J Pharmacol Exp Ther 207:899–905, 1978.

Frederickson RCA: Enkephalin pentopeptides — A review of current evidence for a physiological role in vertebrate neurotransmission. Life Sci 21:23–42, 1977.

Greenberg S, Palmer GC: Biochemical basis of analgesia: Metabolism, storage, regulation and action. Dent Clin North Am 22:31–46, 1978.

Handley SL, Spencer PSJ: Analgesic activity after intracerebral injection in the mouse. Br J Pharmacol 35:361P–362P, 1969.

Janssen PAJ, Niemegeers CJE, Dony JGH: The inhibitory effect of fentanyl and other morphine-like analgesics on the warm water induced tail withdrawal reflex in rats. Arzneim Forsch 13:502–507, 1963.

Kerr FWL: Neuroanatomical substitutes of nociception in the spinal cord. Pain 1:325–356, 1975.

Lipman JL, Spencer PSJ: Further evidence for a central site of action for the antinociceptive effects of clonidine-like drugs. Neuropharmacology 18:731–733, 1979.

Litchfield JT, Wilcoxon F: A simplified method of evaluating dose effect experiments. J Pharmacol Exp Ther 96:99–113, 1949.

Lobatz MA, Proudfit HK, Anderson EG: Effects of noxious stimulation, iontophoretic morphine and norepinephrine on neurons in nucleus raphe magnus. Pharmacologist 18:213, 1976.

Margalit D, Segal M: A pharmacologic study of analgesia produced by stimulation of the nucleus locus coeruleus. Psychopharmacology 62:169–173, 1979.

Miksic S, Lal H: Tolerance to morphine produced discriminative stimuli and analgesia. Psychopharmacology 54:217–221, 1977.

Paalzow G, Paalzow L: Clonidine antinociceptive activity: Effects of drugs influencing central monaminergic and cholinergic mechanisms in the rat. Naunyn Schmiedeberg's Arch Pharmacol 292:119–126, 1976.

Paalzow G: Development of tolerance to the analgesic effect of clonidine in rats, cross-tolerance to morphine. Naunyn Schmiedeberg's Arch Pharmacol 304:1–4, 1978.

Paalzow L: Analgesia produced by clonidine in mice and rats. J Pharm Pharmacol 26:361–363, 1974.

Pepeu G: In Bonica JJ, Albe-Fressard D (eds): "Involvement of Central Transmitters in Narcotic Analgesia in Advances in Pain Research and Therapy," Vol 1. New York: Raven Press, 1976, pp 595–600.

Price TC, Fibiger HC: Ascending catecholamine systems and morphine analgesia. Brain Res 99:189–193, 1975.

Randall LO, Selitto JJ: A method for measurement of analgesic activity on inflamed tissue. Arch Int Pharmacodyn Ther 111:409–414, 1957.

Reddy S, Yaksh T: Spinal noradrenegic terminal system mediates antinociception. Brain Res 189:391–401, 1980.

Redmond DE: Alterations in the functions of the nucleus locus coereleus: A possible model for studies of anxiety. In Manin I, Usdin E (eds): "Animal Models in Psychiatry and Neurology." New York: Pergamon Press, 1977, pp 293–304.

Schmitt H, LeDouarec JC, Petillot N: Antinociceptive effects of some α-sympathomimetic agents. Neuropharmacology 13:289–294, 1974.

Sewell RDE, Spencer PSJ: Possible involvement of norepinephrine and 5-hydroxytryptamine in the antiociceptive activity of narcotic analgesics. In Bonica JJ, Albe-Fessard D (eds): "Advances in Pain Research and Therapy," Vol 1. New York: Raven Press, 1976, pp 607–614.

Siegmund E, Damus R, Lu G: A method for evaluating both nonnarcotic and narcotic analgesics. Proc Soc Exp Biol Med 95:729–731, 1957.

Spaulding TC, Venafro JJ, Ma MG, Fielding S: The dissociation of the antinociceptive effect of clonidine from supraspinal structures. Neuropharmacology 18:103–105, 1979a.

Spaulding TC, Fielding S, Venafro JJ, Lal H: Antinociceptive activity of clonidine and its potentiation of morphine analgesia. Eur J Pharmacol 58:19–25, 1979b.

Starke K: Influence of extracellular noradrenaline on the stimulation evoked secretion of noradrenaline from sympathetic nerves: Evidence for an α-receptor-mediated feedback inhibitor of noradrenaline release. Naunyn Schmiedeberg's Arch Pharmacol 275:11–23, 1972.

Svensson TH, Bunny BS, Aghajanian GK: Inhibition of both noradrenergic and serotonergic neurons in brain by the α-adrenergic agonist clonidine. Brain Res 92:291–306, 1975.

Takagi H, Dio T, Akaike A: Microinjection of morphine into the medial part of the bulboreticular formation in rabbit and rat: Inhibitory effects on lamina V cells of spinal dorsal horn and behavioral analgesia. In Kosterlitz HW (ed): "Opiates and Endogenous Opioid Peptides." New York: Elsevier, 1976, pp 191–198.

Takagi H, Shoimi H, Kursishi Y, Fukui K, Ueda H: Pain and the bulbospinal noradrenergic system: Pain-induced increase in normetanephrine content in the spinal cord and its modification by morphine. Eur J Pharmacol 54:99–107, 1979.

Takemori AE: Pharmacologic factors which alter the action of narcotic analgesics and antagonists. Ann NY Acad Sci 281:262–272, 1976.

Timmermans P, Brands A, Van Zwietan PA: Lipophilicity and brain disposition of clonidine and structurally related imidazolines. Naunyn Schmiedeberg's Arch Pharmacol 300:217–226, 1977.

Yaksh T, Reddy S: Studies in the primate of the analgetic effects associated with intrathecal actions of opiates, alpha-adrenergic agonists, and baclofen. Anesthesiology 54:451–467, 1981.

Yaksh TL, Rudy TA: Narcotic analgesics: CNS sites and mechanisms of action as revealed by intracerebral injection techniques. Pain 4:299–359, 1978.

Zemlan FP, Corrigan SA, Pfaff DW: Noradrenergic and serotonergic mediation of spinal analgesia mechanisms. Eur J Pharmacol 61:111–124, 1980.

Psychopharmacology of Clonidine, pages 243–258
© 1981 Alan R. Liss, Inc., 150 Fifth Avenue, New York, NY 10011

Antinociceptive Mechanism and Acute and Chronic Behavioral Effects of Clonidine

Mario D. Aceto and Louis S. Harris

I. INTRODUCTION

Reports that clonidine may be useful in the rapid withdrawal of patients from methadone [Gold et al, 1978] and that it has antinociceptive properties not antagonized by naloxone [Fielding et al, 1978; Paalzow, 1974; Paalzow and Paalzow, 1976] led us to examine this compound in our laboratory. This drug was found to produce physical dependence unlike that induced by morphine in humans [Hokfelt et al, 1970] and animals [Dix and Johnson, 1977]. Tolerance developed to its sedative [Laverty and Taylor, 1969] and analgesic effects [Paalzow, 1978]. It was also found to suppress some withdrawal signs in morphine-dependent rats [Fielding et al, 1978].

In preliminary studies [Aceto et al, 1979], we found that the drug was active in the mouse tail-flick and phenylquinone antinociceptive tests, that it showed no antagonistic properties when tested versus morphine-induced antinociception, that it did not inhibit the stereospecific binding of ^{3}H-dihydromorphine in mouse brain homogenates, and that it substituted partially for morphine in highly addicted rhesus monkeys.

These findings convinced us that a thorough study of this remarkable compound was in order. We were especially interested in finding common underlying mechanisms of these actions.

II. METHODS

A. Mouse Antinociception Tests

Male Swiss-Webster mice in the weight range of 22–30 gm were used. All drugs were dissolved in distilled water and administered in a volume of 0.1 ml/10 gm of body weight. All doses were expressed as salts. At least three doses per curve were tested and 6–10 animals per dose were used. ED_{50}s and 95% confidence limits were calculated by the method of Litchfield and Wilcoxin [1949].

1. Mouse tail flick tests. The procedure used was essentially that of D'Amour and Smith [1941] as modified by Dewey et al [1970]. The mouse tail was placed in a groove containing a slit under which a photoelectric cell was located. When the heat source or noxious stimulus was turned on, it focused on the tail and the animal responded by flicking its tail out of the groove. Thus light passed through the slit and activated the photocell, which in turn stopped the recording timer. The apparatus was calibrated so that control mice would flick their tails in 2–4 seconds. Mice were given the drug subcutaneously and tested 20 minutes later. Vehicle controls were also tested. In the antagonism experiments, the antagonists were administered subcutaneously 10 minutes before an agonist was given and the animals were tested 20 minutes later.

2. Phenylquinone abdominal stretching test. The procedure used has previously been described by Pearl et al [1968]. The mice received the drugs SC and 10 minutes later received 2 mg/kg of p-phenylquinone solution intra-peritoneally. The mice were then placed in mouse cages in groups of two. Ten minutes after the p-phenylquinone injection, the total number of stretches per group was counted within 1 minute. A stretch was characterized by an elongation of the mouse body, development of tension in the muscles in the abdominal region, and an extension of the forelimbs. The antinociceptive response was expressed as the percent inhibition of the p-phenylquinone-induced stretching response. Appropriate controls were tested.

B. Rat Continuous Infusion Test

This method has been described by Teiger [1974]. Semirestrained male Sprague-Dawley rats were medicated with clonidine by continuous infusion through indwelling intraperitoneal cannulas for 6 days. The rats were anesthetized and each was fitted with a specially prepared cannula that was passed subcutaneously from the nape of the neck to the lateral side of the lower abdomen and then inserted in the peritoneal cavity. The cannula was anchored at both ends with silk sutures and attached to a flow-through swivel mechanism that allowed the animal to move about in the cage and eat and drink normally. The swivel was connected to a syringe, which was attached to a syringe pump. The animals received a volume of 7–10 ml of solution every 24 hours. After the drugs had been given for 6 days, they were abruptly withdrawn, and the animals were observed for changes in body weight, water consumption, and behavioral signs of withdrawal for half an hour at 6, 24, 48, and 72 hours and in one study at 96 hours after withdrawal.

C. Rhesus Monkey Single-Dose Suppression Test (SDS)

For the most part, the recommendations of Seevers [1936] and Seevers and Deneau [1963] were followed. A brief description of the procedure including modifications reported by Aceto et al [1979] follows: Male and female rhesus monkeys [M. mulatta] in the weight range of 3.8–6.5 kg were used. Groups of five animals each were housed in pens and received 3 mg/kg of morphine SC every 6 hours. This dose schedule, according to Seevers and Deneau [1963], induces maximal physical dependence. All the animals had received morphine for at least 6 months. A minimal 2-week washout and recuperation period was allowed for each animal between tests. The SDS test was initiated by subcutaneous injection of clonidine or control substances (morphine and vehicle/H_2O) into a group of animals that had not received morphine for 14–15 hours and showed definite signs of withdrawal. Each animal was randomly allocated to one of five treatments: 1) one of three doses of clonidine; 2) morphine, 3.0 mg/kg; 3) vehicle, 1 ml/kg. The animals were scored for suppression of withdrawal signs during a 2½-hour observation period. The observer was blinded to the allocation of treatments. At the end of the study the data were grouped according to dose and drug, and the results were analyzed by the Mann-Whitney U-Test [Siegel, 1956].

D. Rhesus Monkey Primary Physical Dependence Test (PPD)

Essentially, the same procedure was used as described above in the SDS test except that the number of animals was five, the test substance was given every 6 hours, and the observer was aware of the dose and drug given. At intervals of 16, 31, and 39 days the drugs were abruptly withdrawn. A naloxone challenge was also given on day 16 and at the end of the study.

E. Materials

Atropine SO_2; clonidine HCl; morphine $H_2SO_4 \cdot 5H_2O$; naloxone HCl; oxotremorine sesquifumarate; and yohimbine HCl.

III. RESULTS

As shown in Table I, clonidine has potent antinociceptive properties as compared with morphine in the phenylquinone test and the more rigorous tail-flick test. However, exact potency estimates were not made because the slopes of the dose-response curves were not parallel. We also demonstrated that clonidine is devoid of opiate-antagonistic properties, as indicated by its lack of activity versus morphine-induced antinociception over a wide dose range.

The results presented in Table II are also revealing. Naloxone antagonized morphine, as expected, and the AD_{50} is 0.03 (0.01–0.9) mg/kg. It is partially active as an oxotremorine antagonist (38%) at 10.0 mg/kg, and is inactive versus clonidine in doses up to 15.0 mg/kg. Atropine antagonized oxotremorine, as has been shown many times [AD_{50} is 0.76 (0.34–1.6) mg/kg], and

TABLE I. Effects of Clonidine and Morphine in the Mouse Tail Flick and Phenylquinone Tests

	Results ED_{50} (95% confidence limits) mg/kg SC	
Test	Clonidine	Morphine
1) Tail flick	1.2 (0.2–6.7)	5.8 (5.7–5.9)
2) Tail flick antagonism	Inactive at 0.3, 1.0, and 30.0	
3) Phenylquinone	0.005 (0.001–0.02)	0.23 (0.20–0.25)

TABLE II. The Antinociceptive-Antagonistic Properties of Naloxone, Yohimbine, and Atropine in the Tail Flick Test

	Results (antagonists) AD_{50} (95% confidence limits) or % effect, mg/kg SC		
Agonists	Yohimbine	Atropine	Naloxone
Morphine	5.6 (2.7–11.5)	55% at 5.0	0.03 (0.01–0.9)
Clonidine	7.1 (4.1–12.0)	42% at 10.0	0% at 30.0
			10% at 1.0
Oxotremorine	9.7 (7.2–13.2)	0.8 (0.3–1.7)	38% at 10.0

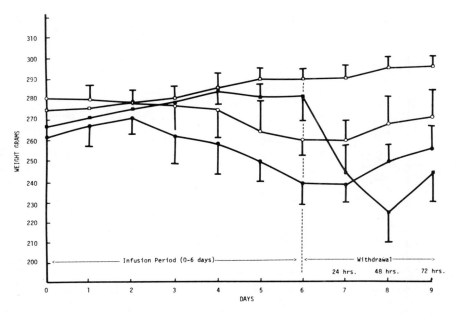

Fig. 1. Weight changes in rats continuously treated with infusions of clonidine, morphine, and dextrose. The dose regimen and number of animals for each drug were as follows:

————□———— 5% Dextrose
7.5 mg/24 hrs (N = 11)

————■———— Morphine
mg/kg/24 hrs (N = 9)
1st day 50 mg
2nd day 100 mg
Days 3–6 200 mg

————○———— Clonidine
mg/kg/24 hrs (N = 6)
1st day 0.1
2nd day 0.5
Days 3–6 1.0

————●———— Clonidine
mg/kg/24 hrs (N = 7)
1st day 0.1
2nd day 0.5
Days 3–6 5.0

it only partially antagonized the agonist activity of both morphine and clonidine. With yohimbine, on the other hand, the antinociceptive actions of all three agonists were antagonized at approximately the same doses (5.6–9.7 mg/kg). In addition, yohimbine also antagonized the locomotor stimulation and aggression produced by clonidine.

In the rat infusion experiments, the results in the clonidine-treated rats contrasted markedly with those obtained with either the morphine-treated or the dextrose controls. As shown in Figure 1, the clonidine-treated animals

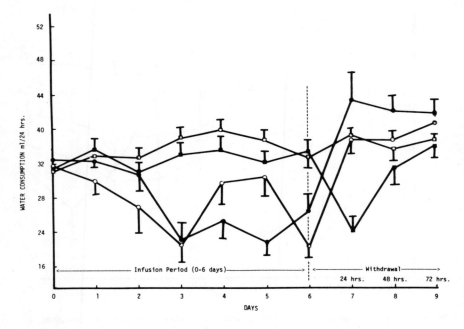

Fig. 2. Water consumption in rats continuously treated with infusions of clonidine, morphine, and dextrose. The dose regimen and number of animals for each drug were as follows:

──────□────── 5% Dextrose 7.5 mg/24 hrs (N = 11)	──────■────── Morphine mg/kg/24 hrs (N = 9) 1st day 50 mg 2nd day 100 mg Days 3–6 200 mg
──────○────── Clonidine mg/kg/24 hrs (N = 6) 1st day 0.1 2nd day 0.5 Days 3–6 1.0	──────●────── Clonidine mg/kg/24 hrs (N = 7) 1st day 0.1 2nd day 0.5 Days 3–6 5.0

lost weight to a dose-related extent during administration of drug. The animals also were excitable, aggressive, and easily startled at this time. When the drug was abruptly withdrawn on day 6, weight loss ceased and the weight gradually returned to normal. Behavioral signs also returned to normal. In sharp contrast, the morphine-treated animals initially appeared drowsy and later appeared normal. Upon abrupt withdrawal of morphine, they lost weight during the first 48 hours, became aggressive and hypersensitive, and

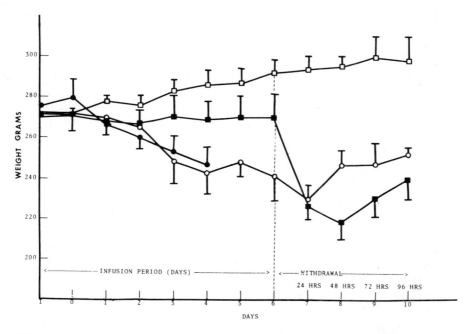

Fig. 3. Another study showing weight changes in rats treated with clonidine, morphine, H₂O, and clonidine + morphine. The dose regimen and number of animals for each drug were as follows:

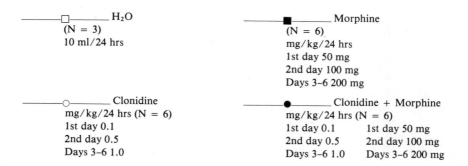

then began to recover. The results obtained with morphine have been described before [Dewey and Patrick, 1975; Teiger, 1974]. The dextrose-treated rats showed a small but steady rise in weight throughout the study. There were marked contrasts in water consumption, as shown in Figure 2. The clonidine-treated animals drastically reduced their water consumption.

TABLE III. Cumulative Number of Wet-Dog Shakes, Rubbing, and Chewing Actions of Rats (Number of Episodes per ½ hour) After Abrupt Withdrawal

Time (Hours)	Drug (No. of animals)		
	Clonidine N = 4	Morphine N = 5	Vehicle (H$_2$O) N = 3
6	89	44	0
24	33	28	2
48	95	116	0
72	64	144	0
96	37	83	2

When these animals were subjected to abrupt withdrawal, water consumption rose dramatically. By contrast, the morphine-treated animals drank water in normal amounts until morphine was withdrawn. During the first 24–48 hours after abrupt withdrawal, water consumption dropped, but it was nearly back to normal by 72 hours. The dextrose-treated rats drank the usual amount of water throughout the study. Because we believed that it was important to study the interaction of clonidine and morphine when given together, additional infusion studies were initiated. The lowest doses of clonidine used in the first infusion study were administered along with the normal doses of morphine. The results in the vehicle controls, clonidine controls, and morphine controls were similar to those reported above. However, the combination of morphine and clonidine was lethal. By day 3, two of the animals had died, and by day 5 all the animals that had received the combination were dead. The weight data are presented in Figure 3. Behavioral signs following abrupt withdrawal were not remarkable in the vehicle controls. Some of the clonidine controls still showed hypersensitivity to touch and squealed when handled at 6 hours. One animal was still hypersensitive at 24 hours, but no such signs were noted at 48, 72, and 96 hours. The morphine controls began to show hypersensitivity and squealed when handled at 6 hours. All showed these signs at 24 hours, and by 96 hours two animals still showed a minimal degree of hypersensitivity and squealed when handled. We have summarized the results of the behavioral signs commonly seen after abrupt withdrawal. These signs are not as reliable as weight loss and hypersensitivity and squealing, and their frequency can vary from day to day. They are shown in Table III. The significance of the differences between total scores was assessed by the Mann-Whitney U-test; the calculated probability values are given in Table IV.

The results of the single-dose suppression test (SDS) in withdrawn monkeys are also instructive (Tables V and VI). It is obvious that water did not

TABLE IV. Probability Values[a] Calculated for Various Comparisons Between Data in Columns of Table III by the Mann-Whitney U-Test

Hour		Clonidine	Morphine
6	Vehicle	0.02	0.01
	Morphine	0.05	—
24	Vehicle	0.31	0.01
	Morphine	0.54	—
48	Vehicle	0.05	0.01
	Morphine	0.2	—
72	Vehicle	0.02	0.01
	Morphine	0.45	—
96	Vehicle	0.57	0.01
	Morphine	0.36	—

[a]One-tailed test.

TABLE V. Single-Dose Substitution Study of Clonidine and Controls in Morphine-Dependent Monkeys (Incidence of Withdrawal Signs)

Treatment	Clonidine			Morphine	H_2O
Dose: mg/kg SC	0.065	0.125	0.25	3.0	1.0 ml/kg
No. of animals	6	6	6	6	6
Slowing	2	4	3	—	—
Lying on side or abdomen	1	3	1	1	15
Drowsiness	22	24	23	2	10
Fighting	—	2	1	—	2
Avoiding contact	5	5	9	5	4
Vocalizing	2	4	4	—	2
Crawling and rolling	—	—	4	—	2
Restlessness (pacing)	5	5	6	9	24
Ptosis	3	8	6	—	—
Tremors	3	5	6	1	4
Retching	5	5	6	1	24
Vomiting	—	3	3	—	3
Coughing	—	—	1	—	2
Vocalizing on palpation of abdomen	17	18	18	1	30
Rigid abdomen	15	15	15	—	30
Wet-dog shakes	4	1	2	2	14
Masturbation	3	—	—	—	6
Total	87	102	108	22	172
Average	14.5	17	18	3.7	28.7

TABLE VI. Single-Dose Suppression Test Probabilities[a] Calculated for Various Comparisons Between Data in Table V by the Mann-Whitney U-Test

	Clonidine 0.065 mg/kg	Clonidine 0.125 mg/kg	Clonidine 0.250 mg/kg	Morphine 3.0 mg/kg
Vehicle (H_2O)	0.001	0.032	0.032	0.001
Clonidine 0.065	—	0.469	0.066	0.002
Clonidine 0.125	—	—	0.531	0.008
Clonidine 0.250 mg/kg	—	—	—	0.001

[a]One-tailed test.

TABLE VII. Summary of Results of the Primary Physical Dependence Study in Rhesus Monkeys

Day	Dose (SC) mg/kg in 96 hrs	Overt behavior principal signs (N = 5)
1–15	0.01–0.24	Drowsy, ptosis, slowing
16 a.m. Abrupt withdrawal		Fighting, yawning, wet-dog shakes
p.m. Precipitated withdrawal (naloxone)	0.1 mg/kg/SC	Same as abrupt withdrawal
17–24	0.32–0.58	Drowsy, ptosis, slowing
25–30	0.64–3.0,	Drowsy, ptosis
31a–38	4.2–14.4	Drowsy, fighting, tremors, staring, stopped eating, slowing
39 a.m. Abrupt withdrawal		Fighting, crawling, tremors, scratching, wet-dog shakes, yawning
p.m. Precipitated withdrawal (naloxone)	1.0 mg/kg SC	Same as abrupt withdrawal

[a]Although the animals were subjected to abrupt withdrawal, the results were not recorded.

substitute for morphine. Equally obvious is the fact that morphine completely suppressed the withdrawal syndrome. Clonidine substituted partially at all doses when compared with the vehicle. It is noteworthy that clonidine increased drowsiness, whereas morphine nearly suppressed this sign. If clonidine had acted like morphine by actually suppressing the drowsiness accompanying withdrawal, the total scores would certainly have been lower. In any case, clonidine diminished the incidence of many individual withdrawal signs such as lying on the side or abdomen, crawling and rolling, restlessness, retching, wet-dog shakes, and vocalizing on palpation of the abdomen. We hasten to add that partial substitution does not necessarily mean that the drug has morphine-like properties.

The results of the primary physical dependence test are summarized in Table VII. Briefly, five naive monkeys were given clonidine (mg/kg SC) as indicated every 6 hours. At the lowest dose (0.01) they became restless. The dose was doubled on day 2 and restlessness was apparent again. At 0.04 and 0.08 mg/kg, drowsiness, eyelid ptosis, and slowing were seen. On day 8, the dose was raised to 0.1 mg/kg and by day 15 the dose was 0.25 mg/kg. The same signs that were noted on days 3–7 were consistently present during this period. The animals were subjected to abrupt withdrawal on day 16, after which fighting, yawning, and wet-dog shakes developed. Later, a naloxone challenge (0.1 mg/kg SC) was given, and the signs noted during abrupt withdrawal were observed again. After the dose had again been increased to 3.0 mg/kg by day 30, drowsiness, ptosis, and slowing were observed consistently, and fighting was noted occasionally. The animals were subjected to abrupt withdrawal but, because of a misunderstanding, the results were not recorded. On days 32, 33, and 34, the dose was 6.6 mg/kg, and drowsiness, fighting, and tremors were recorded. The dose was raised to 12.6 mg/kg on day 36 and raised again to 14.4 the next day; it was reduced to 12.6 on day 38 because, in addition to the effects noted above, the animals stopped eating and were staring. The animals were subjected to abrupt withdrawal on day 39. The only signs noted were residual drowsiness, fighting, avoidance of contact, restlessness, wet-dog shakes, scratching, and yawning. A naloxone challenge (1.0 mg/kg SC) did not produce any significant change from the signs noted during abrupt withdrawal. Apparently, a high degree of tolerance but a very low degree of physical dependence on this agent developed. It does not appear to induce a significant degree of morphine-like physical dependence.

IV. DISCUSSION

A report by Paalzow and Paalzow [1976] that yohimbine antagonized clonidine-induced antinociception provided us with a lead in our search for a common mechanism for action of clonidine and morphine. We posed the question of whether or not yohimbine would also antagonize morphine-induced antinociception. Yohimbine did indeed antagonize the effects of both drugs in the tail flick test. Another important lead was provided by the suggestion of Paalzow and Paalzow [1976] that presynaptic α-adrenoreceptors in the central nervous system might be involved in the analgesic effect and locomotor depression caused by clonidine. There is evidence that clonidine is more potent in reducing norepinephrine release during nerve stimulation than in stimulating the postsynaptic α-adrenoreceptors [Starke et al, 1975a, b]. The drug appeared to be more potent on α-presynaptic than on postsynaptic receptors. Although yohimbine has commonly been regarded as an adrenergic blocking agent [Nickerson and Hollenberg, 1967; Bolme et al, 1974], it was found to be more potent in blocking presynaptic α receptors in the rabbit [Starke et al, 1975a, b].

Among other presynaptic receptors believed to be present at noradrenergic nerve endings, muscarinic-inhibitory receptors have been described [Langer, 1977; Steinsland et al, 1973]. Oxotremorine and several other drugs with cholinergic properties [Harris et al, 1969; Paalzow and Paalzow, 1976; Pedigo et al, 1975] showed antinociceptive activity in the tail flick test, and this activity was selectively blocked by anticholinergic drugs.

Thus clonidine, morphine, and oxotremorine can act on different presynaptic receptors. By contrast, the actions of naloxone and atropine are relatively specific. Yohimbine blocks all three presynaptic receptors. These observations support the hypothesis that antinociceptive activity in the tail flick test is related, at least in part, to inhibition of norepinephrine release by presynaptic mechanisms. It is also possible that yohimbine acts by interfering with the adrenergic feedback mechanisms postulated by Langer [1977].

When chronically administered to rats in relatively high doses, clonidine produced certain signs reminiscent of those seen in morphine-dependent rats after abrupt withdrawal. Weight loss and aggressive behavior are considered the more reliable signs for evaluating the degree of morphine dependence in the rat infusion technique [Dewey and Patrick, 1975; Teiger, 1974]. When clonidine administration was discontinued, the animals reverted back to their normal behavior; that is, they resumed drinking normal amounts of water, began regaining weight, and became much less aggressive and hypersensitive.

In one abrupt withdrawal study, we noticed that the incidence of wet-dog shakes, chewing, and rubbing was significantly higher in the clonidine and morphine controls than in the vehicle controls, but we have not been able to show this consistently. Perhaps other studies with a larger number of animals are indicated.

Aggressive behavior has been observed after single doses of clonidine in mice [Morpurgo, 1968; Razzak et al, 1971] and after chronic administration in rats [Dix and Johnson, 1977]. All of these workers believed that the mechanism is central and one thought that it is not related to systemic toxicity [Morpurgo, 1968]. It has been shown that chronic treatment with clonidine leads to an increased responsiveness of postsynaptic central α-adrenoreceptors and that clonidine activated these receptors at high doses [Svensson and Strombom, 1975]. Very low doses were required to produce cardiovascular and sedative effects [Strombom, 1975] or to inhibit firing of brain NE neurons through activation of adrenergic receptors [Svensson et al,

1971]. The hyperexcitability and increased aggressiveness noted during chronic administration of relatively high doses of clonidine and after abrupt withdrawal of morphine from dependent rats may be the result of a facilitated brain noradrenergic mechanism. While we were not able to show that high doses of clonidine alter the development of morphine dependence when these two drugs are given together, we did find that this combination is lethal in rats, and we therefore suggest that caution be exercised whenever the two drugs are given to humans concomitantly.

Whether or not the observed suppression of drinking and weight loss by clonidine and morphine can be explained by another common mechanism remains to be shown. Clonidine suppresses renin release in many animal species [Hokfelt et al, 1970; Onesti et al, 1971]. This suppression of renin release has been attributed to a centrally mediated decrease in sympathetic tone [Onesti et al, 1971], but peripheral effects on α-adrenoreceptors in the kidney have been reported as well [Chevillard et al, 1978]. A physiological role of the renin-angiotension system in thirst and drinking and release of pituitary hormones has been proposed [Severs and Daniels-Severs, 1975]. The weight loss and suppression of drinking during the administration of clonidine and after the abrupt withdrawal of morphine may indeed have a common neuroendocrine or neurochemical mechanism.

Our results with monkeys were also revealing. Clonidine substituted partially for morphine. This observation may be relevant to reports by Gold et al [1978, 1980] that clonidine is effective in opiate-dependent patients. It is important to note that partial substitution in rhesus monkeys does not necessarily mean that the drug has an opiate-like tendency to induce dependence. That clonidine substituted partially rather than completely may be related to the high degree of addiction of the monkeys used in this study: Some had received 3.0 mg/kg of morphine SC every 6 hours for over 3 years. We wonder if clonidine would substitute partially rather than fully in highly addicted human subjects. We plan to reevaluate clonidine in monkeys dependent on much lower doses of morphine to see if it will substitute for them completely.

Although some signs of withdrawal were noted, clonidine did not produce a significant degree of morphine-like physical dependence in monkeys on an escalating SC dose schedule starting at 0.01 mg/kg and extending to 14.4 mg/kg every 6 hours for 39 days. This finding is in accord with clinical observations [Hokfelt et al, 1970; Pettinger, 1975] that it does not produce opiate-like physical dependence in humans.

In summary, there is substantial evidence that presynaptic receptors play a significant role in the antinociceptive actions of clonidine and morphine. In addition, clonidine given in high doses has certain effects that may be related to actions on α-adrenergic postsynaptic receptors or to neuroendocrine events. That clonidine produces less dependence than morphine may be related to its direct action on α-adrenoreceptors. These receptors play a physiological role in norepinephrine transmission and are associated with regulatory feedback mechanisms. Morphine, on the other hand, acts directly on opiate receptors to modify norepinephrine transmission directly. Opiate receptors may be predominantly of pharmacological importance and may be less subject to feedback regulation.

V. ACKNOWLEDGMENTS

This work has been supported in part by a contract (DA-271-77-3404) and grant (DA-00490) from the National Institute of Drug Abuse. We wish to thank Mr. F.T. Grove, Mr. R. Jones, Mr. D. Miller, and Mrs. S. Welch for their technical assistance. We are also indebted to Dr. A. Jacobson at NIH and Dr. W. Smith at A.H. Robins Co. for their generous supplies of clonidine HCl and yohimbine HCl.

VI. REFERENCES

Aceto MD, Carchman RA, Harris LS, Flora R: Caffeine elicited withdrawal signs in morphine-dependent rhesus monkeys. Eur J Pharmacol 50:203–207, 1978.

Aceto MD, Dewey WL, Harris LS, Chau-Pham TT, Kramer CM: Analgesic properties and dependence liability of clonidine. Fed Proc 38:853, 1979.

Bolme P, Corrodi H, Fuxe K, Hokfelt T, Lidbrink P, Goldstein H: Possible involvement of central adrenaline neurons in vasomotor and respiratory control: Studies with clonidine and its interactions with piperoxane and yohimbine. Eur J Pharmacol 28:89–94, 1974.

Chevillard C, Pasquier R, Duchene N, Alexander J: Mechanism of inhibition of renin release by clonidine in rats. Eur J Pharmacol 48:451–454, 1978.

D'Amour FE, Smith DL: A method for determining loss of pain sensation. J Pharmacol Exp Ther 72:74–79, 1941.

Dewey WL, Harris LS, Howes JF, Nuite JA: The effects of various neurohumoral modulators on the activity of morphine and the narcotic antagonists in the tail-flick and phenylquinone tests. J Pharmacol Exp Ther 175:435–443, 1970.

Dewey WL, Patrick GA: Narcotic antagonist in the rat infusion technique. Proceedings from 37th Annual Meeting, Committee on Problems of Drug Dependence, NRC-NAC, USA, 1975, pp 64-73.

Dix RK, Johnson EM Jr: Withdrawal syndrome upon cessation of chronic clonidine treatment in rats. Eur J Pharmacol 44:153–159, 1977.

Fielding S, Wilker J, Hynes M, Szewezak M, Novick WJ, Lal H: A comparison of clonidine with morphine for antinociceptive and antiwithdrawal actions. J Pharmacol Exp Ther 207:899–905, 1978.

Gold MS, Pottash AC, Sweeney DR, Kleber HD: Opiate withdrawal using clonidine: A safe, effective, and rapid nonopiate treatment. JAMA 243:343–346, 1980.

Gold MS, Redmond DE Jr, Kleber HD: Clonidine blocks acute opiate withdrawal symptoms. Lancet 2:599–602, 1978.

Hansson L, Hunyor SN, Julius S, Hoobler SW: Blood pressure crisis following withdrawal of clonidine (catapres, catapresan) with special reference to arterial and urinary catecholamine levels and suggestions for acute management. Am Heart J 85:605–610, 1973.

Harris LS, Dewey WL, Howes JF, Kennedy JS, Pars H: Narcotic-antagonists analgesics, interactions with cholinergic mechanisms. J Pharmacol Exp Ther 169:17–22, 1969.

Hokfelt B, Hedeland H, Dymling JF: Studies on catecholamines, renin and aldosterone following catapresan (2-(2,6-dichlorophenylamino)-2-imidazoline hydrochloride) in hypertensive patients. Eur J Pharmacol 10:389–397, 1970.

Langer SZ: Presynaptic receptors and their role in the regulation of transmitter release. Br J Pharmacol 60:481–497, 1977.

Laverty R, Taylor KM: Behavioral and biochemical effects of (2-(2,6-dichlorophenylamino)-2-imidazoline hydrochloride) (St 155) on the central nervous system. Br J Pharmacol 35:253–264, 1969.

Lipmen JJ, Spencer SJ: Clonidine and opiate withdrawal. Lancet 2:521, 1978.

Litchfield ST, Wilcoxon FA: A simplified method of evaluating dose-effect experiments. J Pharmacol Exp Ther 96:99–113, 1949.

Meyer DR, El R, Zhary A, Bierer DWS, Hansen SK, Robbins MS, Sparber SB: Tolerance and dependence after chronic administration of clonidine on the rat. Pharmacol Biochem Behav 7:227–231, 1977.

Montel H, Starke R, Weber F: Influence of morphine and naloxone on the release of noradrenaline from rat brain cortex slices. Naunyn Schmiedeberg's Arch Pharmacol 283:357–369, 1974.

Morpurgo C: Aggressive behavior induced by large doses of (2-(2,6-dichlorophenylamino)-2-imidazoline hydrochloride) (St 155) in mice. Eur J Pharmacol 3:374–377, 1968.

Nickerson M, Hollenberg K: Blockade of α-adrenergic receptors. In Root WS, Hofmann FG (eds): "Physiological Pharmacology." New York, London: Academic Press, 1967, pp 243–305.

Onesti G, Schwartz AB, Kim KE, Paz-Martinea V, Swartz C: Antihypertensive effect of clonidine. Circ Res 28, 29, Suppl II; 53–69, 1971.

Paalzow G: Development of tolerance to the analgesic effect of clonidine in rats cross-tolerance to morphine. Naunyn Schmiedeberg's Arch Pharmacol 304:1–4, 1978.

Paalzow G, Paalzow L: Clonidine antinociceptive activity: Effects of drugs influence on central monoaminergic and cholinergic mechanisms in the rat. Naunyn Schmiedeberg's Arch Pharmacol 292:119–126, 1976.

Paalzow L: Analgesia produced by clonidine in mice and rats. J Pharm Pharmacol 20:361–363, 1974.

Pearl J, Aceto MD, Harris LS: Prevention of writhing and other effects of narcotic and narcotic antagonists in mice. J Pharmacol Exp Ther 160:217–230, 1968.

Pearl J, Harris LS: Inhibition of writhing by narcotic antagonists. J Pharmacol Exp Ther 154:319–323, 1966.

Pedigo NW, Dewey WL, Harris LS: Determination and characterization of the antinociceptive activity of intraventricularly administered acetylcholine in mice. J Pharmacol Exp Ther 193:845–852, 1975.

Pettinger W: Clonidine, a new hypertensive drug. N Engl J Med 293:1179–1180, 1975.

Razzak A, Fujiwara M, Oishi R, Euki S: Possible involvement of a central noradrenergic system in automutilation induced by clonidine in mice. Jpn J Pharmacol 27:145–152, 1977.

Seevers MH: Opiate addiction in the monkey. I. Methods of study. J Pharmacol Exp Ther 56:147–156, 1936.

Seevers MH, Deaneau GA: Physiological aspects of tolerance and physical dependence. In Root WS, Hofmann FG (eds): "Physiological Pharmacology," Vol I. New York: Academic Press, 1963, pp 565–670.

Severs MB, Daniels-Severs AE: Effects of angiotensin on the central nervous system. Pharmac Rev 25:415, 1973.

Siegel S: "Nonparametric Statistics for the Behavioral Sciences." New York: McGraw-Hill, 1956, pp 116–127.

Starke K, Borowski E, Endo T: Preferential blockade of presynaptic α-adrenoceptors to yohimbine. Eur J Pharmacol 34:385–388, 1975a.

Starke K, Endo T, Taube HD: Relative pre and post synaptic potencies of α-adrenoceptors agonists in the rabbit pulmonary artery. Naunyn Schmiedeberg's Arch Pharmac 291:55–78, 1975b.

Steinsland DS, Furchgott RF, Kirpekar SM: Inhibition of adrenergic neurotransmission by parasympathomimetics in the rabbit ear artery. J Pharmacol Exp Ther 184:346–356, 1973.

Strombom J: Effects of low doses of catecholamine receptor agonists on exploration in mice. J Neural Transmission 37:229–235, 1975.

Svensson TH, Bunney BS, Aghajanian GK: Inhibition of both noradrenergic and serotonergic neurons in brain by the α-adrenergic agonist clonidine. Brain Res 92:291–306, 1975.

Svensson TH, Strombom J: Discontinuation of chronic clonidine treatment: Evidence for facilitated brain noradrenergic neurotransmission. Naunyn Schmiedeberg's Arch Pharmacol 299:8387, 1977.

Teiger DG: Induction of physical dependence on morphine, codeine and meperidine in the rat by continuous infusion. J Pharmacol Exp Ther 196:408–415, 1974.

Psychopharmacology of Clonidine, pages 259–276
© 1981 Alan R. Liss, Inc., 150 Fifth Avenue, New York, NY 10011

Self-Administration of Clonidine by the Rat

Gary T. Shearman, Martin Hynes, and Harbans Lal

Clonidine is a specific α-2-adrenergic agonist [Young and Kuhar, 1981] that reduces the activity of the neurons in the locus coeruleus (LC) [Svenson et al, 1975], a noradrenergic nucleus containing 40% of all norepinephrine neurons of the rat brain [Swanson and Hartman, 1975]. The efferent input into the LC emanates from many neurotransmitter systems, among them the recently discovered opioid-peptidergic nerve terminals. The densest population of opiate receptors is found in the LC [Pert et al, 1975], where many enkephalin-containing nerve terminals synapse with the NE-containing dendrites [Pickel et al, 1979]. The opioid-peptide containing nerve terminals in the LC are the first of a recently identified nerve tract which originates in the arcuate nucleus [Bloom et al, 1978]. The opioid antagonist naloxone blocks the inhibition of LC firing caused by stimulation of the arcuate nucleus [Strahlendorf et al, 1979]. An opioid-noradrenergic interaction is further suggested by reports that the hypotensive effect of clonidine is reversed by naloxone in the rat [Farsang and Kunos, 1979] and in humans [Resnick et al, 1980]. No similar reversal of effect has been observed with the peripherally acting drugs hydralazine or diazoxide [Elko et al, 1981].

Both opioid and noradrenergic sites have been implicated in the brain reward system. Since the opioid and noradrenergic neurons interact in the LC and most of the psychopharmacological effects of clonidine are produced by its action on the LC [for review see Redmond, 1981; Lal and Shearman, 1981b; Fielding and Lal, 1981], we made a study to determine whether clonidine would be self-administered by the rat. In order to elucidate the mechanism of such self-administration, it was compared with self-administration of a narcotic analgesic, fentanyl.

I. METHODS

Male hooded rats of the Long-Evans strain (Charles River Breeding Laboratories, Wilmington, Massachusetts) weighing 300–400 grams at the beginning of the investigation were used. Throughout the experiment the rats were allowed continuous access to food and water. The animals were surgically prepared with chronic intravenous (jugular) catheters according to the method described before [Lal and Neuman, 1976]. After surgery, combiotic (60,000 units) was injected intramuscularly to provide protection against infection. The animals were placed in velcro harnesses to which a saddle was attached. The catheter was passed through the harness via a protective metal coil attached to the harness. The animals were allowed 1–2 days to recover from the surgical stress and were then placed in the self-administration apparatus.

A. Apparatus

The self-administration apparatus consisted of conventional Plexiglas operant chambers (26 × 20 × 26cm) enclosed in light-proof, ventilated, sound-attenuating chambers. The outer chambers contained a house light that was turned on between 8:00 a.m. and 8:00 p.m. A response lever, 4 cm wide, extended 3 cm into the operant chamber 3.5 cm above the floor through the center of the front wall. As the catheter emerged from the protective metal coil, it was passed through the roof of the operant chamber and through the roof of the outer chamber to a point at which it was eventually connected to a pneumatically driven Hamilton Precision Liquid Dispenser (PLD) syringe. Depression of the response lever activated the pump to deliver in less than 1 second a constant volume (100 μg/kg) of a drug solution into the jugular vein of the animal. The number of lever presses was recorded at the same time each day.

B. Drugs

Clonidine hydrochloride (Boehringer Ingelheim Ltd., Ridgefield, Connecticut), fentanyl citrate (McNeil Laboratories, Inc., Fort Washington, Pennsylvania), and naloxone hydrochloride (Endo Laboratories, Inc.,

Garden City, New York) were dissolved in 0.9% sodium chloride. Haloperidol and azaperone (Janssen Pharmaceutica N.V., Beerse, Belgium) were dissolved in 0.3% tartaric acid.

C. Experimental Design

The rats were allowed to self-administer clonidine (15 mg/kg/injection), fentanyl (0.1 or 1 μg/kg/injection), or saline on a continuous reinforcement (CRF) schedule until a stable rate of lever pressing was reached.

In one clonidine-administering rat, the response requirement for obtaining each clonidine injection was progressively increased to a fixed ratio (FR) of 3 and then to a FR-10 schedule of clonidine reinforcement.

In ten rats self-administering fentanyl, the fentanyl solution was replaced by a clonidine (1 or 15 μg/kg/injection) or saline solution as soon as a stable rate (variation less than 10% from the moving average for at least 2 days) of fentanyl self-administration was attained. The rats were allowed to self-administer these solutions for an additional 4 days.

In the remaining rats self-administering clonidine (15μg/kg/injection) or fentanyl (1 μg/kg/injection) at stable rates naloxone, haloperidol, or azaperone was added to the standard self-administration solutions. After self-administration of the drug mixture for 2 consecutive days, the animals were again allowed to self-administer only clonidine or fentanyl.

II. RESULTS

A. Acquisition of Clonidine Self-Administration

As shown in Figure 1, the rats began to self-administer clonidine (15 μg/kg/injection) readily when an intravenous injection of this drug was made contingent upon lever pressing. A significant increase in clonidine injections was observed from day 1 to day 3, after which the self-administration rate became stabilized. It is also seen that the other rats did not self-administer saline. The rate of clonidine self-administration was significantly higher than that of saline self-administration, which did not differ from random lever pressing under similar conditions.

When the FR requirement for obtaining each clonidine injection was increased from FR-1 to FR-3, a small but significant ($P < 0.05$; Tukey test) increase in the frequency of lever pressing was observed (Fig. 2). However, the total daily clonidine intake (Table I) on the FR-3 schedule was decreased significantly ($P < 0.05$; Tukey test) from the FR-1 schedule. On the other hand, when the FR requirement was increased from FR-3 to FR-10, a significant increase ($P < 0.05$; Tukey test) in the frequency of lever pressing (Fig. 2) to obtain clonidine injections was observed so that the total daily intake of clonidine on the FR-3 and FR-10 schedules of clonidine reinforcement re-

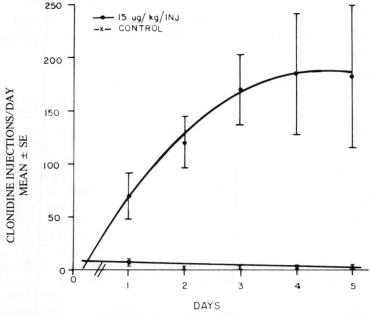

Fig. 1. Acquisition of clonidine self-administration in drug-naive rats when clonidine (15 µg/kg/injection) was delivered on a continuous reinforcement (CRF) schedule, and failure of acquisition of self-administration when a saline (N = 3) control was delivered on a CRF schedule. Each value represents the mean ± SE number of lever presses for the number of subjects indicated in parentheses.

mained approximately the same (N.S., Tukey test) with both schedules (Table I). Clonidine intake on the FR-3 and FR-10 schedules of reinforcement was significantly below (P < 0.05; Tukey test) that observed on the FR-1 schedule.

B. Acquisition of Fentanyl Self-Administration

As shown in Figure 3, rats began to self-administer fentanyl (1µg/kg/injection) readily when an intravenous injection of this drug was made contingent on lever pressing. From day 1 to day 5 there was a gradual increase in lever pressing to obtain fentanyl injections, after which the rate of self-administration became stabilized. It is also seen that the rats did not self-administer a lower dose (0.1 µg/injection) of fentanyl.

C. Substitution of Clonidine for Fentanyl

As shown in Figure 4, the substitution of clonidine for the 15 µg/kg/injection but not for the 1 µg/kg/injection did not change the self-

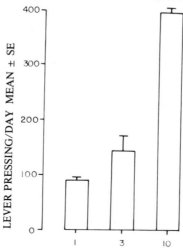

FIXED RATIO REQUIREMENT

Fig. 2. Effect of increasing the fixed ratio (FR) requirement on the rate of clonidine self-administration in one rat. A significant increase in lever pressing to obtain each clonidine injection was observed when the FR requirement was increased from FR-1 to FR-3 ($P < 0.05$; Tukey test) and from FR-3 to FR-10 ($P < 0.001$; Tukey test). Values are the mean ± SE for 3 days at each required FR.

TABLE I. Effect of Increasing the Fixed Ratio (FR) Requirement on the Total Daily Clonidine Intake of One Rat

Fixed ratio requirement	Clonidine intake/day[a] (mg/kg)
1	1.28 ± 0.17
3	0.71 ± 0.13[b]
10	0.60 ± 0.01[b, c]

[a]Values are the mean ± SE for 3 days at each required FR.
[b]Significantly different ($P < 0.05$; Tukey test) from clonidine intake at FR-1.
[c]Not significantly different ($P > 0.05$; Tukey test) from clonidine intake at FR-3.

administration behavior in rats that previously self-administered fentanyl (1 µg/kg/injection). One rat died within 11 hours after the substitution of clonidine (15 µg/kg/injection). The substitution of either clonidine at the lower dose level or of saline for the fentanyl solution resulted in cessation of the self-administration activity.

D. Effect of Specific Antagonists

As shown in Table II, addition of naloxone at 64 µg/kg/injection to the fentanyl solution produced a significant decrease ($P < 0.05$; Scheffe's test)

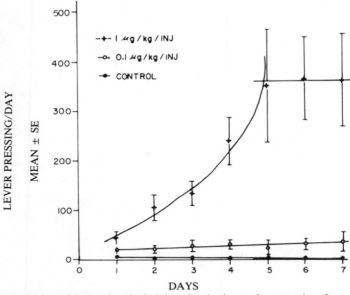

Fig. 3 Acquisition of fentanyl self-administration in drug-naive rats when fentanyl (1 μg/kg/injection) was delivered on a continuous reinforcement (CRF) schedule. No acquisition of self-administration when 0.1 μg/kg/injection fentanyl or saline (N = 3) was delivered on a CRF schedule. Each value represents the mean ± SE number of lever presses for the number of subjects indicated in parentheses.

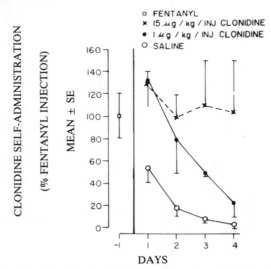

Fig. 4. Effect of substituting clonidine and saline on rate of self-administration in rats previously self-administering fentanyl (1 μg/kg/injection) on a CRF schedule. The square at day 1 is the mean ± SE of the 3 days prior to substitution for all subjects. Substitution of clonidine (15 μg/kg/injection) N = 4; (1 μg/kg/injection) N = 2; saline N = 3. Values are expressed as percent of the mean ± SE of day 1.

TABLE II. Effect of Naloxone, Haloperidol, and Azaperone on Clonidine and Fentanyl Self-Administration.

Self-administration group	Test drug[a]	Self-administration responses[b] /24 hr, % control, $\bar{X} \pm$ SE (N)				
		Predrug	During drug		Post drug	
			1	2	1	2
Clonidine	Naloxone	100 ± 9 (3)[c]	119 ± 19 (3)	153 (2)	173 (2)	—
Fentanyl	Naloxone	100 ± 2 (3)	25 ± 10 (3)	6 ± 2 (3)	34 ± 13 (3)	88 ± 88 (3)
Clonidine	Haloperidol	100 ± 2 (8)	18 ± 3 (8)	16 ± 2 (5)	58 ± 7 (3)	90 ± 22 (3)
Fentanyl	Haloperidol	100 ± 6 (5)	18 ± 5 (5)	27 ± 6 (3)	46 ± 4 (3)	103 ± 3 (3)
Clonidine	Azaperone	100 ± 4 (3)	28 ± 3 (3)	31 ± 5 (3)	67 (2)	90 (2)
Fentanyl	Azaperone	100 ± 3 (5)	35 ± 6 (5)	44 ± 6 (5)	92 ± 5 (3)	—

[a]Test drugs (64 μg/kg/injection) were added to clonidine (15 μg/kg/injection) or fentanyl (1 μg/kg/injection) solution for self-administration of the drug mixture.
[b]Predrug values were obtained by taking the mean $\pm$ SE of the percentage of the mean of the 2 days prior to adding test drugs. Other values are means $\pm$ SE and are expressed as percent of the predrug rate for the number of rats indicated in parentheses. Only the mean is given when N was less than 3. A decrease of N was the result of technical difficulties.
[c]Values in parentheses give number of rats listed.

in the self-administration rates, but failed to affect the self-administration rates of rats that previously self-administered clonidine ($P < 0.05$). Removal of naloxone from the fentanyl solution (postnaloxone) resulted in a return to the prenaloxone rates of self-administration. The postnaloxone self-administration rates were not significantly different ($P < 0.05$; Scheffe's test) from the rates recorded before the addition of naloxone (prenaloxone) in this case.

The addition of haloperidol or azaperone to the clonidine or fentanyl solutions resulted in a significant decrease (Scheffe's test, $P < 0.05$) in the self-administration rates of the rats that previously self-administered either clonidine or fentanyl. The self-administration rates remained significantly below (Scheffe's test, $P < 0.05$) the prehaloperidol or preazaperone rates as long as these drugs were mixed with the clonidine or fentanyl solutions. Upon removal of haloperidol or azaperone from the clonidine or fentanyl solutions, self-administration returned to the pre-antagonist rates (Scheffe's test, $P < 0.05$).

III. DISCUSSION

Most of the evidence indicates that clonidine acts as an α-noradrenergic agonist in the central nervous system and, depending on the dose administered, may stimulate either pre- or postsynaptic noradrenergic receptors. Low doses (4–8 μg/kg IV) have been reported to inhibit the firing of the noradrenergic neurons of the locus coeruleus [Svensson et al, 1975], an action suggesting a presynaptic locus of action, whereas higher doses (100 μg/kg IP) have appeared to stimulate postsynaptic noradrenergic receptors.

When an intravenous injection of clonidine (15 μg/kg) was made contingent on lever pressing, drug-naive rats readily began to press the lever to obtain injections of the drug. The number of times the lever was pressed to produce clonidine injections gradually increased over the first 3 days of self-administration from a mean of 69 ± 22 (N = 23) lever presses on day 1 to a mean of 169 ± 32 (N = 13) by day 3. The mean number of lever presses to produce clonidine injections remained approximately the same from day 3 to day 5. The average daily intake of clonidine on these 3 days was 2.8 mg/kg.

It cannot be stated with certainty whether or not the dose of clonidine that was self-administered by rats stimulates pre- or postsynaptic noradrenergic receptors; however, behavioral and sympathomimetic signs shown by the rats indicate that clonidine may stimulate postsynaptic noradrenergic receptors. If clonidine stimulated presynaptic noradrenergic receptors, this would inhibit the release of norepinephrine from noradrenergic nerve endings and so reduce impulse transmission in the noradrenergic system. It has been suggested that an action on presynaptic receptors could account for the depressant effect of clonidine on locomotor and/or exploratory activity [Laverty and Taylor, 1969; Maj et al, 1972; Strombom, 1976; Tilson et al, 1977]. However, the rats self-administering clonidine were highly excitable and made erratic movements when disturbed, leaping up to the roof of the operant chambers. If the door of the operant chamber was left open, the subjects would try desperately to escape, thus demonstrating that locomotor and/or exploratory activity was not decreased. In fact, exploration or escape attempts may actually have increased, since rats self-administering saline or fentanyl did not try to escape from the chamber when the door was left open. Clonidine has been reported to potentiate escape attempts induced by naloxone in morphine-dependent rats [Tseng et al, 1975], and to induce hyperactivity in mice after intraperitoneal administration of a large (5–30 mg/kg) dose [Razzak et al, 1975].

While self-administering clonidine, the subjects exhibited marked sympathomimetic signs such as exophthalmos and piloerection. These and other sympathomimetic signs such as horripilation, tremor, and hyperactivity have been observed [Hoefke and Kobinger, 1966; Morpurgo, 1968; Razzak et al, 1975] when doses of 30–100 μg/kg IV or 1–30 mg/kg IP were administered to mice. Morpurgo [1968] reported that administration of the α-noradrenergic receptor blocker phentolamine reversed the sympathomimetic signs. The antidiarrheal effect of clonidine is well known [Lal and Shearman, 1981a; Lal et al, 1981]. Animals self-administering clonidine became constipated, as evidenced by the absence of fecal matter on the wood shavings under the floor of the operant chamber.

Clonidine has been reported to produce irritability and aggression in mice and rats [Morpurgo, 1968; Laverty and Taylor, 1969; Dix and Johnson, 1977] and also to intensify morphine withdrawal signs and apomorphine-induced aggression in rats [Gianutsos et al, 1976]. Rats self-administering clonidine assumed an attack posture and showed aggressiveness towards the experimenter when a gloved hand was introduced into the operant chamber. Morpurgo [1968] noted that the clonidine-induced aggression was blocked by dopamine receptor antagonists such as haloperidol but was poorly antagonized by norepinephrine receptor blockers, and he therefore concluded that the aggressiveness was independent of the sympathomimetic effects of clonidine.

Deneau et al [1969] reported that monkeys with unlimited access to cocaine would self-administer the drug until convulsions and death occurred, usually within 30 days. Similarly, approximately 22% of subjects self-administering clonidine did so until death, which invariably occurred on the first day of self-administration. Profuse salivation and complete loss of eye pigmentation were noted in these subjects. Since clonidine will maintain behavior leading to its administration in rats, it can be said to act as a positive reinforcer. To judge from the behavioral and sympathomimetic signs shown by rats self-administering clonidine, the drug stimulates postsynaptic noradrenergic receptors.

Intravenous administration of drugs of several pharmacological classes, including narcotic analgesics, narcotic antagonists, barbiturates, benzodiazepines, dissociative anesthetics, and psychomotor stimulants has been found to maintain responding by laboratory animals on FR schedules of reinforcement [for review see Spealman and Goldberg, 1978]. An intravenous clonidine injection sustained responding in drug-naive rats when the drug was delivered on an FR-1 schedule of reinforcement. When the FR requirement for obtaining each clonidine injection was increased from 1 to 3 responses per reinforcement, the total daily intake of clonidine decreased, even though a significant increase in responding was observed. When the FR requirement was further increased to FR-10, however, responding increased so that the total daily clonidine intake was the same on the FR-3 and FR-10 schedules of reinforcement. Similar observations were made by Weeks [1962], who examined morphine intake on different FR schedules of reinforcement. When the FR requirement for each morphine injection was increased from 1 to 5, morphine intake decreased even though responding to obtain the drug increased. However, when the FR requirement was increased to 10, the response rate doubled from its FR-5 level so that morphine intake remained the same on the FR-5 and FR-10 schedules of reinforcement.

Goldberg et al [1971] increased the FR requirement for rhesus monkeys to obtain each intravenous injection of pentobarbital from 1 to 3 to 5 to 10 and observed a corresponding decrease in both response rate and total pentobar-

bital intake as the FR requirement was increased. Even though both clonidine [Nickerson and Ruedy, 1975] and pentobarbital [Harvey, 1975], therefore, cause central nervous system depression, the effect of increasing the FR
requirement for clonidine self-administration does not resemble the effect of
increasing the FR requirement for pentobarbital self-administration. These
differential results may mean that different neurochemical mechanisms un-
derlay the reinforcing properties of clonidine and pentobarbital.

When the psychomotor stimulants cocaine [Pickens, 1968; Pickens and
Thompson, 1968; Goldberg et al, 1971] and amphetamine [Pickens and Harris, 1968] are delivered on FR schedules of reinforcement, an increase in responding is observed as the FR requirement is increased so that the total intake of these drugs remains constant. Therefore, in some respects the effect
of increasing the FR requirement for obtaining clonidine injections resem-
bles the effect of increasing the FR requirement for obtaining psychomotor
stimulants: Increasing the FR requirement for each clonidine injection from
3 to 10 resulted in an increase in responding so that the total clonidine intake
remained the same.

Fentanyl is a synthetic narcotic that is approximately 80 times more potent as an analgesic than morphine [Jaffe and Martin, 1975]. We have reported previously [Lal et al, 1977] that when an intravenous injection of fentanyl (1 μg/kg/injection) was made contingent on lever pressing, drug-naive
rats readily began to press the lever to obtain an injection of this drug. Lever
pressing to obtain fentanyl injections gradually increased in frequency over
the first 5 days from a mean of 44 ± 12 (N= 21) lever presses on day 1 of
self-administration to a mean of 350 ± 114 (N = 17) by day 5. The mean
number of lever presses for injection of fentanyl remained approximately the
same for day 5 to day 7. The average daily intake of fentanyl on these 3 days
was 358 μg/kg. It has been shown that fentanyl (1 μg/kg/injection) will function as a positive reinforcer; ie, it will sustain behavior leading to its
administration.

When the intravenous injection of a lower dose (0.1 μg/kg) of fentanyl
was made contingent on lever pressing, the subjects did not acquire self-
administration behavior. This dose of fentanyl thus appears not to be
reinforcing. That rates of self-administration for fentanyl (0.1
μg/kg/injection) were not significantly different from those of saline
supports this conclusion.

It has been reported that clonidine and morphine have similar
pharmacological effects on noradrenergic neurons [Gomes et al, 1976;
Redmond, 1977]. Both clonidine and morphine inhibit the firing of the
noradrenergic nucleus locus coeruleus [Svenson et al, 1975; Korf et al, 1974],

and opiate receptors have been localized on locus coeruleus cell bodies [Kuhar et al, 1974].

Recently, Redmond [1977] reported that the effects of electrical or pharmacological activation of the locus coeruleus in monkeys were strikingly similar to those noted after opiate withdrawal in humans (anxiety state). Both clonidine and morphine blocked the effects of activation of the locus coeruleus [Redmond, 1977], and the time course of this blockade correlated with the decreased neuronal activity in the locus coeruleus [Svenson et al, 1975; Cedarbaum and Aghajanian, 1977] and the decreased norepinephrine release [Maas et al, 1976] due to these drugs. Clonidine has been shown to decrease the incidence of certain narcotic withdrawal signs, such as body shakes, induced by discontinuation of narcotic administration [Fielding et al, 1977, 1978] or by administration of narcotic antagonists [Tseng et al, 1975; Vetulani and Bednarczyk, 1977] in morphine-dependent rats. Gold et al [1978] have reported a study in which clonidine eliminated opiate withdrawal signs in narcotic addicts, all of the subjects noting a dramatic relief of distress. In an earlier study in humans, Bjorkqvist [1975] found that clonidine decreased the sweating, tremor, and anxiety accompanying alcohol withdrawal.

Also of interest are the findings that clonidine produces analgesia in rats and mice [Paalzow, 1974; Paalzow and Paalzow, 1976; Fielding et al, 1977, 1980] and that the antinociceptive effects of clonidine are not reversed by naloxone [Paalzow and Paalzow, 1976; Fielding et al, 1980], which suggests that clonidine is not bound by opiate receptors.

The above reports may suggest a resemblance between clonidine and narcotics, particularly in view of the fact that self-administration behavior was maintained in rats self-administering the narcotic fentanyl when clonidine (15 μg/kg/injection) was substituted for the fentanyl solution. However, since clonidine itself is self-administered and since there is no evidence of a narcotic nature of clonidine, it cannot be determined whether this self-administration was a substitution or a new acquisition. Nor is it possible to establish whether clonidine was self-administered for its reinforcing action or as a means of blocking fentanyl withdrawal.

In general, all drugs that are abused by man are self-administered by laboratory animals, but the reverse is not always true. There are no reports of clonidine abuse among people. It is very interesting that the heroin addicts who choose to be maintained on clonidine rather than methadone have not reported any euphoriant effect of clonidine. Also, clonidine does not generalize to morphine in rats trained to discriminate between morphine and saline [Lal et al, 1977, Miksic et al, 1978]. Clonidine may not produce the same subjective effects as narcotics since these effects are considered related to their discriminative stimulus properties [Lal and Gianutsos, 1976; Lal et al, 1977].

One subject died within 11 hours of the substitution of clonidine (15μg/kg/injection) for fentanyl. Complete loss of eye pigmentation (eye white) was noted. In another rat the substitution of clonidine (15/μg/kg/injection) was followed by self-mutilation of the forelimbs. Razzak [1975] reported that intraperitoneal administration of a large dose (50 mg/kg) of clonidine led to self-mutilation in mice. Rats that had previously self-administered fentanyl did not continue to do so when a lower dose of clonidine (1 μg/kg/injection) or saline was substituted for the fentanyl solution.

Narcotic antagonists are effective in preventing and reversing the pharmacological effects of opiates, and can elicit narcotic withdrawal signs in opiate-dependent organisms. Naloxone can be considered a relatively pure opiate antagonist that produces no discriminable subjective effect when administered to non-opiate-dependent subjects [Jaffe and Martin, 1975].

As mentioned earlier, clonidine exerts several pharmacologic effects similar to those of narcotics. Therefore, it was of interest to study the effect of naloxone on clonidine and fentanyl self-administration. When added to the clonidine solution, naloxone did not decrease the rate of self-administration.

The above findings agree with the results of recent studies by Paalzow and Paalzow [1976] and Fielding et al [1980] which showed that clonidine-induced analgesia is not antagonized by naloxone. They are also consistent with the report by Meyer et al [1977] that at doses capable of suppressing operant behavior, causing body weight loss and other symptoms of withdrawal in morphine-dependent rats [Gellert and Sparber, 1977], naloxone failed to disrupt operant behavior in clonidine-dependent rats. Therefore, the reinforcing effects of clonidine do not appear to be mediated by an interaction at the opiate receptor.

When naloxone was added to the fentanyl solution, there was a significant decrease in self-administration rates. The response rate remained significantly below the prenaloxone rate while naloxone remained in the fentanyl solution but it gradually returned to the prenaloxone value when naloxone was removed from the fentanyl solution. Similar results were obtained by Woods et al [1975], who examined the effect of response-contingent naloxone injections on codeine-reinforced responding in rhesus monkeys. Naloxone caused a dose-dependent decrease in codeine-reinforced responding when added to the codeine solution for self-administration. Furthermore, codeine-reinforced responding remained suppressed while naloxone remained in the codeine solution; it gradually returned to prenaloxone rates over three sessions following removal of naloxone. Woods et al [1975] suggest that response-contingent naloxone injections function as a punishing stimulus that decreases self-administration (lever pressing) behavior. Decreased fentanyl-reinforced responding after addition of naloxone to the fentanyl solution may also be explained by the punishing effects of response-contingent naloxone injections. Haloperidol has been reported [Pozuelo and Kerr, 1972; Glick and Cox, 1975] to decrease morphine self-administration by laboratory animals. Karkalas and Lal [1973] found that haloperidol suppresses heroin abstinence and reduces craving for the drug.

The lever pressing rates of rats previously self-administering clonidine or fentanyl alone significantly decreased when haloperidol or azaperone was added to the clonidine and fentanyl solutions. The addition of haloperidol or azaperone did not preferentially affect clonidine- or fentanyl-reinforced responding; rather, haloperidol caused a similar reduction in lever pressing when added to either drug solution. Suppression of clonidine- and fentanyl-reinforced responding remained stable while haloperidol or azaperone remained in the drug solutions. Fentanyl- and clonidine-reinforced responding returned to pre-haloperidol and preazaperone rates upon removal of these drugs from the clonidine and fentanyl solutions.

To our knowledge, previous animal studies have only measured the effect of subcutaneous or intraperitoneal administration of neuroleptics on self-administration of narcotics and psychomotor stimulants. Therefore, a direct comparison with the effect exerted on clonidine- and fentanyl-reinforced responding by the neuroleptics added in this study is difficult. This addition of haloperidol or azaperone to the clonidine and fentanyl solutions could have decreased the response rates in rats previously self-administering these drugs for three reasons:

First, investigations of the neurochemical basis for reinforcement resulting from the self-administration of narcotics [Davis and Smith, 1972, 1973a; Glick et al, 1972] and psychomotor stimulants [Davis and Smith, 1972, 1973b] have implicated central catecholaminergic brain mechanisms. In view of the known anticatecholaminergic activity of haloperidol and azaperone, it could be assumed therefore that decreased rates of self-administration in rats previously self-administering either clonidine or fentanyl alone resulted from attenuation of the reinforcing property associated with the action of these drugs.

Second, neuroleptics are well known to cause sedation and motor deficits. Consequently, reduced lever pressing after addition of haloperidol and azaperone may be due to a motor performance deficit. Wise [1978] has reviewed evidence that neuroleptics interfere with reward processes at doses that do not cause any significant impairment of performance. Wise noted that "data from studies of intravenous stimulant reward suggest the use of moment-to-moment analysis of the pattern of neuroleptics effects." This type of analysis is designed to avoid the incorrect observations that can result when response rates are measured over an entire test session. For example, Yokel and Wise [1975, 1976] observed that low doses of the neuroleptic drugs pimozide and (+)-butaclamol increased lever pressing for intravenous amphetamine injections. Higher doses produced an initial increase in lever pressing followed by cessation of responding. Yokel and Wise suggest that low doses of neuroleptics decrease the rewarding effects of amphetamine, and that animals increase lever pressing to overcome the neuroleptic attenuation of the rewarding effects. Higher doses were given to block the rewarding effects completely, and after an initial burst of complete cessation, a gradual decline of lever pressing was observed. A response pattern similar to this appears when saline solution is substituted for a drug reinforcer. Had response rates been averaged over the entire session, however, Yokel and Wise would not have made the same observations. In our studies the response rates were depressed throughout the test session. Since the effect of added haloperidol or azaperone on the lever pressing rate in rats that previously self-administered either clonidine or fentanyl alone was measured over a 24-hour period, an initial increase in the response rate (an indicator of reward attenuation) would have been masked. Therefore, it is not certain whether haloperidol was decreasing the reinforcing powers of clonidine and fentanyl or was causing sedation and motor deficits.

Finally, neuroleptics of the butyrophenone and phenothiazine types are well known to have dysphoric effects in non-schizophrenic humans [Janke and Debus, 1968]. Furthermore, both types of neuroleptics have been shown to maintain behavior leading to termination or absence of self-administration (ie, to act as negative reinforcers) in rhesus monkeys [Hoffmeister, 1975, 1977; Hoffmeister and Wuttke, 1975]. By definition, punishment is considered to have occurred when the probability of future behavior leading to delivery of the punishing stimulus is reduced [Azrin and Holz, 1966]. Perhaps the best explanation for the decreased response rates after addition of haloperidol or azaperone to the clonidine or fentanyl solutions is that addition of these drugs creates a punishing, aversive stimulus, which tends to reduce lever pressing activity.

In summary, we have demonstrated that laboratory rats will self-administer the α-noradrenergic receptor agonist clonidine when delivery of a dose of 15 μg/kg is linked to a continuous reinforcement schedule. That clonidine was self-administered for its positive reinforcing effect and not because of the drug's nonspecific behavioral effects is indicated by the fact that the response rate increased as the response requirement for obtaining each clonidine injection was increased. In rats self-administering fentanyl (1 μg/kg/injection), substitution of clonidine (15 but not 1 μg/kg/injection) for the fentanyl solution maintained the self-administration activity.

Addition to the narcotic antagonist naloxone to the clonidine or fentanyl solutions resulted in a significant decrease in fentanyl-reinforced, but not in clonidine-reinforced, responding. This finding suggests that clonidine reinforcement is mediated by opioid-independent mechanisms. It was also observed that addition of haloperidol or azaperone to the clonidine or fentanyl solutions led to a decrease in clonidine- and fentanyl-reinforced responding; however, the exact nature of this effect was unclear.

Self-administration of the α-noradrenergic receptor agonist clonidine and its continuation despite the increased lever pressing required to obtain each clonidine injection show that stimulation of α-adrenergic receptors can result in positive reinforcement.

IV. REFERENCES

Azria NH, Holz WC: Punishment. In Honig WK (ed): "Operant Behavior: Areas of Research and Application." New York: Appleton-Century-Crofts, 1966, pp 380–447.

Bjorkqvist SE: Clonidine in alcohol withdrawal. Acta Psych at Scand 52:256–263, 1975.

Bloom FE, Rossier J, Battenberg EL, Bayon A, French E, Henrickson SJ, Siggens GR, Segal D, Brone R, Long N, Guilliem R: Beta-endorphin: Cellular localization, electrophysiological, and behavioral effect. Adv Biochem Pharmacol 18:89–109, 1978.

Cedarbaum JM, Aghajanian GK: Catecholenergic receptors on locus coerulus neurons: Pharmacological characteristics. Eur J Pharmacol 44:375–385, 1977.

Davis WM, Smith SF: Alpha-methyl-tyrosine to prevent self-administration of morphine and amphetamine. Curr Ther Res 14:814–819, 1972.

Davis WM, Smith SG: Blocking of morphine based reinforcement by alpha-methyltyrosine. Life Sci 12:185–191, 1973a.

Davis WM, Smith SG: Blocking effect of alpha-methyltyrosine on amphetamine based reinforcement. J Pharm Pharmacol 25:174–177, 1973b.

Deneau, G, Yangita T, Seevers MH: Self-administration of psychoactive substances by the monkey. A measure of psychological dependence. Psychopharmacologia 16:30–48, 1969.

Dix RK, Johnson EM: Withdrawal syndrome upon cessation of chronic clonidine treatment in rats. Eur J Pharmacol 44:153–159, 1977.

Elko E, Bennet D, DeFeo J, Lal H: Differential reversal by naloxone of centrally and not peripherally mediated hypotension. Fed Proc 40:712, 1981.

Farsang C, Kunos G: Naloxone reverses the antihypertensive effect of clonidine. Br J Pharmacol 67:161–164, 1979.

Fielding S, Lal H: Clonidine: New research in psychotropic drug. Pharmacology Medicinal Research Reviews Vol. 1(1):97–123, 1981.

Fielding S, Wilker J, Hynes M, Szewzak M, Novick W, Lal H: Antinociceptive and withdrawal actions of clonidine: A comparison with morphine. Fed Proc 36:1024, 1977.

Fielding S, Wilker J, Hynes M, Szewezak M, Novick W, Lal H: A comparison of clonidine with morphine for antinociceptive and antiwithdrawal actions. J Pharmacol Exp Ther 207:899–905, 1978.

Gellert VF, Sparber SB: A comparison of the effects of naloxone upon body weight loss and suppression of fixed-ratio operant behavior in morphine-dependent rats. J Pharmacol Exp Ther 201:44–54, 1977.

Gianutsos G, Hynes MD, Lal H: Enhancement of morphine-withdrawal and apomorphine-induced aggression by clonidine. Psycho Pharm Comm 2:165–171, 1976.

Glick SD, Cox RO: Dopaminergic and cholinergic influences on morphine self-administration in rats. Clin Pathol Pharmacol 12:17–24, 1975.

Glick SD, Greenstein S, Zimmerberg B: Facilitation of recovery by alpha-methyl-para-tyrosine after lateral hypothalamic damage. Science 177:534–535, 1972.

Gold MS, Redmond DE Jr, Kleber HD: Clonidine blocks acute opiate withdrawal symptoms. Lancet 2:599–602, 1978.

Goldberg SR, Woods JH, Schuster CR: Nalorphine-induced changes in morphine self-administration in Rhesus monkeys. J Pharmacol Exp Ther 76:464–471, 1971.

Gomes C, Svensson TH, Trolin G: Effects of morphine on central catecholamine turnover, blood pressure and heart rate in the rat. Naunyn-Schmiedebergs Arch Pharmacol 294:141–147, 1976.

Hoefke W, Kobinger W: Pharmacological effects of 2-(2,6 dichlorophenylamine) 2-imidazoline-hydrochloride, a new antihypertensive substance. Arzneim Forsch 16:1038–1050, 1966.

Hoffmeister F: Negative reinforcing properties of some psychotropic drugs in drug-naive Rhesus monkeys. J Pharmacol Exp Ther 192:468–477, 1975.

Hoffmeister F: Reinforcing properties of perphenazine, naloperidol and amitryptiline in Rhesus monkeys. J Pharmacol Exp Ther 200:516–522, 1977.

Hoffmeister F, Wuttke W: Psychotropic drugs as negative reinforcers. Pharmacol Rev 27:419–428, 1975.

Jaffe JH, Martin WR: Narcotic analgesics and antagonists. In Goodman LS, Gilman A (eds): "The Pharmacological Basis of Therapeutics." New York: MacMillan Publishing Co, 1975, pp 245–283.

Janke W, Debus G: Experimental studies on antianxiety agents with normal subjects: Methodological considerations and review of main effect. In Efron EH (ed): Psychopharmacology. A Review of Progress, 1957-1967. U.S. Government Printing Office, Washington, D.C., 1968, pp 205–230.

Karkalas J, Lal H: A comparison of haloperidol with methadone in blocking heroin-withdrawal symptoms. Pharmacopsychiat 8:248–251, 1973.

Korf J, Bunney BS, Aghajanian GK: Noradrenergic neurons: Morphine inhibition of spontaneous activity. Eur J Pharmacol 25:165–169, 1974.

Kuhar MJ, Pert CB, Snyder SH: Regional distribution of opiate receptor binding in monkey and human brain. Nature 245:447–450, 1973.

Lal H, Gianutsos G: Discriminable stimuli produced by narcotic analgesics. Psychopharmacol 2:311–314, 1976.

Lal H, Neuman R: Blockade of morphine-withdrawal body shakes by haloperidol. Life Sci 18:163–168, 1976.

Lal H, Shearman G: A comparison of the antidiarrheal and some other pharmacological effects of clonidine, lidamidine, and loperamide in the rat. Drug Devel Res 1:37–41, 1981a.

Lal H, Shearman G: Psychotropic actions of clonidine. In: Lal H, Fielding S (eds): "Psychopharmacology of Clonidine" New York: Alan R. Liss Inc, 1981b.

Lal H, Shearman GT, Fielding S, Dunn R, Kruse H, Theurer K: Evidence that GABA mechanisms mediate the anxiolytic action of benzodiazepines: A study with valproic acid. Neuropharmacol 19:785–789, 1980.

Laverty R, Taylor KM: Behavioral and biochemical effects of 2-(2,6-dichlorophenylamine)-2-imidazoline hydrochloride (ST 155) on the central nervous system. Brit J Pharmacol 35:253–264, 1969.

Maas JW, Hattox SE, Landis DH, Roth RH: The determination of a brain arteriovenous difference for 3-methyl-4-hydroxyphenethyleneglyclol (MHPG). Brain Res 118:167–173, 1976.

Maj J, Grabowska M, Gajda L: Effect of apomorphine on motility in rats. Eur J Pharmacol 17:208–214, 1972.

Meyer DR, El-Azhary R, Bierer DWS, Hanson SK, Robbins MS, Sparber SB: Tolerance and dependence after chronic administration of clonidine to the rat. Pharmacol Biochem Behav 7:277–231, 1977.

Miksic S, Shearman G, Lal H: Generalization study with some narcotic and non-narcotic drugs in rats trained for morphine-saline discrimination. Psychopharmacol 60:103–104, 1978.

Morpurgo C: Aggressive behavior induced by large doses of 2-(2,6-dichlorophenylamino)-2-imidazoline hydrochloride (ST 155) in mice. Eur J Pharmacol 3:374–377, 1968.

Nickerson M, Ruedy J: Antihypertensive agents and the drug therapy of hypertension. In Goodman LS, Gilman AG (eds): "The Pharmacological Basis of Experimental Therapeutics." New York: MacMillan Publishing Co, 1975, pp 705–726.

Paalzow G, Paalzow L: Clonidine antinociceptive activity: Effects of drugs influencing central monaminergic and cholinergic mechanisms in the rat. Naunyn-Schmiedebergs Arch Pharmacol 292:119–126, 1976.

Paalzow L: Analgesia produced by clonidine in mice and rats. J Pharm Pharmacol 26:361–363, 1974.

Pert CB, Kuhar MJ, Snyder SH: Autoradiographic localization of the opiate receptors in rat brain. Life Sci 16:1849–1854, 1975.

Pickel VM, Joh TH, Reis DJ, Leeman SE, Miller RJ: Electron microscopic localization of substance and enkephalin in axon terminals related to dentrites of catecholaminergic neurons. Brain Res 160:387–400, 1979.

Pickens R: Self-administration of stimulants by rats. Int J Addiction 3:215–221, 1968.

Pickens R, Harris WC: Self-administration of d-amphetamine by rats. Psychopharmacologia 12:158–163, 1968.

Pickens R, Thompson T: Characteristics of stimulant drug reinforcement. In Thompson T, Pickens R (eds): "Stimulus Properties of Drugs." New York: Appleton-Century-Crofts, 1971, pp 177–191.

Pozuelo J, Kerr FW: Suppression of craving and other signs of dependence in morphine-addicted monkeys by administration of alpha-mythyl-para-tyrosine. Mayo Clin Pro 47:621–628, 1972.

Razzak F, Fujiwara M, Veki S: Automutilation induced by clonidine in mice. Eur J Pharmacol 30:356–360, 1975.

Redmond DE Jr: Alterations in the function of the nucleus locus coeruleus: A possible model for studies of anxiety. In: Hanin I, Usdin E (eds): "Animal Models in Psychiatry and Neurology." Oxford: Pergamon Press, 1977, pp 293–305.

Redmond DE Jr: Clonidine and the primate locus coeruleus: Evidence suggesting anxiolytic and anti-withdrawal effects. In: Lal H, Fielding S (eds): "Psychopharmacology of Clonidine." New York: Alan R. Liss, Inc, 1981.

Resnick RB, Washton AM, Lal H: Reversal of clonidine-induced hypotension by opioid antagonists in man. In Way EL (ed): "Endogenoces and Exogenous Opiate Agonists and Antagonists." New York: Pergamon Press, 1980, pp 565–566.

Shearman GT, Ursillo R: Non-narcotic anti-diarrheal action of clonidine and lofexidine in the rat. J Clin Pharmacol 21:16–19, 1981.

Shearman G, Hynes MD, Fielding S, Lal H: Clonidine self-administration in the rat. A comparison with fentaynl self-administration. Pharmacol 19:171, 1977.

Smith RC, David JM: Behavioral evidence for supersensitivity after chronic administration of haloperidol, clozapine, and thioridazine. Life Sci 19:725–732, 1976.

Spealman RD, Goldberg SR: Drug self-administration by laboratory animals: Control by schedules of reinforcement. Ann Rev Pharmacol Toxicol 18:313–339, 1978.

Strahlendorf HK, Strahlendorf JC, Barnes CD: Evidence for endophin modulation of locus coerulus. Neurosci Abstr 5:540, 1979.

Strombom U: Catecholamine receptor agonists. Effects on motor activity and rate of tyrosine hydroxylation in mouse brain. Naunyn-Schmied Arch Pharmacol 292:167–176, 1976.

Svensson TH, Bunney BS, Aghajanian GK: Inhibition of both noradrenergic and serotonergic neurons in brain by the alpha-adrenergic agonist clonidine. Brain Res 92:291–306, 1975.

Swanson LW, Hartman BK: The central adrenergic system: An immunoflourescent study of the location of cell bodies and their efferent connections in the rat using dopamine β-hydroxylase as a marker. J Comp Neurol 163:467–506, 1975.

Tilson HA, Chamberlain JH, Gylys JA, Boyniski JP: Behavioral suppressant effects of clonidine in strains of normotensive and hypertensive rats. Eur J Pharmacol 43:99–105, 1977.

Tseng LF, Loh HH, Wei ET: Effect of clonidine on morphine withdrawal signs in the rat. Eur J Pharmacol 30:93–99, 1975.

Vetulani J, Bednarczyk B: Depression by clonidine of shaking behavior elicited by nalorphine in morphine-dependent rats. J Pharm Pharmacol 29:567–568, 1977.

Weeks JR: Experimental morphine addiction: Method for automatic intravenous injections in unrestrained rats. Science 138:143–144, 1962.

Wise RA: Neuroleptic attenuation of intracranial self-stimulation: Reward or performance deficits? Life Sci 22:535–542, 1978.

Yokel RA, Wise RA: Increased lever pressing for amphetamine after pimozide in rats: Implications for a dopamine theory of reward. Science 187:547–549, 1975.

Yokel RA, Wise RA: Attenuation of intravenous amphetamine reinforcement by central dopamine blockade in rats. Psychopharmacology 48:311–318, 1976.

Young WS, Kuhar MJ: Anatomical mapping of clonidine (alpha-2 noradrenergic) receptors in rat brain. In Lal H, Fielding S (eds): "Psychopharmacology of Clonidine." New York: Alan R. Liss, Inc, 1981.

Psychopharmacology of Clonidine, pages 277–284
© 1981 Alan R. Liss, Inc., 150 Fifth Avenue, New York, NY 10011

The Clinical Use of Clonidine in Outpatient Detoxification From Opiates

Arnold M. Washton and Richard B. Resnick

I. INTRODUCTION

Our interest in clonidine has focused on the clinical use of this medication to help opiate-addicted outpatients detoxify from heroin and methadone. The initial report [Gold et al, 1978] of clonidine's withdrawal-suppressing effects in opiate addicts suggested to us that clonidine might be uniquely suited for use as a transitional treatment between opiate dependence and induction onto the long-acting opiate antagonist, naltrexone [Resnick et al, 1979]. Naltrexone can be useful in preventing relapse to opiate use, but access to this treatment has been seriously limited by the inability of patients to complete the opiate-free period of at least 1 week that is needed before the first dose of naltrexone can be given without precipitating a severe withdrawal reaction. Because clonidine is a nonopiate medication with specific and significant withdrawal-suppressing effects, it can provide symptomatic relief after discontinuation of opiates without postponing the introduction of naltrexone at the earliest possible time to foster continued abstinence.

Portions of this manuscript appeared in *Pharmacotherapy*, Vol. 1, No. 2, 1981.

II. OUTPATIENT STUDIES

Our studies of clonidine have been conducted in an outpatient setting with opiate-dependent volunteers. It was our hope that if outpatients could be detoxified safely and effectively using clonidine, they would have greater access to naltrexone or drug-free modalities without hospital admission. Outpatient detoxification services are generally more cost-effective, and do not exclude patients for whom hospital admission is impractical. Since the inpatient clonidine dose regimen of 17 μg/kg used by earlier researchers [Gold et al, 1980] generated profound sedation and hypotension in some cases, our initial efforts focused on developing safe and effective dosing procedures for ambulatory outpatients before conducting any further evaluations of clonidine's suitability for outpatient use.

Our first study [Washton et al, 1980a] sought to replicate the single-dose findings of Gold et al [1978] in order to gather additional information on the physiological and subjective effects of clonidine in opiate-dependent subjects. A single oral dose of 5 μg/kg clonidine was administered to 12 opiate-dependent outpatients experiencing acute withdrawal from heroin and/or methadone. Blood pressure and ratings for the presence and severity of withdrawal symptoms were taken immediately before clonidine administration and at 2 hours postclonidine. The data showed that clonidine produced a marked and significant reduction in subjective withdrawal severity. The particular symptoms reduced most effectively by clonidine were chills, lacrimation, rhinorrhea, yawning, stomach cramps, sweating, and muscle and joint aches. Marked reductions in anxiety and restlessness were also reported. Side effects were dry mouth, drowsiness, and a decrease of 10–15 mm Hg in systolic and diastolic blood pressure. None of the 12 subjects experienced euphoria or any other opiate-like effects from the clonidine, and none reported unpleasant side effects.

We subsequently explored clonidine's usefulness as an adjunct to methadone dose reductions and also as a transitional treatment during the 10-day period between opiate dependence and naltrexone. In an initial outpatient trial [Washton and Resnick, 1980a] with 20 methadone-dependent volunteers, an attempt was made to determine whether clonidine could be used to prevent emergence of abstinence symptoms during gradual methadone withdrawal. This study addressed the issue of prophylactic blockade of the abstinence syndrome in contrast to the previous studies [Gold et al, 1978, 1980; Washton et al, 1980a] that used clonidine to reduce ongoing withdrawal symptoms. Patients taking 10–50 mg methadone daily were inducted onto clonidine doses of 0.5–0.9 mg per day before initiating methadone dose reductions of 5 or 10 mg per week. All patients had been taking clonidine for at least 2 weeks before the methadone detoxification was begun. Ten of the 20 patients (50%) reached a zero methadone dose and remained opiate-free on clonidine for 10 days before starting naltrexone. Although the patients who successfully completed the detoxification generally complained of less severe and fewer symptoms than the patients who failed, it was evident that clonidine did not totally prevent the emergence of withdrawal symptoms. Patients who complained of intense withdrawal discomfort tended to be those who had been taking clonidine for more than 3 weeks, suggesting the development of tolerance to clonidine's antiwithdrawal effects.

In another outpatient trial [Washton et al, 1980b], clonidine was administered to 88 opiate-dependent volunteers following abrupt discontinuation of methadone or heroin. Forty-three patients had received methadone 5–40 mg daily (mean 15 mg), and the other 45 patients had been taking illicit methadone or heroin in varying doses. On day 1, all patients received placebo methadone and started a self-administered clonidine dose regimen of 0.1 mg qid with gradual increases as needed over succeeding days. The maximum daily clonidine dose averaged 0.8 mg (range 0.3–1.2 mg). On day 10, patients who showed opiate-free urines and denied using any illicit opiates while on clonidine were given a naloxone challenge of 2.0 mg IV to assess their readiness to begin treatment with naltrexone. Seventy-two percent of the 43 methadone maintenance patients and 50% of illicit opiate users completed detoxification and started naltrexone treatment. Those who were on the higher doses of heroin and/or methadone had the greatest difficulty in completing detoxification. All patients reported that clonidine reduced, but did not eliminate, their withdrawal discomfort. Lethargy and insomnia were the most frequent and persistent residual complaints. Most patients experienced some mild dizziness or lightheadedness upon standing, but these side effects were unacceptably severe in only six cases. No single clonidine dose regimen was best for all patients, because sensitivity to clonidine's effects varied widely among individuals. To achieve effective control of withdrawal symptoms without untoward side effects, it was necessary to individualize the clonidine dose regimen according to each patient's blood pressure and symptomatology.

Rawson et al [1980] provided additional evidence of clonidine's effectiveness in outpatient opiate withdrawal, and found that the availability of naltrexone aftercare treatment significantly increased detoxification success rates. Among patients offered clonidine as a transitional treatment between methadone and naltrexone, 9 of 12 (75%) achieved 10 days of opiate abstinence and started naltrexone, whereas only 3 of 12 (25%) in a group offered clonidine but no naltrexone achieved 10 days' abstinence. The differential efficacy of the clonidine detoxification procedure between the two groups of subjects did not appear to result from differences in the degree of symptom relief, but rather from different subject attitudes toward their detoxification. Subjects in the clonidine/naltrexone group perceived the clonidine detoxification as a transitional treatment with a specific goal. Naltrexone induction on day 10 postmethadone was perceived as a clear end point to the detoxification. Subjects in this group frequently expressed the feeling that they had "made it" when they started naltrexone and many reported feeling relief that once on naltrexone they no longer had to struggle with the urges and cravings to use opiates. It appeared that if the clonidine procedure was perceived by subjects as being for a specific number of days with a clear goal and end point such as starting naltrexone, most of them could exert sufficient control to abstain from opiate use for the 10 days postmethadone. Subjects in the clonidine-only group did not view the detoxification process as having a clear end point or goal, and this seemed to contribute to their inability to resist opiate cravings.

Although the clinical studies summarized above were encouraging, none compared clonidine against other detoxification methods. We therefore conducted a double-blind outpatient study [Washton and Resnick, 1980b] in which 26 volunteers dependent on methadone (15–30 mg daily) were randomly assigned to a clonidine or methadone detoxification procedure. The clonidine procedure (N = 13) consisted of abrupt substitution of clonidine for methadone on day 1 of the study. The methadone procedure (N = 13) consisted of methadone dose reductions of 1 mg per day until a zero dose was reached. Both procedures were placebo-controlled with daily dose regimens of clonidine or placebo tablets individualized by a physician who was not aware of the patient's assigned treatment group. No significant difference was found between the clonidine and methadone procedures in terms of the numbers of patients who completed a 10-day opiate-abstinence period after the last dose of active methadone. Four of 13 subjects (38%) were successful with clonidine, and 6 of 13 (46%) were successful with methadone ($P > 0.05$, chi-square test). Major withdrawal symptoms were nearly identical for both groups and consisted mainly of lethargy, restlessness, and insomnia. The clinical course of subjects was distinctly different for the clonidine and methadone procedures, making it impossible to maintain truly double-blind conditions. Subjects taking clonidine reported sedation, dry mouth, occasional dizziness, and onset of withdrawal symptoms within the first 2–3 days of the study. By contrast, subjects taking methadone reported no sedation, dry mouth, or dizziness, and no major withdrawal symptoms until the final week of the procedure when methadone doses were approaching zero.

III. DISCUSSION

Our studies confirm clonidine's potent antiwithdrawal effects and demonstrate that outpatients can be detoxified with clonidine in a safe, acceptable, and effective manner. Our 10-day clonidine detoxification procedure seems to be extremely useful in allowing a rapid switch from opiate dependence to naltrexone without hospital admission. The treatment sequence of clonidine followed as soon as possible by naltrexone induction is highly attractive to outpatients because it offers an opportunity to achieve opiate abstinence rapidly and with minimal discomfort, with the reassuring protection against subsequent relapse to opiate use.

Our clinical experience indicates that sensitivity to clonidine's hypotensive, sedative, and withdrawal-suppressing effects varies widely among individuals. Under the close supervision of an inpatient setting, clonidine has been given in relatively large doses, with profound hypotension and sedation resulting in some cases [Gold et al, 1980]. With outpatients, however, doses must be lower and must be adjusted individually for each patient on a day-to-day basis in order to maximize safety, efficacy, and acceptability. Because the withdrawal-suppressing effects of a single clonidine dose last approximately 4–6 hours (with a peak effect at about 2 hours), a tid or qid dosing schedule is almost always required to maintain consistent relief. When administered for longer than 10–14 days, clonidine's effectiveness in suppressing withdrawal discomfort seems to dissipate. It therefore is preferable to discontinue methadone rapidly when clonidine treatment is started, so that the most intense period of withdrawal discomfort coincides with the period of maximum clonidine effectiveness. It is helpful to mask the exact day when methadone is discontinued by substituting placebo methadone during the postmethadone period. This eliminates an important psychological cue for the onset of withdrawal symptoms.

One way to gauge sensitivity to clonidine is to administer a single oral dose of 0.1 mg under observation, with assessment of blood pressure and side effects at 2 hours. If this dose is well tolerated, without orthostatic hypotension or extreme drowsiness, a dose regimen of 0.1 mg every 4–6 hours during the day with 0.2 mg at bedtime (0.5 mg total for day 1) can be initiated. Patients who are extremely sensitive to clonidine can be started on a smaller dose regimen of 0.05 mg at each dosing interval. Subsequent adjustments in the dose regimen must rely on careful daily assessment of symptoms and side effects. Some patients can tolerate rapid increases to 0.2 or 0.3 mg every 4–6 hours in order to gain sufficient withdrawal relief, but the daily clonidine dose must often be held steady or decreased temporarily in order to compensate for sedation and hypotension. The maximum daily dose rarely exceeds 1.0 mg total. Extreme lethargy, dizziness, or lightheadedness can be signs of clonidine overdose. In some patients it can be extremely difficult to find a dose regimen that provides adequate relief of withdrawal discomfort without undesirable side effects. Insomnia is a highly predictable and troublesome withdrawal symptom that can be severe enough to result in discontinuation of treatment. Clonidine does not adequately relieve withdrawal-related insomnia, and thus ancillary sedative-hypnotic medication used judiciously for 1–2 weeks postmethadone can be extremely helpful in fostering detoxification success. Alcohol use during clonidine treatment should be avoided because it can intensify clonidine's hypotensive action and thereby precipitate severe dizziness or lightheadedness. When discontinuing clonidine treatment, it is preferable to taper the daily dose gradually by 0.1 or 0.2 mg per day in order to avoid possible untoward effects. It is highly inadvisable simply to dispense a prescription for clonidine tablets without providing close ongoing supervision. In order to increase the possibility of frequent contact with the supervising physician, patients should receive at each clinic visit a limited supply of clonidine tablets that will last only until the next scheduled visit.

Heroin addicts are generally less successful with clonidine than patients withdrawing from methadone. Heroin addicts who receive interim stabilization on methadone tend to do better than those who attempt to go directly from heroin to clonidine. The intermediate step of methadone substitution affords an opportunity for the heroin user to adjust to oral dosing and to lower the level of opiate dependence before switching to clonidine. Successful detoxification using clonidine seems to be difficult to accomplish with outpatients on methadone doses over 30 mg per day.

There are several types of patients for whom clonidine treatment might be specifically indicated and preferable to detoxification with methadone. For example, clonidine might be the treatment of choice for addicts with extremely low levels of opiate dependence whose addiction might be increased by the use of methadone, and for individuals with iatrogenic addiction to prescription opiates as well as addicted physicians and other professionals, for whom exposure to methadone or methadone treatment facilities would be inadvisable. In general, clonidine offers an additional treatment option that may be useful whenever detoxification with methadone is inappropriate, unsuccessful, or simply unavailable.

Clonidine's side effects of sedation and hypotension have limited its clinical usefulness with outpatients. Drowsiness and dizziness induced by clonidine can interfere with normal daily activities, leading some patients to find clonidine unacceptable. Additionally, clinicians may hesitate to use clonidine because of the time-consuming daily supervision of the patient that is needed to adjust the clonidine dose regimen properly in order to maximize efficacy and avoid untoward side effects. Clonidine's efficacy in opiate withdrawal has suggested that other α-2 noradrenergic agonists might be equally efficacious in suppressing opiate withdrawal symptoms but without clonidine's undesirable side effects. Lofexidine is a structural analogue of clonidine that has been shown to suppress opiate withdrawal in morphine-dependent rats [Shearman et al, 1980]. Clinical trials of lofexidine in hypertensive patients [Maner et al, 1980, St John LaCorte et al, 1981] suggest that its sedative and hypotensive effects are substantially milder than clonidine's. We have recently conducted an initial open clinical trial [Washton et al, 1981] of lofexidine in methadone detoxification with 15 outpatient volunteers who were switched abruptly to lofexidine from 10–25 mg daily methadone. As in our studies with clonidine, the test of lofexidine's usefulness was conducted on an outpatient basis, with the measure of success defined by induction onto naltrexone. Successful detoxification and induction onto naltrexone was accomplished with 10 of the 15 subjects. All patients rated lofexidine as moderately to extremely effective in reducing most of the commonly experienced withdrawal symptoms: Insomnia, lethargy, and muscle and bone pain were the most frequent residual complaints. None of the 10 subjects reported unacceptable withdrawal symptoms while taking lofexidine. Those who failed to complete the detoxification procedure cited opiate craving rather than withdrawal discomfort as the major reason for returning to opiate use. None reported oversedation, dizziness, or lightheadedness from lofexidine, despite rapid increases in the dose to as much as 1.6 mg per day within the first 5 days. There was no significant lowering of blood pressure even at the maximum lofexidine dose (mean prelofexidine BP 115/74 mm Hg; mean BP at maximum dose 115/76 mm Hg). Dry mouth and mild drowsiness were the most commonly reported side effects. These findings suggest that lofexidine might be safer and more clinically useful than clonidine, especially in outpatient detoxification treatment. Lofexidine might allow opiate-addicted outpatients even greater access to naltrexone or drug-free modalities without hospital admission. Further studies of lofexidine are currently in progress at our treatment facility.

IV. ACKNOWLEDGMENTS

The authors' studies described in this paper were funded by the National Institute on Drug Abuse, Boehringer Ingelheim, Ltd, and Merrell-Dow Pharmaceuticals, Inc, and were conducted in a treatment program at New York Medical College, supported by the New York State Office of Alcoholism and Substance Abuse, Division of Substance Abuse Services.

The authors are grateful to the staff of the Division of Drug Abuse Research and Treatment for clinical support and assistance in data collection. Special thanks to John Garwood, MD, and Dorothy Singletary, RPA.

V. REFERENCES

Gold MS, Pottash AC, Sweeney DR, et al: Opiate withdrawal using clonidine. JAMA 243:343–346, 1980.

Gold MS, Redmond DE, Kleber HD: Clonidine blocks acute opiate-withdrawal symptoms. Lancet 1:599–601, 1978.

Maner T, Mehra J, Johnson C, et al: Comparative efficacy of two centrally acting imidazoline derivatives, clonidine and lofexidine. Clin Res 28:33A, 1980.

Rawson RA, Washton AM, Resnick RB, et al: Clonidine hydrochloride detoxification from methadone treatment: The value of naltrexone aftercare. In Harris LS (ed): "Problems of Drug Dependence." Washington, DC: DHEW, NIDA Research Monograph, 1980.

Resnick RB, Schuyten-Resnick E, Washton AM: Narcotic antagonists in the treatment of opioid dependence: Review and commentary. Comp Psychiatry 20:116–125, 1979.

St John LaCorte W, Jain AK, Ryan JR, et al: Comparative efficacy and tolerability of lofexidine and clonidine given alone or concomitantly with hydrochlorathiazide in hypertensive outpatients. Clin Pharmacol Ther 29:259, 1981.

Shearman GT, Lal H, Ursillo RC: Effectiveness of lofexidine in blocking morphine-withdrawal signs in the rat. Pharmacol Biochem Behav 12:573–575, 1980.

Washton AM, Resnick RB: Clonidine for opiate detoxification: Outpatient clinical trials. Am J Psychiatry 137:1121–1122, 1980a.

Washton AM, Resnick RB: Clonidine versus methadone for opiate detoxification. Lancet 2:1297, 1980b.

Washton AM, Resnick RB, LaPlaca R: Clonidine hydrochloride: A nonopiate treatment for opiate withdrawal. Psychopharm Bull 2:50–52, 1980a.

Washton AM, Resnick RB, Perzel JF, et al: Lofexidine, a clonidine analogue effective in opiate withdrawal. Lancet 1:991–992, 1981.

Washton AM, Resnick RB, Rawson RA: Clonidine for outpatient opiate detoxification. Lancet 1:1078–1079, 1980b.

Psychopharmacology of Clonidine, pages 285–298
© 1981 Alan R. Liss, Inc., 150 Fifth Avenue, New York, NY 10011

Neuroanatomical Sites of Action of Clonidine in Opiate Withdrawal: The Locus Coeruleus Connection

Mark S. Gold, A. Carter Pottash, Irl L. Extein, and Herbert D. Kleber

I. INTRODUCTION

Imidazoline derivative clonidine has been demonstrated to be an effective nonopiate treatment for opiate withdrawal [Gold et al 1978a, b, 1979a, b, c]. Clonidine, a presynaptic α-adrenergic agonist, in acute double-blind studies, reversed both the affective and physiological symptoms and signs of methadone [Gold et al, 1978a, b] and other opiate withdrawal [Gold et al, 1979c]. In a 14-day inpatient study, clonidine was also demonstrated to be effective as a rapid nonopiate treatment for moderate dose methadone withdrawal which enabled patients to be opiate- and clonidine-free in less than 14 days [Gold et al 1979d, 1980]. These clinical data suggested that chronic methadone treatment could be abruptly discontinued without the expected severe affective or physiological consequences. We suggested that the opiate withdrawal syndrome itself might be better understood from the point of view of the critical (symptom-generating) neurobiological events. The critical neuroanatomical events and sites we were most interested in were those that follow the discontinuation of chronic opiate administration and directly result in clinical signs and symptoms [Gold et al 1979a, b]. In this chapter we review the rodent, primate, and human data that supported an endorphin–locus coeruleus (LC) disinhibition hypothesis for opiate withdrawal [Gold et al 1978a, 1979a, c]. This norepinephrine (NE) hyperactivity hypothesis can explain a large body of clinical and preclinical data and may be useful in predicting newer and more effective nonopiate treatments [Gold et al, 1979b]. The neuroanatomy of clonidine's efficacy is important in that clonidine will be but the first in a series of noradrenergic-inhibitor medications that will become available for rapid and safe nonopiate detoxification.

II. ENDORPHIN–LC CONNECTION

The effects of opiates on catecholamine neurons have been reported elsewhere [Eidelberg, 1976; Lal, 1975; Roberts et al, 1978], but have tended to show that opiates can decrease NE activity and turnover [Herz et al, 1974; Korf et al, 1974]. Studies of the brain's major noradrenergic nucleus, nucleus locus coeruleus (LC) [Dahlstrom and Fuxe, 1964; Loisou, 1969; Morrison et al, 1979], have clearly demonstrated that the opiate morphine causes a marked reduction in the normal LC neuronal firing rate [Korf et al, 1974]. These LC neurons are known to respond to a painful stimulus with an increased firing rate and this pain-induced effect can be blocked by morphine [Korf et al, 1974]. These data demonstrated an important opiate–NE interaction, and suggested the possibility that some of the effects of opiates might be medicated by opiate-induced decreases in LC activity and NE release [Korf et al, 1974; Basbaum and Fields, 1978].

The discovery of specific opiate receptors in the brain [Gold and Byck, 1978; Hughes, 1975], the data by Pert et al [Pert et al, 1975] and Simon [Simon, 1975] demonstrating very dense opiate receptor accumulations in the LC, and the use of naloxone reversal in electrophysiological studies as a means of identifying effects that could be attributable to opiate receptor stimulation [Gold and Byck, 1978; Kleber and Gold, 1978; Svensson et al, 1975; Kuhar, 1978] allowed LC–endorphin, LC–enkephalin, and LC–opiate interactions to be expanded and more clearly understood. Investigators using single neuronal recording techniques and microiontophoresis reported that the endogenous opiates and exogenous opiates decreased LC firing rates, and that this effect was specifically reversed by the opiate antagonist naloxone [Kleber and Gold, 1978; Svensson et al, 1975; Kuhar, 1978]. These data suggested that the specific opiate receptors on the LC that might normally utilize endorphins as a natural neurotransmitter inhibit LC firing rate and modulate ascending NE activity and release [Gold et al, 1979b]. Naloxone only antagonized opiate and enkephalin effects but did not, by itself, produce an increase in LC activity [Kuhar, 1978]. These data suggested that this LC–opiate interaction was not tonic; that is, endorphins do not tonically inhibit LC activity, but rather endorphin is released in response to neural or environmental events. These data suggested to us that a critical endorphin–LC connection might exist and be related to some opiate effects and possibly play a critical role in opiate withdrawal [Gold et al, 1978a, 1979b], as chronic exogenous opiate administration tonically inhibits the LC.

The existence of LC cell body receptors for norepinephrine (NE) and epinephrine (E) were also suggested by single neuronal electrophysiological and microiontophoretic studies by Cedarbaum and Aghajanian [1976a, b] and confirmed in binding-affinity studies [Greenberg et al, 1976]. LC neurons responded to the α-2 adrenergic agonist clonidine with a decrease in LC firing [Cedarbaum and Aghajanian, 1976a, 1977] resulting in a marked decrease in NE release [Schmitt et al, 1971; Starke, 1977] and turnover [Bertilsson et al, 1977; Strombom, 1975] in whole brain, cortex, and more recently arteriovenous-difference studies [Maas et al 1976, 1979]. This depressant effect of clonidine on LC neurons could be reversed by the α-2 adrenergic antagonist piperoxane but not other drugs (B-blockers, naloxone) without specificity for this α receptor [Cedarbaum and Aghajanian, 1976a, 1977]. These data suggested that LC activity may be tonically modulated, under normal physiological conditions, by presynaptic NE or E release. These studies clearly demonstrated that, in very low doses, clonidine decreased LC activity by their interaction with inhibitory α-2 adrenergic on the LC [Cedarbaum and Aghajanian, 1976a, 1977]. In higher doses this specifically is lost, and clonidine has effects on postsynaptic NE and other receptors [Anden et al, 1970; Sastuy and Phillis, 1977].

III. ACTIVATION OF THE LC: A MODEL FOR DRUG WITHDRAWAL AND NATURALLY OCCURRING PANIC STATES

Piperoxane was given to nonhuman primates [Gold and Redmond, 1977] in doses (1 mg/kg; 2.5 mg/kg) previously shown to increase noradrenergic activity in rats [Kuhar, 1978] and turnover in these nonhuman primates [Gold and Redmond, 1977]. Piperoxane produced a behavioral syndrome that resembled spontaneous opiate withdrawal [Gold and Redmond, 1977]. A virtually identical primate "panic" syndrome was evoked by yohimbine, a drug similar in neurochemical action to piperoxane [Gold et al, 1979e]. Piperoxane administration studies suggested that noradrenergic augmentation might be a model system for studying the neuroanatomy, neurophysiology, and neurochemistry of opiate withdrawal which related to specific physiological and affective parameters. We also demonstrated that piperoxane-induced increase in these specific monkey behaviors and physiological signs could be reversed by morphine through an opiate receptor-medicated mechanism, as assessed by naloxone reversal. The synthetic M-Enkephalin FK 33-824 had a similar effect on this pharmaco-logical NE-augmentation primate model system [Extein et al, 1979]. Clonidine was also demonstrated to block or reverse the effects of piperoxane [Gold and Redmond, 1977]. This effect was not antagonized by naloxone. These behavioral data suggested that the noradrenergic LC is under the dual control of inhibitory α-2 and opiate receptors. This conclu-sion was supported by our demonstration that yohimbine (2.5 mg/kg) produced a similar behavioral syndrome in the monkey that could be blocked or reversed by morphine or clonidine [Redmond et al, 1978].

These primate drug studies led to the hypothesis that the effects of piperoxane and yohimbine mimicked the majority of opiate withdrawal signs and symptoms. We attributed the "panic syndrome" to NE effects, and suggested that a common noradrenergic hyperactivity mediates the behaviors observed after piperoxane, yohimbine, or discontinuation of chronic opiate administration (see Fig. 1) [Gold and Redmond, 1977].

To test these hypotheses, we more specifically increased noradrenergic activity by electrical stimulation (biphasic, bipolar 0.2–0.4 MA, 0.5 msec, 5–50 HZ) of the locus coeruleus. Electrical stimulation produced a behav-ioral syndrome with physiological changes that were very similar to that produced by piperoxane [Redmond et al, 1977, 1978]. Electrical stimulation-induced changes could be completely blocked or reversed by opiate receptor stimulation as assessed by naloxone reversal of the effects of morphine or FK 33-824 [Extein et al, 1979; Redmond et al, 1977, 1978]. These electrical stimulation changes could also be blocked or reversed by clonidine [Gold and Redmond, 1977; Redmond et al, 1977]. These data suggested to us that increases in NE release resulting from NE hyper-activity could be reversed by clonidine [Gold and Redmond, 1977; Red-mond et al, 1977]. These data again suggested to us that increases in NE release resulting from NE hyperactivity could be reversed by exogenous and endogenous opiates and clonidine.

IV. LC: OPIATE WITHDRAWAL HYPOTHESIS

We hypothesized that chronic exogenous opiate administration might cause a decrease in endogenous opiate release and synthesis as well as a decrease in opiate receptor sensitivity [Gold et al 1978a, 1979b]. Abrupt discontinuation of chronic opiate administration would, according to our model system, result in the absence of exogenous opiate-mediated inhibi-tion of ascending NE activity. As a result of this release from chronic exogenous inhibition and absence of adequate inhibitory neurotransmitters at the level of the NE nucleus [Gold et al, 1979b], there would be a resultant large increase in NE activity, release, and turnover [Gold et al, 1978a, 1979c]. Attempts to use endorphin stores to autoregulate this profound LC

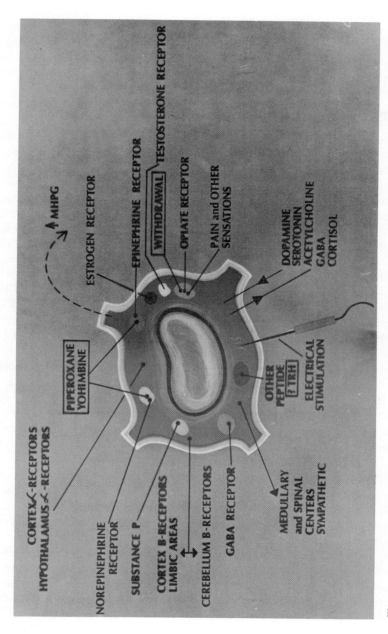

Fig. 1. Receptors on the locus coeruleus: increasing activity and NE release produces monkey panic behaviors which are phenomenologically similar to opiate withdrawal behaviors. LC or NE augmentation may be a model for opiate withdrawal.

firing increase would be too little too late, as the stores of available endogenous opiates would be of insufficient quantity, and the receptor sensitivity would be too low to augment the available endorphins. In addition, it is likely that other available inhibitory presynaptic neurotransmitters such as E and NE would be of insufficient quantity and would interact with receptors that are themselves abnormal to reverse the NE "rebound" release from opiate-mediated inhibition [Gold et al, 1979b].

V. TESTS OF THE HYPOTHESIS IN MAN

We tested the efficacy of clonidine in opiate withdrawal not only to demonstrate that clonidine might be a new and important treatment for addicts but also to see which physiological and affective variables would be clonidine-reversible and thereby attributable to clonidine's agonistic effects on presynaptic α-2 receptors on the LC. We had speculated that clonidine would reverse in man the behaviors and affective state produced by electrical or pharmacological activation of the LC as we had demonstrated in primates. However, we did not perform the critical studies actually comparing opiate withdrawal, piperoxane, yohimbine, and electrical stimulation of the LC in nonhuman primates. Our LC or NE hyperactivity hypothesis was supported by knowledge of LC neuroanatomy. The known anatomical connections of the LC suggested an important role for this structure in the wide variety of behaviors and physiological changes which accompany drug withdrawal and spontaneous panic states. The LC also receives afferents from serotonergic, adrenergic, peptidergic, and noradrenergic neurons, and the hypothalamus, and may have transducer cells to receive and relay hormonal messages [Jones et al, 1977; Sakai et al, 1977]. This LC neuroanatomy supports an important neuromodulatory or "tone" role for the LC and does not necessitate the direct involvement of numerous brain systems in the feeling state, cardiovascular sympathetic, parasympathetic, and many other manifestations of opiate withdrawal states [Gold et al, 1978a, 1979b].

After we administered 5 μg/kg of clonidine and placebo double-blind, orally in matching vehicles to five male opiate (methadone) addicts, we recognized that clonidine was effective for the full spectrum of withdrawal signs, symptoms, and affects. In a study of 11 methadone addicts [Gold et al, 1978b] and a study of five male heroin and five male methadone addicts [Gold et al, 1979c], we demonstrated that clonidine reversed the signs, symptoms, and affects of opiate withdrawal. Clonidine effectively reversed withdrawal in patients addicted to high doses of methadone for many years [Gold et al, 1978b]. Finally, in two well-controlled studies, one small [Gold et al, 1980] followed by another large [Gold et al, 1979d] inpatient study, we delineated a safe and 100% effective protocol for rapid nonopiate detoxification with clonidine that demonstrated that clonidine blocked and reversed acute withdrawal and continued (nearly completely) to suppress the reemergence of withdrawal symptoms after abrupt discontinuation of chronic opiate addiction. This series of studies demonstrated that clonidine could be substituted for opiates and discontinued without withdrawal signs of its own.

VI. SUPPORT FOR THE HYPOTHESIS

All of this clinical data [Gold et al 1978a, b, 1979c, 1980] served to offer strong support for an important Endorphin-LC interaction and NE hyperactivity as the most critical event in the generation of withdrawal symptoms on the basis of clonidine's known effects on the LC and NE activity when given in low doses. After the report of clonidine's efficacy in withdrawal, the hypothesis could be directly investigated only in animal studies. In rodent and primate studies it was demonstrated that clonidine decreased NE activity, release, and turnover as assessed by changes in the brain's major NE metabolite MHPG [Maas et al, 1979]. Morphine and endogenous opiates were found to have a similar effect through interaction with LC opiate receptors as assessed by naloxone reversal. Finally, Aghajanian [1978] demonstrated that chronic exogenous opiate administration produced tolerance of LC neurons to suppression. He also demonstrated that tolerance develops in the LC inhibition response to chronic opiates (in opiate addiction) and that naloxone-precipitated withdrawal was accompanied by the predicted [Gold et al, 1978a, b] noradrenergic hyperactivity [Aghajanian, 1978]. He demonstrated in single neuronal electrophysiological and microiontophoresis that this NE hyperactivity could be reversed by clonidine [Aghajanian, 1978]. This study confirmed the hypothesized LC activity in withdrawal, and supported our notion that NE was the important neurotransmitter in the generation of withdrawal symptoms. Our studies and others in the literature [Gold et al, 1978a, b, 1979b; Ary et al, 1977] did not exclude an important or at least significant role for other brain monoamine nuclei and neurotransmitters in opiate withdrawal.

VII. DA VERSUS NE HYPERACTIVITY: DA

To investigate neurotransmitter changes in withdrawal we conducted indirect neuroendocrine and direct MHPG studies in methadone addicts. While we had proposed a NE hyperactivity hypothesis to explain the signs and symptoms of withdrawal, a dopaminergic (DA) hyperactivity hypothesis has also been proposed and supported in basic studies [Ary et al, 1977; Lal and Hynes, 1978]. Serum prolactin (PRL) is predominantly controlled in vivo and in vitro by an inhibitory DA mechanism [Clemens et al, 1974].

Consistent with this control mechanism, augmentation of DA function results in increases in serum PRL [Gold et al, 1978c, 1979f]. To investigate the relation of opiate withdrawal symptoms to serum PRL and by inference to assess the role of DA in acute withdrawal symptom generation and relief, we measured serum PRL in duplicate by radioimmunoassay [Gold et al, 1978d]. Fourteen days after being clonidine- and opiate-free (drug-free baseline), during the peak of opiate withdrawal and after clonidine-induced suppression, we collected samples for serum PRL. PRL was significantly reduced from a preclonidine mean ($\pm$ SEM) of 10.8 ng/ml $\pm$ 1.0 to 8.2 $\pm$ 0.8 at 60 minutes and 7.0 $\pm$ 0.8 at 120 minutes after clonidine administration (paired t = 3.92; P < 0.02). Serum PRL was significantly reduced during the peak of opiate withdrawal to a mean of 10.2 $\pm$ 0.7 ng/ml compared to a mean of 13.6 $\pm$ 0.9 ng/ml when the patient had been opiate- and clonidine-free for 14 days (t = 3.50 P < 0.02).

Dopaminergic hyperactivity has been both postulated and reported in withdrawal. Significant decreases in serum PRL are normally attributable to direct stimulation of DA receptors [Ary et al, 1977; Lal and Hynes, 1978] or increased DA release or neurotransmission [Clemens et al, 1974; Gold et al, 1979f]. The decreased serum PRL for patients in withdrawal supports underlying DA hyperactivity in withdrawal [Lal and Hynes, 1978]. These data were consistent with animal studies showing decreases in PRL in opiate withdrawal [Lal et al, 1977]. However, in our studies the serum PRL levels did not return to baseline after clonidine-induced amelioration of symptoms. This suggested that DA hyperactivity continues even though clonidine markedly relieves symptoms. Therefore we have suggested that DA hyperactivity is present but is not related to symptoms or symptom relief.

VIII. NE–MHPG IN MAN

Direct testing of a NE hyperactivity hypothesis has been difficult because of the methodological problems in measuring plasma 3-methoxy-4-hydroxyphenyl glycol (MHPG). Our laboratory has recently developed a method for the rapid analysis of free MHPG levels. Using this technique we have been able to reproducibly measure high picogram quantities of MHPG and related fluorescent compounds. In a pilot study of three patients in spontaneous withdrawal, we have demonstrated increasing plasma-free MHPG levels that correlate with the increase in signs and symptoms with increasing time of abstinence. In addition, clonidine caused a significant decrease in withdrawal symptoms and plasma MHPG. These pilot data offer tentative support for the hypothesized NE hyperactivity and relationship of NE activity to symptom generation and relief. These data are supported by recent data in rodents and primates that demonstrate increases in MHPG in withdrawal and clonidine reversal of the MHPG increases [Crawley et al, 1979; Redmond et al, 1979].

Recent data reported in the literature also support a NE hypothesis [Gold et al, 1979h]. For example, clonidine withdrawal itself has significant phenomenological similarities to opiate withdrawal [Hansson et al, 1973; Hunyor et al, 1973], and would be expected to result, in part, from chronic exogenous inhibition of the LC through α-2 receptor stimulation. Clonidine withdrawal results in increases in MHPG and may be treatable with clonidine or opiates [Tang et al, 1979]. Clonidine, while not an opiate drug and having no apparent affinity for opiate receptors [Simon, personal communication, 1979], has a number of opiate-like properties including analgesia, miosis, hypotension, sedation, antianxiety, and decreased respiration [Paazlow, 1974; Koss, 1979; Kobinger, 1975]. These data suggest that the effects of exogenous α-2 or opiate agonists that tonically inhibit brain areas like the LC may be responsible for tolerance and the development of withdrawal symptoms after abrupt discontinuation of chronic administration.

IX. IMPLICATIONS OF THE LC NEUROANATOMY HYPOTHESIS

What would be important from the neurotransmitter hypothesis and clinical point of view would be the development of an α-2 agonist like clonidine, which decreases LC activity and NE release but which does not produce extreme sedation and severe hypotension. However, it may be that potent α-2 nonopiate drugs that reverse withdrawal from high doses of chronic opiate administration must produce sedation and decrease blood pressure. The NE hyperactivity or LC hypothesis would predict that other drugs, which specifically inhibit the LC by an action at specific presynaptic LC receptors, will be found to have marked antiwithdrawal efficacy in man. Known drugs we believe inhibit NE activity at the level of the LC and which may have antiwithdrawal efficacy are shown in Figure 2. Therefore, non-α adrenergic drugs and neural peptides may be found to be safe for use in humans, and to decrease LC activity. These medications may be safely developed for use in withdrawal. Nonaddicting opiate receptor agonists, vasopressin, or GABA agonists like baclofen may be found to have potent antiwithdrawal efficacy, but without hypotensive effects and with significantly less sedation than clonidine. These drugs would be without α-2 activity, but might be expected to have antiwithdrawal activity by decreasing LC activity. These new possibilities would thus provide additional tests for the NE hyperactivity hypothesis for opiate withdrawal as well as possibly adding new, safe, and effective nonopiate treatments to the treatment armamentarium.

Finally, it should be mentioned that the discovery of opiate receptors, their density in the LC, the parallel function of α-2 and opiate receptor

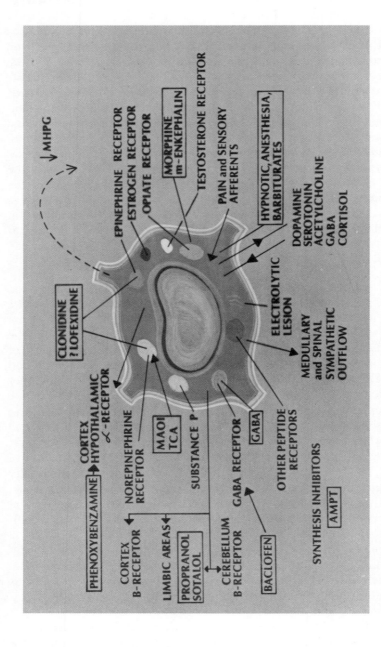

Fig. 2. Strategies to use existing LC receptors to find new treatments. The main implication of clonidine is this model neuron. With the LC hyperactivity theory, presynaptic mechanisms which stimulate specific LC receptors to inhibit LC activity and NE release should have marked antiwithdrawal effects.

stimulation at the level of the LC have suggested the efficacy of clonidine in withdrawal, and the possibility that NE hyperactivity may be responsible for the affects—anxiety and panic—as well as the physiological changes associated with withdrawal. This raises the question of naturally occurring panic and anxiety states and whether these states share LC hyperactivity as a final common neurobiological pathway [Gold et al, 1979a]. NE hyperactivity might then also provide a model for studying natural and drug-related panic states and lead to a neural construct for these states that could predict new treatment possibilities including opiates, endorphins, and clonidine [Gold et al, 1979a, c, g; Washton et al, 1978]. Studies in progress utilizing serial plasma clonidine [Christersson et al, 1979] levels may establish a plasma level–response relationship that may simplify and increase the margin of safety in the clinical use of clonidine in withdrawal.

Our studies [Gold et al, 1979a, b] and studies reported by other groups in rodents [Aghajanian, 1978; Fielding et al, 1977, 1978; Meyer and Sparber, 1976; Spaulding et al, 1977; Tseng et al, 1975] strongly support the clinical data [Gold et al, 1978a, b, 1980; Washton et al, 1978] reporting opiate-like efficacy for the nonopiate clonidine in opiate withdrawal. These clinical and basic data offer new hope for addicts as well as for the role of basic science in developing new and useful treatments in medicine.

X. REFERENCES

Aghajanian GK: Tolerance of locus coeruleus neurones to morphine and suppression of withdrawal response by clonidine. Nature 276:136–188, 1978.

Anden NE, Corrodi H, Fuxe K, Hokfelt B, Hokfelt T, Rydin C, Svensson T: Evidence for a central noradrenaline receptor stimulation by clonidine. Life Sci 9:513–523, 1970.

Ary M, Cox B, Lomax P: Dopaminergic mechanisms in precipitated withdrawal in morphine-dependent rats. J Pharmacol Exp Ther 200:271–276, 1977.

Basbaum AI, Fields HL: Endogenous pain control mechanisms: Review and hypothesis. Ann Neurol 4:451–462.

Bertilsson L, Haglund K, Ostman J, Rawlins MD, Ringberger VA, Sjoqvist F: Monoamine metabolites in cerebrospinal fluid during treatment with clonidine or alprenolol. Eur J Clin Pharmacol 11:125–128, 1977.

Cedarbaum JM, Aghajanian GK: Noradrenergic neurons of the locus coeruleus: Inhibition by epinephrine and activation by the alpha-antagonist piperoxane. Brain Res 112:413–419, 1976a.

Cedarbaum JM, Aghajanian GK: Characterization of catecholamine receptors on noradrenergic neurons of the locus coeruleus. Neurosci Abstr 2:683, 1976b.

Cedarbaum JM, Aghajanian GK: Catecholamine receptors on locus coeruleus neurons: Pharmacological characteristics. Eur J Pharmacol 44:375–385, 1977.

Christersson S, Frisk-Holmberg M, Paalzow L: Steady state plasma concentration of clonidine and its relation to the effects on blood pressure in normotensive and hypertensive rats. J Pharm Pharmacol 3:418–419, 1979.

Clemens JA, Smalstig EB, Sawyer BD: Antipsychotic drugs stimulate prolactin release. Psychopharmacologia 40:123–127, 1974.

Crawley JN, Laverty R, Roth RH: Clonidine reversal of increased norepinephrine metabolite levels during morphine withdrawal. Eur J of Pharmacol 57:2–3, 1979.

Dahlstrom A, Fuxe K: Evidence for the existence of monoamine containing neurons in the central nervous system. 1. Demonstration of monoamine in the cell bodies of brain stem neurons. Acta Physiol Scand (Suppl) 232:1, 1964.

Eidelberg E: Possible action of opiates upon synapes. Prog Neurobiol 6:81–102, 1976.

Extein I, Goodwin FK, Lewy AJ, Schoenfeld RI, Fakhuri L, Gold MS, Redmond DE: Behavioral and biochemical effects of FK 33-824, a parenterally and orally active enkephalin analogue. In Usdin E (ed): "Endorphins in Mental Health Research." London: Macmillan, 1979, pp 279–292.

Fielding S, Wilker J, Hynes M, Szewszak M, Novick W, Lal H: Antinociceptive and antiwithdrawal actions of clonidine: A comparison with morphine. Fed Proc 36:1024, 1977.

Fielding S, Wilker J, Hynes M, Szewczak M, Novick WJ, Lal H: A comparison of clonidine with morphine for antinoceptive and antiwithdrawal actions. J Pharmacol Exp Ther 207:899–905, 1978.

Gold MS, Byck R: Endorphins, lithium, and naloxone: Their relationship to pathological and drug-induced manic-euphoric states. NIDA Research Monograph No 19, pp 192–209, 1978.

Gold MS, Redmond DE Jr: Pharmacological activation and inhibition of nonadrenergic activity alter specific behaviors in nonhuman primates. Neurosci Abs 3:250, 1977.

Gold MS, Redmond DE Jr, Kleber HD: Clonidine blocks acute opiate-withdrawal symptoms. Lancet 2:599–602, 1978b.

Gold MS, Redmond DE Jr, Donabedian RK, Goodwin FK, Extein I: Increase in serum prolactin by exogenous and endogenous opiates: Evidence for antidopamine and antipsychotic effects. Am J Psychiatry 135:1415–1416, 1978c.

Gold MS, Donabedian RK, Redmond DE Jr: Effect of piperoxane on serum prolactin: Possible role of epinephrine-mediated synapses in the inhibition of prolactin secretion. Endocrinology 102:1183–1189, 1978d.

Gold MS, Byck R, Sweeney DR, Kleber HD: Endorphin locus coeruleus connection mediates opiate action and withdrawal. Biomedicine 30:1–4, 1979b.

Gold MS, Redmond DE Jr, Kleber HD: Noradrenergic hyperactivity in opiate withdrawal supported by clonidine reversal of opiate withdrawal. Am J Psychiatry 136:100–102, 1979c.

Gold MS, Pottash ALC, Sweeney DR, Kleber HD: Clonidine detoxification: A fourteen day protocol for rapid opiate withdrawal. NIDA Research Monograph, pp 226–232, 1979d.

Gold MS, Donabedian RK, Redmond DE Jr: Further evidence for alpha-2 andrenergic receptor mediated inhibition of prolactin secretion: The effect of yohimbine. Psychoneuroendocrinology 3:253–260, 1979e.

Gold MS, Redmond DE Jr, Donabedian RK: The effects of opiate agonist and antagonist on serum prolactin in primates: Possible role for endorphins in prolactin regulation. Endocrinology: 105:284–289, 1979f.

Gold MS, Pottash ALC, Sweeney DR, Kleber HD, Redmond DE Jr: Rapid opiate detoxification: Clinical evidence of antidepressant and antipanic effects of opiates. Am J Psychiatry 136:982–983, 1979g.

Gold MS, Sweeney DR, Pottash ALC, Kleber HD: Decreased serum prolactin in opiate withdrawal and dopaminergic hyperactivity. Am J Psychiatry 136:849–850, 1979h.

Gold MS, Pottash ALC, Sweeney DR, Kleber HD: Clonidine: A safe, effective, and rapid nonopiate treatment for opiate withdrawal. JAMA 243:4, 1980.

Greenberg DA, U'Prichard DC, Snyder SH: Alpha-noradrenergic receptor binding in mammalian brain. Life Sci 19:69–76, 1976.

Hansson L, Hunyor SN, Julius S, Hoobler SW: Blood pressure crisis following withdrawal of clonidine with special reference to arterial and urinary catecholamine levels, and suggestions for acute management. Am Heart J 85:605–610, 1973.

Herz A, Blasig J, Papeschi R: Role of catecholaminergic mechanisms in the expression of the morphine abstinence syndrome in rats. Psychopharmacologia 39:121–143, 1974.

Hughes J: Isolation of an endogenous compound in brain with pharmacological properties similar to morphine. Brain Res 88:295–308, 1975.

Hunyor SN, Hansson L, Harrison TS, Hoobler SW: Effects of clonidine withdrawal: Possible mechanisms and suggestions for management. Br Med J 2:209–211, 1973.

Jones BE, Halaris AE, McIlhany M, Moore RY: Ascending projections of the locus coeruleus in the rat: I & II. Brain Res 127:1–21, 23–53, 1977.

Kleber HD, Gold MS: Use of psychotropic drugs in treatment of methadone maintained narcotic addicts. Ann NY Acad Sci 311:81–1978.

Kobinger W: Central cardiovascular actions of clonidine. In Davies DS, Reid JL (eds): "Central Action of Drugs in Blood Pressure Regulation." Baltimore: University Park Press, 1975, p 181.

Korf J, Bunney BS, Aghajanian GK: Noradrenergic neurons: Morphine inhibition of spontaneous activity. Eur J Pharmacol 25:165–169, 1974.

Kuhar MJ: Opiate receptors: Some anatomical and physiological aspects. NY Acad Sci 311:35–48, 1978.

Koss MD: Topical clonidine produces mydriasis by a central nervous system action. Eur J pharmacol 55:305–310, 1979.

Lal H: Narcotic dependence, narcotic action and dopamine receptors. Life Sci 17:483–496, 1975.

Lal H, Brown W, Drawbaugh R, Hynes M, Brown G: Enhanced prolactin inhibition following chronic treatment with haloperidol and morphine. Life Sci 20:101–106, 1977.

Lal H, Hynes MD: Effectiveness of butyrophenones and related drugs in narcotic withdrawal. In Deniker P et al (eds): "Neuropsychopharmacology." Elmsford, New York: Pergamon Press, 1978, pp 289–295.

Loisou LA: Projections of the nucleus locus coeruleus in the albino rat. Brain Res 15:563, 1969.

Maas JW, Hattox SE, Landis DH, Roth RH: The determination of a brain arteriovenous difference for 3-methoxy-4-hydroxyphenethylene glycol (MPHG). Brain Res 118:167–173, 1976.

Maas JW, Greene NM, Hattox SE, Landis DH: Neurotransmitter metabolite production by human brain. In Usdin E, Kopin IJ, Barchas J (eds): "Catecholamines: Basic and Clinical Frontiers." Elmsford, New York: Pergamon Press, 1979, pp 1878–1880.

Meyer DR, Sparber SB: Clonidine antagonized body weight loss and other symptoms used to measure withdrawal in morphine pelleted rats given naloxone. Pharmacologist 18:236, 1976.

Morrison JH, Molliver ME, Grazanna R: Noradrenergic innervation of cerebral cortex: Widespread effects of local cortical lesions. Science 205:313–316, 1979.

Paalzow L: Analgesia produced by clonidine in mice and rats. J Pharm Pharmacol 26:361–363, 1974.

Pert CB, Kuhar MJ, Snyder SH: Autoradiographic localization of the opiate receptor in rat brain. Life Sci 16:1849–1854, 1975.

Redmond DE Jr, Hunag YH, Gold MS: Anxiety: The locus coeruleus connection. Neurosci Abstr 3:258, 1977.

Redmond DE Jr, Hunag YH, Gold MS: Evidence for the involvement of a brain norepinephrine (NE) system in anxiety. Proc 4th Int Catecholamine Symposium, Pacific Grove, California, 1978.

Redmond DE Jr, Roth RH, Hattox SE, Stogin JM, Baulu J: 3-Methyoxy-4-hydroxy-phenethylene glycol (MHPG) in monkey brain, CSF, and plasma during naloxone precipitated morphine abstinence. Neurosci Abstr 5:1160, 1979.

Roberts DCS, Mason S, Fibiger HC: 6-OHDA Lesions to the dorsal noradrenergic bundle alters morphine-induced locomotor activity and catalepsy. Eur J Pharmacol 52:209–214, 1978.

Sakai K, Touret M, Salvert D, Leger L, Jouvet M: Afferent projections to the cat locus coeruleus as visualized by the horseradish peroxidase technique. Brain Res 119:21–41, 1977.

Sastuy B, Phillis J: Evidence that clonidine can activate histamine H^2-receptors in rat cerebral cortex. Neuropharmacology 16:223–225, 1977.

Schmitt H, Schmitt H, Fenard S: Evidence for an alpha-sympathomimetic component in the effects of Catapresan on vasomotor centres: Antagonism by piperoxane. Eur J Pharmacol 14:98–100, 1971.

Simon EJ: Opiate receptor binding with 3H-etorphine. Neurosci Res Program Bull 13:43–50.

Spaulding TC, Venafro JJ, Ma MG, Fielding S: The dissociation of the antinociceptive effect of clonidine from supraspinal structures. Neuropharmacology 18:103–105, 1977.

Starke K: Regulation of noradrenaline release by presynaptic receptor systems. Rev Physiol Biochem Pharmacol 77:1–124, 1977.

Strombom U: On the functional role of pre- and postsynaptic catecholamine receptors in brain. Acta Physiol Scand (Suppl) 431:1–43, 1975.

Svensson TH, Bunney BS, Aghajanian GK: Inhibition of both nonadrenergic and serotonergic neurons in brain by the alpha-adrenergic antagonist clonidine. Brain Res 92:291–306.

Tang LF, Lal H, Wei E: Effects of clonidine withdrawal on total 3-methoxy-4-hydroxyphenethylene glycol in the rat brain. Psychopharmacology 61:11–12, 1979.

Tseng LF, Lal H, Wei E: Effects of clonidine on morphine withdrawal signs in the rat. Eur J Pharmacol 30:93–99, 1975.

Washton AM, Resnick RB, La Placa R: Clonidine hydrochloride — A nonopiate treatment for opiate withdrawal. Maui, Hawaii: American College of Neuropsychopharmacology, 1978.

Psychopharmacology of Clonidine, pages 299–306

Clinical Utility of Clonidine in Opiate Withdrawal: A Study of 100 Patients

Mark S. Gold and Herbert D. Kleber

I. INTRODUCTION

We have previously reported that a single dose of 5 μg/kg of clonidine caused a rapid and significant decrease in opiate withdrawal signs and symptoms in patients addicted to methadone [Gold et al, 1978a]. More recently, we confirmed these findings with other synthetic opiates and heroin [Gold et al, 1979]. These initial studies suggested a new use for clonidine, an imidazoline drug widely used in the treatment of hypertension [Schmitt and Schmitt, 1970; Schmitt et al, 1971; Svensson and Strombom, 1977]. We proposed after an open outpatient study that treatment with a nonopiate such as clonidine, which could control symptoms during the acute phase of opiate withdrawal and provide symptomatic relief during detoxification, could enable patients to transfer to other treatment modalities, especially maintenance with the long-acting opiate antagonist naltrexone. Clonidine detoxification appeared to be superior to the usual treatment of opiate withdrawal [Gold et al, 1978a]. During clonidine detoxification the patients experience a few mild opiate withdrawal symptoms, and many of them are able to discontinue their methadone treatment. While our previous studies [Gold et al, 1978a, b, 1979] offered considerable promise, their evaluation was complicated by the small number of patients studied; moreover, in the outpatient study phase patients discharged from the hospital found it difficult to refrain from use of other drugs.

Results of studies in rodents and primates have suggested that the neurotransmitter norepinephrine is involved in opiate withdrawal [Gold et al, 1978b; Gold and Redmond, 1977; Gold et al, 1979a, b, d; Kuhar, 1978; Meyer and Sparber, 1976; Paalzow and Paalzow, 1976; Redmond et al, 1977, 1978]. Our early experience with the α-2-adrenergic agonist clonidine [Gold et al, 1978a, 1979c], which reduces noradrenergic brain activity, provided presumptive pharmacological evidence that in man noradrenergic hyperactivity mediates the opiate withdrawal syndrome [Gold et al, 1978a, 1979a, c]. In a new study we administered clonidine acutely in doses of 6 μg/kg and chronically in a daily dose of 17 μg/kg in an inpatient setting to 100 opiate addicts after withdrawal from 10–80 mg of chronic methadone treatment. Our results are presented below.

II. SUBJECTS AND METHODS

The subjects were 100 patients who had been addicted to opiates for periods up to 15 years. The average methadone dose was 42 mg/day. Eighty-seven of the patients were employed. They all expressed interest in discontinuing the methadone treatment and gave informed consent to a study that required an abrupt withdrawal from methadone 3 days after admission to the Evaluation and Research Unit and at least 36 hours with no opiate administration. All patients had previously made unsuccessful attempts at opiate detoxification. All had objective signs of opiate withdrawal. The patients were observed hourly for the presence or absence of withdrawal signs and symptoms by a research nurse-clinician, beginning at 8 a.m., while they rested in bed during the day of clonidine administration [Gold et al, 1978b]. The nurse rated 21 items associated with withdrawal [Gold et al, 1978b] as present or absent [Aghajanian, 1978]; the total score then gave a measure of withdrawal severity. The symptoms and signs were opiate craving, anxiety, yawning, perspiration, lacrimation, rhinorrhea, yen sleep, mydriasis, goose flesh, tremors, hot and cold flashes, aching bones and muscles, anorexia, increased blood pressure, insomnia, increased temperature, increased respiratory rate and depth, increased pulse rate, restlessness, nausea and vomiting, and diarrhea. All patients completed self-rating Addiction Research Center Inventory (ARCI) WOW scales [Gold et al, 1978b] every hour from 9 a.m. on to assess their opiate withdrawal symptoms. After the first day of clonidine administration, the patients were given clonidine 16 μg/kg/day in divided doses, and their opiate withdrawal symptoms were rated three times a day, before administration, by a research nurse-clinician. In addition, all patients completed self-rating analogue scales. These analogue rating scales were used to assess changes in nervousness, feeling high, unpleasantness, energy, irritability, fear and anger. They were completed every hour from 9 a.m. on

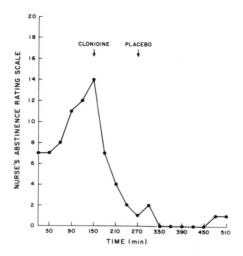

Fig. 1.   The effect of Clonidine (6 μg/kg) and placebo on acute methadone withdrawal in man.

the first day of administration and three times a day prior to administration on subsequent days. On the first day, the patients were given 6 μg/kg of clonidine or placebo orally in matching vehicles so that the effect of clonidine on opiate withdrawal signs and symptoms and the changes in blood pressure produced by this dose of clonidine might be determined. After the initial clonidine and placebo administration, patients without precipitous blood pressure declines were given clonidine 17 μg/kg/day for at least 9 days. The clonidine dose was gradually decreased to zero by day 14. Naloxone (1.2 mg) was then given intravenously to assess the patients' readiness for this medication. Patients who had a history of cardiac arrhythmias, hypotension, vasomotor instability, or psychiatric illness or hospitalization were excluded from the study [Gold et al, 1979b].

III. RESULTS

The number of opiate withdrawal signs increased during the baseline period to a peak of 13.7 ± 0.6 SEM. Clonidine, 6 μg/kg, produced a rapid and significant decrease in the incidence of opiate withdrawal signs and symptoms to 1.5 ± 1.0 at 90 minutes and to 0.9 ± 0.5 at 120 minutes (paired t-test, P < 0.01). Examples of this acute effect are shown in Figures 1 and 2. Opiate withdrawal ratings remained unchanged for an additional 240 minutes. Systolic blood pressure was significantly reduced (P < 0.01) from pretreatment readings to 104.0 ± 5.2 mm Hg at +120 minutes. Diastolic blood pressure was also significantly reduced to mean of 65.7 ± 4.8 mm Hg

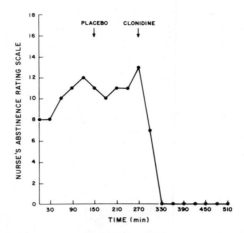

Fig. 2.   The effect of Clonidine (6 μg/kg) and placebo on acute methadone withdrawal in man.

120 minutes after clonidine administration (P < 0.01). The blood pressure was not significantly changed over the next 240 minutes. ARCI ratings were also significantly (P < 0.01) reduced from a pretreatment mean of 12.2 ± 1.2 to 6.8 ± 0.4 120 minutes after clonidine administration. The relief of subjective and objective distress was significant.

On the self-rating analogue scales, on which 70 is the highest score, there were significant (P < 0.01) decreases in self-rated nervousness, irritability, "uninvolved," and "angry" scales at 120 minutes. No significant changes were noted in the self-rating analogue scales for energy or feeling "high." All patients stated that they needed their methadone and that they were "kicking" immediately before clonidine administration. Two hours after clonidine administration, four of the patients stated that they felt the need for methadone or had the sensation of "kicking." Placebo had no significant effects on any of the above measurements or ratings. The effects of clonidine on patients addicted to either low or moderate doses of methadone did not differ significantly.

All 100 patients continued to receive clonidine in a hospital setting. None of the patients chose a return to methadone after their first dose of clonidine. On the first day of clonidine administration, the patients were given 6 μg/kg as a test dose and then 6 μg/kg at bedtime. Thereafter, 17 μg/kg/day of clonidine was given in divided doses of 7 μg/kg at 8 a.m., 3 μg/kg at 4 p.m., and 7 μg/kg at 11 p.m. Each day vital signs were monitored and nurses' abstinence ratings and self-ratings given as described previously [Gold et al, 1978b]. There were no significant changes in the abstinence ratings during this 10-day inpatient trial. Seventy-one patients, however, complained of difficulty in falling asleep. Dry mouth, sluggishness, depression, and occasional bone pain were less frequent complaints. The mean incidence of opiate withdrawal symptoms and signs at noon was 1.2 ± 0.4 on day 2, 1.0 ± 0.2 on day 3, 0.6 ± 0.2 on day 4, 0.3 ± 0.1 on day 5, and 0.3 ± 0.1 on day 6. Systolic and diastolic blood pressure remained significantly decreased throughout the 9 days during which 17 μg/kg of clonidine was administered. There were no significant increases or decreases in self-rated nervousness, irritability, "uninvolved," angry, fear, "high," or energy. Clonidine was withheld in some instances because of severe hypotension. In 41 cases the clonidine dose was decreased to compensate for oversedation or hypotension.

On days 11, 12, and 13, the clonidine dose was decreased by 50%. On day 14 the patients received no clonidine whatsoever. None of them showed any increase in opiate withdrawal signs or symptoms, nor did any clonidine withdrawal symptoms develop. One patient eloped from the hospital on day 5 of the study. On day 14 all patients were given naloxone (1.2 mg) intravenously to assess residual opiate dependence. All naloxone tests were negative. All but one of the 100 patients completed the 14-day inpatient study and were ready for naltrexone.

IV. DISCUSSION

In contrast to our previous studies [Gold et al, 1978a, b, 1979c], the data reported here were not confounded by small sample size, difficulties in compliance, or use of other drugs. All patients in this study were successfully detoxified from chronic methadone addiction in an inpatient setting, and all but one had abstained from opiates for 14 days or more at the time of discharge from the hospital. This detoxification success rate greatly exceeds our experience and literature data concerning methadone detoxification groups. Significant and potentially serious decreases in systolic and diastolic blood pressure were successfully managed in the hospital, without the emergence of additional opiate withdrawal symptoms, by frequent monitoring of vital signs and bed rest. Finally, the risk of illicit drug use adding to the hypotensive effect of clonidine was avoided in this inpatient study.

We have shown that clonidine is a safe and effective nonopiate medication for opiate withdrawal, which suppresses its symptoms and signs as well as the affective changes associated with opiate withdrawal. Such associated affects as anxiety, irritability, and anger were in fact rapidly reduced after clonidine administration. Clonidine is therefore extremely useful as a noneuphorigenic treatment for detoxification. This 14-day inpatient clonidine detoxification protocol could be useful in the treatment of selected opiate addicts. For example, clonidine detoxification would be linked to maintenance with long-acting opiate antagonists such as naltrexone. Clonidine, being a nonopiate, allows the patient to discontinue opiate administration abruptly and to remain free of opiates long enough to initiate maintenance treatment with naltrexone. Clonidine may allow the detoxification of patients maintained on methadone whose previous attempts at detoxification failed owing to the morbidity associated with current slow detoxification practices. Clonidine is also potentially useful in the treatment of added iatrogenic symptoms and the protracted abstinence syndrome, in which it may lessen the risk of exposure to opiates.

We have tested the efficacy of clonidine in opiate withdrawal on the basis of studies reported in the literature [Bednarczyk and Vetulani, 1978; Bolme et al, 1974; Fielding et al, 1977; Kuhar, 1978; Meyer and Sparber, 1976; Paalzow and Paalzow, 1976; Schmitt and Schmitt, 1970; Schmitt et al, 1971; Svensson and Strombom, 1977] and of our studies of the major noradrenergic nucleus, the locus coeruleus (LC), in monkeys. The effects of electrical or pharmacological activation of this nucleus were found to produce changes resembling those seen in opiate withdrawal [Gold and Redmond, 1977; Gold et al, 1979a, b]. Morphine and clonidine blocked the effects of the electrical and pharmacological activation of the LC in primates [Gold and Redmond, 1977; Gold et al, 1979a, b]. This observation indicated that opiate withdrawal may be due, in part, to increased noradrenergic neural activity in areas such as the LC which are susceptible to the action of opiates through opiate receptors as well as to the action of clonidine through α-2-adrenergic receptors [Gold et al, 1978a]. This hypothesis is supported by the similarity of the vital signs and mood characteristic of both clonidine and opiate withdrawal and by the noradrenergic hyperactivity seen in clonidine withdrawal [Svensson and Strombom, 1977].

Opiates administered systemically and microiontophoretically inhibit the activity of the locus coeruleus by stimulation of inhibitory opiate receptor sites; this effect can be reversed by the opiate antagonist naloxone [Gold et al, 1979d; Kuhar, 1978]. Clonidine, too, inhibits the LC, but does so by stimulation of a different, α-2-adrenergic receptor. This effect in turn is reversed by specific α-2-adrenergic antagonists such as piperoxan [Cedarbaum and Aghajanian, 1976]. Although morphine and endogenous opiates and clonidine appear to act upon independent receptors within the LC, they have in common a similar depressant effect on overall LC activity [Aghajanian, 1978; Cedarbaum and Aghajanian, 1976; Kuhar, 1978]. These observations by Aghajanian are consistent with the hypothesis that the α-2 agonist clonidine suppresses certain signs and symptoms of opiate withdrawal by means of a parallel but independent action on LC activity. These and other data [Gold et al, 1979a; Kuhar, 1978] suggest the possibility that opiate interactions with noradrenergic areas such as the LC, regulated by both α-2 adrenergic and opiate receptors, become activated in panic states related to opiate withdrawal and perhaps also in naturally occurring panic states.

To sum up, the effects of clonidine on opiate withdrawal in man [Gold et al, 1978a, b, 1979c] and rodents [Aghajanian, 1978; Bednarczyk and Vetulani, 1978; Fielding et al, 1977; Gold et al, 1979a; Meyer and Sparber, 1976] provide pharmacological evidence in support of the hypothesis implicating noradrenergic hyperactivity in the opiate withdrawal syndrome. It appears that clonidine reverses opiate withdrawal symptoms by replacing opiate-mediated inhibition with α-2-adrenergic inhibition of noradrenergic brain activity. Additional basic and clinical tests of this hypothesis are needed. Our own studies and studies by Washton et al [1978] have already demonstrated that clonidine detoxification is a safe and rapid procedure that may afford alternatives to the current, standard treatment of the opiate addict. Our data make it probable that clonidine detoxification allows the vast majority of the addicts to achieve freedom from both opiates and clonidine within 14 days, although maintenance treatment with naltrexone and group therapy may be necessary to maintain this state.

V. REFERENCES

Aghajanian GK: Tolerance of locus coeruleus neurons to morphine and suppression of withdrawal response by clonidine. Nature 276:186–188, 1978.

Bednarczyk B, Vetulani J: Antagonism of clonidine to shaking behavior in morphine abstinence syndrome and to head twitches produced by serotonergic agents in the rat. Pol J Pharmacol Pharm 30:307–322, 1978.

Bolme P, Corrodi H, Fuxe K, Hokfelt T, Lidbrink P, Goldstein M: Possible involvement of central adrenaline neurons in vasomotor and respiratory control: Studies with clonidine and its interactions with piperoxan and yohimbine. Eur J Pharmacol 28:89–94, 1974.

Cedarbaum JM, Aghajanian GK: Noradrenergic neurons of the locus coeruleus: Inhibition by epinephrine and activation by the antagonist piperoxane. Brain Res 112:413–419, 1976.

Fielding S, Wilker J, Hynes M, Szewszak M, Novick W, Lal H: Antinociceptive and antiwithdrawal actions of clonidine: A comparison with morphine. Fed Proc 36:1024, 1977.

Gold, MS, Redmond DE Jr, Kleber HD: Clonidine in opiate withdrawal. Lancet 1:929–930, 1978a.

Gold MS, Redmond DE Jr, Kleber HD: Clonidine blocks acute opiate withdrawal symptoms. Lancet 2:599–602, 1978b.

Gold MS, Redmond DE Jr: Pharmacological activation and inhibition of noradrenergic activity alter specific behaviors in nonhuman primates. Neurosci Abstr 3:250, 1977.

Gold MS, Redmond DE Jr, Kleber HD: Noradrenergic hyperactivity in opiate withdrawal supported by clonidine reversal of opiate withdrawal. Am J Psychiatry 136:100–102, 1979c.

Gold MS, Byck R, Sweeney DR, Kleber HD: Endorphin–locus coeruleus connection mediates opiate action and withdrawal. Biomedicine 30:1–4, 1979a.

Gold MS, Pottash ALC, Sweeney DR, Kleber HD, Redmond DE Jr: Rapid opiate detoxification: Clinical evidence of antidepressant and antipanic effects of opiates. Am J Psychiatry 136:982–983, 1979b.

Gold MS, Sweeney DR, Pottash ALC, Kleber HD: Decreased serum prolactin in opiate withdrawal and dopaminergic hyperactivity. Am J Psychiatry 136:849–850, 1979d.

Kuhar MJ: Opiate receptors: Some anatomical and physiological aspects. NY Acad Sci 311:35–48, 1978.

Meyer DR, Sparber SB: Clonidine antagonized body weight loss and other symptoms used to measure withdrawal in morphine-pelleted rats given naloxone. Pharmacologist 18:236, 1976.

Paalzow G, Paalzow L: Clonidine antinociceptive activity: Effects of drugs influencing central monoaminergic and cholinergic mechanism in the rat. Naunyn Schmiedeberg's Arch Pharmacol 292:119–126, 1976.

Redmond DE Jr, Hwang YH, Gold MS: Anxiety: The locus coeruleus connection. Neurosci Abstr 3:258, 1977.

Redmond DE Jr, Gold MS, Hwang YH: Enkephalin acts to inhibit locus coeruleus mediated behaviors. Neurosci Abstr 4:413, 1978.

Schmitt H, Schmitt H: Interactions between 2-(2,6-dichlorophenylamino)-2-imidazoline hydrochloride (St 155, Catapresan) and 2-adrenergic blocking drugs. Eur J Pharmacol 9:7–13, 1970.

Schmitt H, Schmitt H, Fenard S: Evidence for an 2-sympathomimetic component in the effects of Catapresan on vasomotor centres: Antagonism by piperoxane. Eur J Pharmacol 14:98–100, 1971.

Svensson TH, Strombom U: Discontinuation of chronic clonidine treatment: Evidence for facilitated brain noradrenergic neurotransmission. Naunyn Schmeidberg's Arch Pharmacol 299:83–87, 1977.

Washton A, Renick R, La Placa R: Clonidine hydrochloride—A nonopiate treatment for opiate withdrawal. Maui, Hawaii: Am Coll Neuropsychopharmacol, 1978.

Index

PROGRESS IN CLINICAL AND BIOLOGICAL RESEARCH

Series Editors
Nathan Back
George J. Brewer

Vincent P. Eijsvoogel
Robert Grover
Kurt Hirschhorn

Seymour S. Kety
Sidney Udenfriend
Jonathan W. Uhr

321